Fundamentals and Principles of Ophthalmology

BASIC AND CLINICAL SCIENCE COURSE

Section 2

2011–2012

(Last major revision 2009–2010)

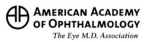

AMERICAN ACADEMY OF OPHTHALMOLOGY
The Eye M.D. Association

LEO

LIFELONG
EDUCATION FOR THE
OPHTHALMOLOGIST®

The Basic and Clinical Science Course is one component of the Lifelong Education for the Ophthalmologist (LEO) framework, which assists members in planning their continuing medical education. LEO includes an array of clinical education products that members may select to form individualized, self-directed learning plans for updating their clinical knowledge. Active members or fellows who use LEO components may accumulate sufficient CME credits to earn the LEO Award. Contact the Academy's Clinical Education Division for further information on LEO.

The American Academy of Ophthalmology is accredited by the Accreditation Council for Continuing Medical Education to provide continuing medical education for physicians.

The American Academy of Ophthalmology designates this enduring material for a maximum of 15 *AMA PRA Category 1 Credits*™. Physicians should claim only credit commensurate with the extent of their participation in the activity.

The Academy provides this material for educational purposes only. It is not intended to represent the only or best method or procedure in every case, nor to replace a physician's own judgment or give specific advice for case management. Including all indications, contraindications, side effects, and alternative agents for each drug or treatment is beyond the scope of this material. All information and recommendations should be verified, prior to use, with current information included in the manufacturers' package inserts or other independent sources, and considered in light of the patient's condition and history. Reference to certain drugs, instruments, and other products in this course is made for illustrative purposes only and is not intended to constitute an endorsement of such. Some material may include information on applications that are not considered community standard, that reflect indications not included in approved FDA labeling, or that are approved for use only in restricted research settings. **The FDA has stated that it is the responsibility of the physician to determine the FDA status of each drug or device he or she wishes to use, and to use them with appropriate, informed patient consent in compliance with applicable law.** The Academy specifically disclaims any and all liability for injury or other damages of any kind, from negligence or otherwise, for any and all claims that may arise from the use of any recommendations or other information contained herein.

Cover image courtesy of Thomas A. Weingeist, PhD, MD.

Basic and Clinical Science Course

Gregory L. Skuta, MD, Oklahoma City, Oklahoma, *Senior Secretary for Clinical Education*

Louis B. Cantor, MD, Indianapolis, Indiana, *Secretary for Ophthalmic Knowledge*

Jayne S. Weiss, MD, Detroit, Michigan, *BCSC Course Chair*

Section 2

Faculty Responsible for This Edition

K. V. Chalam, MD, PhD, *Chair,* Jacksonville, Florida

Balamurali K. Ambati, MD, Salt Lake City, Utah

Hilary A. Beaver, MD, Iowa City, Iowa

Sandeep Grover, MD, Jacksonville, Florida

Lawrence M. Levine, MD, Jacksonville, Florida

Tony Wells, MD, *Consultant,* Wellington, New Zealand

Edward K. Isbey, III, MD, Asheville, North Carolina
   Practicing Ophthalmologists Advisory Committee for Education

Financial Disclosures

The authors state the following financial relationships:

Dr Beaver: Genzyme, lecture honoraria recipient

Dr Wells: Alcon, consultant; Allergan, consultant

The other authors state that they have no significant financial interest or other relationship with the manufacturer of any commercial product discussed in the chapters that they contributed to this publication or with the manufacturer of any competing commercial product.

Recent Past Faculty

Gerhard W. Cibis, MD

Karla Johns, MD

Shalesh Kaushal, MD, PhD

James C. Tsai, MD

In addition, the Academy gratefully acknowledges the contributions of numerous past faculty and advisory committee members who have played an important role in the development of previous editions of the Basic and Clinical Science Course.

American Academy of Ophthalmology Staff

Richard A. Zorab, *Vice President, Ophthalmic Knowledge*

Hal Straus, *Director, Publications Department*

Christine Arturo, *Acquisitions Manager*

Stephanie Tanaka, *Publications Manager*

D. Jean Ray, *Production Manager*

Brian Veen, *Medical Editor*

Steven Huebner, *Administrative Coordinator*

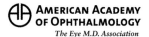

AMERICAN ACADEMY
OF OPHTHALMOLOGY
The Eye M.D. Association

655 Beach Street
Box 7424
San Francisco, CA 94120-7424

Contents

PART IV   Biochemistry and Metabolism 233

General Introduction

The Basic and Clinical Science Course (BCSC) is designed to meet the needs of residents and practitioners for a comprehensive yet concise curriculum of the field of ophthalmology. The BCSC has developed from its original brief outline format, which relied heavily on outside readings, to a more convenient and educationally useful self-contained text. The Academy updates and revises the course annually, with the goals of integrating the basic science and clinical practice of ophthalmology and of keeping ophthalmologists current with new developments in the various subspecialties.

The BCSC incorporates the effort and expertise of more than 80 ophthalmologists, organized into 13 Section faculties, working with Academy editorial staff. In addition, the course continues to benefit from many lasting contributions made by the faculties of previous editions. Members of the Academy's Practicing Ophthalmologists Advisory Committee for Education serve on each faculty and, as a group, review every volume before and after major revisions.

Organization of the Course

The Basic and Clinical Science Course comprises 13 volumes, incorporating fundamental ophthalmic knowledge, subspecialty areas, and special topics:

1 Update on General Medicine
2 Fundamentals and Principles of Ophthalmology
3 Clinical Optics
4 Ophthalmic Pathology and Intraocular Tumors
5 Neuro-Ophthalmology
6 Pediatric Ophthalmology and Strabismus
7 Orbit, Eyelids, and Lacrimal System
8 External Disease and Cornea
9 Intraocular Inflammation and Uveitis
10 Glaucoma
11 Lens and Cataract
12 Retina and Vitreous
13 Refractive Surgery

In addition, a comprehensive Master Index allows the reader to easily locate subjects throughout the entire series.

References

Readers who wish to explore specific topics in greater detail may consult the references cited within each chapter and listed in the Basic Texts section at the back of the book. These references are intended to be selective rather than exhaustive, chosen by the BCSC faculty as being important, current, and readily available to residents and practitioners.

Related Academy educational materials are also listed in the appropriate sections. They include books, online and audiovisual materials, self-assessment programs, clinical modules, and interactive programs.

Study Questions and CME Credit

Each volume of the BCSC is designed as an independent study activity for ophthalmology residents and practitioners. The learning objectives for this volume are given on page 1. The text, illustrations, and references provide the information necessary to achieve the objectives; the study questions allow readers to test their understanding of the material and their mastery of the objectives. Physicians who wish to claim CME credit for this educational activity may do so by mail, by fax, or online. The necessary forms and instructions are given at the end of the book.

Conclusion

The Basic and Clinical Science Course has expanded greatly over the years, with the addition of much new text and numerous illustrations. Recent editions have sought to place a greater emphasis on clinical applicability while maintaining a solid foundation in basic science. As with any educational program, it reflects the experience of its authors. As its faculties change and as medicine progresses, new viewpoints are always emerging on controversial subjects and techniques. Not all alternate approaches can be included in this series; as with any educational endeavor, the learner should seek additional sources, including such carefully balanced opinions as the Academy's Preferred Practice Patterns.

The BCSC faculty and staff are continuously striving to improve the educational usefulness of the course; you, the reader, can contribute to this ongoing process. If you have any suggestions or questions about the series, please do not hesitate to contact the faculty or the editors.

The authors, editors, and reviewers hope that your study of the BCSC will be of lasting value and that each Section will serve as a practical resource for quality patient care.

Objectives

Upon completion of BCSC Section 2, *Fundamentals and Principles of Ophthalmology,* the reader should be able to

- identify the bones making up the orbital walls and the orbital foramina

- identify the origin and pathways of cranial nerves I–VII

- identify the origin and insertions of the extraocular muscles and use CT and MRI studies to point out the extraocular muscles, optic nerve, and lacrimal gland in axial and coronal views of the orbit

- describe the distribution of the arterial and venous circulations of the orbit and optic nerve

- summarize the structural-functional relationships of the outflow pathways for aqueous humor of the eye

- delineate the events of early embryogenesis that are important for the subsequent development of the eye and orbit

- identify the roles of growth factors, homeobox genes, and neural crest cells in the genesis of the eye

- describe the sequence of events in the differentiation of the ocular tissues during embryonic and fetal development of the eye

- describe the stages in the development of the eye and the correlation between congenital ocular disorders and the timing of an insult to the embryo

- describe the organization of the human genome and the role of genetic mutations in health and disease

- explain how DNA can be manipulated in the laboratory to map and to clone genes, to identify genes from surrounding DNA, and to create transgenic and knockout animals

- demonstrate how appropriate diagnosis and management of genetic diseases can lead to better patient care

- assess the role of the ophthalmologist in the provision of genetic counseling

- identify the biochemical composition of the various parts of the eye and the eye's secretions

- discuss new concepts regarding the interaction between membrane proteins and G proteins and the effects of this interaction on ocular functions, such as rhodopsin with transducin in the conversion of "light-stimulus" to "electric-signal"

- discuss the biochemical derangements in diabetes mellitus and the way in which they lead to the disease's ocular complications, such as diabetic retinopathy and cataract formation

- list the varied functions of the retinal pigment epithelium such as phagocytosis and vitamin A metabolism and their relationship to retinal diseases

- summarize the role of free radicals and antioxidants

- describe the features of the eye that facilitate or impede drug delivery

- cite the basic principles underlying the use of autonomic therapeutic agents in a variety of ocular conditions

- list the indications, contraindications, mechanisms of action, and side effects of various drugs in the management of glaucoma

- describe the mechanisms of action of antibiotics, antivirals, and antifungal medications: their indications, dosages, and side effects

- discuss the anesthetic agents used in ophthalmology, their dosages and adverse effects

- discuss therapeutic drugs on the horizon and in the process of being introduced into clinical practice in the immediate future

PART I

Anatomy

CHAPTER 1

Orbit and Ocular Adnexa

Orbital Anatomy

Orbital Volume

The eyes lie within 2 bony orbits; the volume of each adult orbit is slightly less than 30 cm^3. Each orbit is pear-shaped, with the optic nerve representing the stem. The orbital entrance averages about 35 mm in height and 45 mm in width. The maximum width is located about 1 cm behind the anterior orbital margin. In adults, the depth of the orbit varies from 40 to 45 mm from the orbital entrance to the orbital apex. Both race and sex affect each of these measurements.

Bony Orbit

Seven bones make up the bony orbit (Fig 1-1; see also Fig 1-5):

1. frontal
2. zygomatic
3. maxilla (or maxillary bone)
4. ethmoid (or ethmoidal bone)
5. sphenoid
6. lacrimal
7. palatine

Orbital Margin

The orbital margin forms a quadrilateral spiral (Fig 1-2) whose superior margin is formed by the frontal bone, which is interrupted medially by the supraorbital notch. The medial margin is formed above by the frontal bone and below by the posterior lacrimal crest of the lacrimal bone and the anterior lacrimal crest of the maxillary bone. The inferior margin derives from the maxillary and zygomatic bones. Laterally, the zygomatic and frontal bones complete the rim.

Orbital Roof

The orbital roof is formed from both the orbital plate of the frontal bone and the lesser wing of the sphenoid bone (Fig 1-3). The fossa for the lacrimal gland, lying anterolaterally

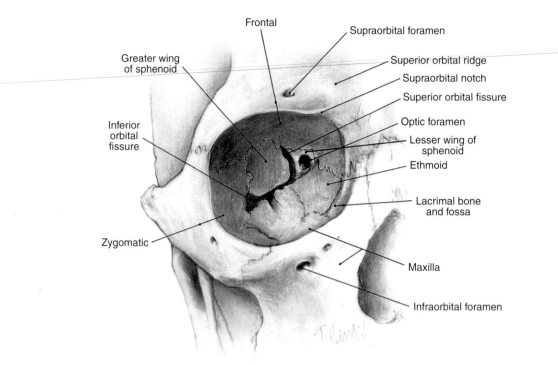

Figure 1-1 Frontal view of bony right orbit. *(Reproduced with permission from Doxanas MT, Anderson RL. Clinical Orbital Anatomy. Baltimore: Williams & Wilkins; 1984.)*

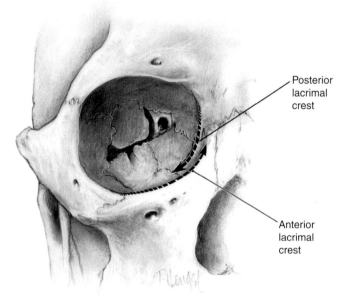

Figure 1-2 Right orbital margin. The orbital rim forms a quadrilateral spiral *(arrows)*. Note the relationship between the anterior lacrimal crest of the maxillary bone and the posterior lacrimal crest of the lacrimal bone. *(Reproduced with permission from Doxanas MT, Anderson RL. Clinical Orbital Anatomy. Baltimore: Williams & Wilkins; 1984.)*

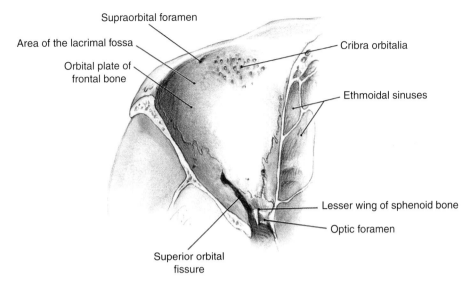

Supraorbital foramen

Area of the lacrimal fossa

Orbital plate of
frontal bone

Cribra orbitalia

Ethmoidal sinuses

Lesser wing of sphenoid bone

Optic foramen

Superior orbital
fissure

Figure 1-3 View from below, looking up into the orbital roof (superior orbital wall). *(Reproduced with permission from Doxanas MT, Anderson RL. Clinical Orbital Anatomy. Baltimore: Williams & Wilkins; 1984.)*

behind the zygomatic process of the frontal bone, resides within the orbital roof. Medially, the trochlear fossa is located on the frontal bone approximately 4 mm from the orbital margin and is the site of the pulley of the superior oblique muscle, where the trochlea, a curved plate of hyaline cartilage, is attached.

> Helveston EM, Merriam WW, Ellis FD, Shellhamer RH, Gosling CG. The trochlea. A study of the anatomy and physiology. *Ophthalmology.* 1982;89(2):124–133.

Medial Orbital Wall

The medial wall of the orbit is formed from 4 bones (Fig 1-4):

1. frontal process of the maxilla
2. lacrimal bone
3. orbital plate of the ethmoid
4. lesser wing of the sphenoid

The ethmoidal bone makes up the largest portion of the medial wall. The lacrimal fossa is formed by the frontal process of the maxillary and the lacrimal bone. Below, the lacrimal fossa is continuous with the bony nasolacrimal canal, which extends into the inferior meatus (the space beneath the inferior turbinate) of the nose. The paper-thin structure of the medial wall is reflected in its name, *lamina papyracea.*

Orbital Floor

The floor of the orbit, which is the roof of the maxillary antrum, or sinus, is composed of 3 bones (Fig 1-5):

1. maxilla

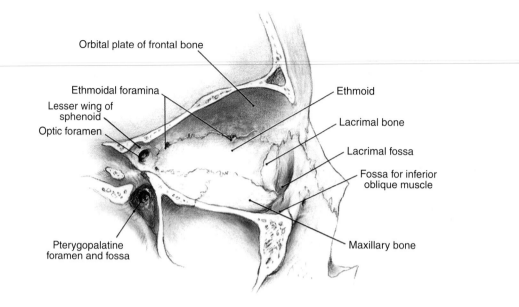

Figure 1-4 Right medial orbital wall as viewed from lateral side. *(Reproduced with permission from Doxanas MT, Anderson RL. Clinical Orbital Anatomy. Baltimore: Williams & Wilkins; 1984.)*

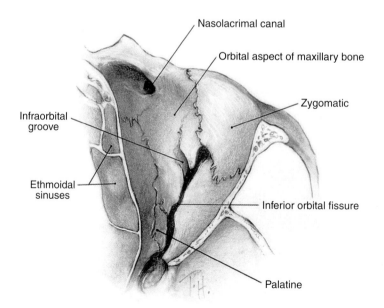

Figure 1-5 Right orbital floor and inferior orbital fissure. *(Reproduced with permission from Doxanas MT, Anderson RL. Clinical Orbital Anatomy. Baltimore: Williams & Wilkins; 1984.)*

2. palatine
3. orbital plate of the zygomatic

The infraorbital groove traverses the floor and descends anteriorly into a canal. It exits as the infraorbital foramen, below the orbital margin of the maxillary bone. Arising from the floor of the orbit just lateral to the opening of the nasolacrimal canal is the inferior oblique muscle, the only extraocular muscle that does not originate from the orbital apex. The floor of the orbit slopes downward approximately 20° from posterior to anterior.

Lateral Orbital Wall

The thickest and strongest of the orbital walls, the lateral wall of the orbit is formed from 2 bones (Fig 1-6): the zygomatic and the greater wing of the sphenoid.

The lateral orbital tubercle (the *Whitnall tubercle*), a small elevation of the orbital margin of the zygomatic bone, lies approximately 11 mm below the frontozygomatic suture. This important landmark is the site of attachment for the following:

- check ligament of the lateral rectus muscle
- suspensory ligament of the eyeball (Lockwood suspensory ligament)
- lateral palpebral ligament
- aponeurosis of the levator muscle
- Whitnall ligament

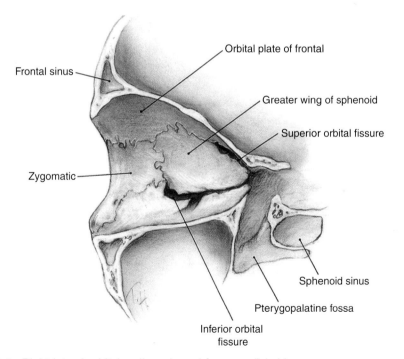

Figure 1-6 Right lateral orbital wall as viewed from medial side. *(Reproduced with permission from Doxanas MT, Anderson RL. Clinical Orbital Anatomy. Baltimore: Williams & Wilkins; 1984.)*

Orbital Foramina, Ducts, Canals, and Fissures

Foramina

The *optic foramen* leads from the middle cranial fossa to the apex of the orbit. It is directed forward, laterally, and somewhat downward and conducts the optic nerve, the ophthalmic artery, and sympathetic fibers from the carotid plexus (Fig 1-7). The optic foramen passes through the lesser wing of the sphenoid bone. The *supraorbital foramen* (in some people, it is a notch instead of a foramen) is located at the medial third of the superior margin of the orbit. It transmits blood vessels and the supraorbital nerve, which is a branch of the ophthalmic division (V_1) of cranial nerve V (CN V, trigeminal). The *anterior ethmoidal foramen* is located at the frontoethmoidal suture and transmits the anterior ethmoidal vessels and nerve. The *posterior ethmoidal foramen* lies at the junction of the roof and the medial wall of the orbit and transmits the posterior ethmoidal vessels and nerve through the frontal bone. The *zygomatic foramen* lies in the lateral aspect of the zygomatic bone and contains zygomaticofacial and zygomaticotemporal branches of the zygomatic nerve and the zygomatic artery.

Nasolacrimal duct

The nasolacrimal duct travels inferiorly from the lacrimal fossa into the inferior meatus of the nose.

Infraorbital canal

The infraorbital canal continues anteriorly from the infraorbital groove and exits 4 mm below the inferior orbital margin, where it transmits the infraorbital nerve, which is a branch of V_2 (the maxillary division of CN V).

Fissures

The *superior orbital fissure* (Fig 1-8) is located between the greater and the lesser wings of the sphenoid bone and lies below and lateral to the optic foramen. It is about 22 mm long and is spanned by the common tendinous ring of the rectus muscles *(annulus of Zinn)*. Above the ring, the superior orbital fissure transmits the

- lacrimal nerve of CN V_1
- frontal nerve of CN V_1
- CN IV (trochlear)
- superior ophthalmic vein

Within the ring or between the 2 heads of the rectus muscle are the following:

- superior and inferior divisions of CN III (oculomotor)
- nasociliary branch of CN V_1
- sympathetic roots of the ciliary ganglion
- CN VI (abducens)

Occasionally, the inferior ophthalmic vein is below the ring.

The *inferior orbital fissure* lies just below the superior fissure between the lateral wall and the floor of the orbit, giving access to the pterygopalatine and inferotemporal fossae. Hence, it is close to the foramen rotundum and the pterygoid canal. It transmits the

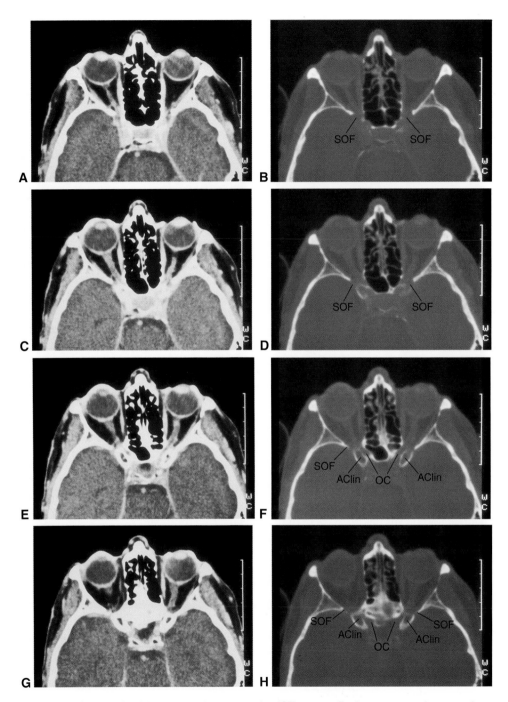

Figure 1-7 Series of axial computed tomography (CT) scans. Each compares tissue and corresponding bone-window density through the optic canal *(OC)* and superior orbital fissure *(SOF)*. The SOF passes above and below the plane of the OC and is commonly mistaken for the OC. The OC lies in the same plane as the anterior clinoid processes *(AClin)* and may be cut obliquely in scans so that the entire canal length does not always appear in 1 section. Four different planes of section are shown in this series: **A–B,** Plane 1 is below the canal; **C–D,** Plane 2 is just under the canal; **E–F,** Plane 3 is at the canal; **G–H,** Plane 4 is just at the top of and above the canal.

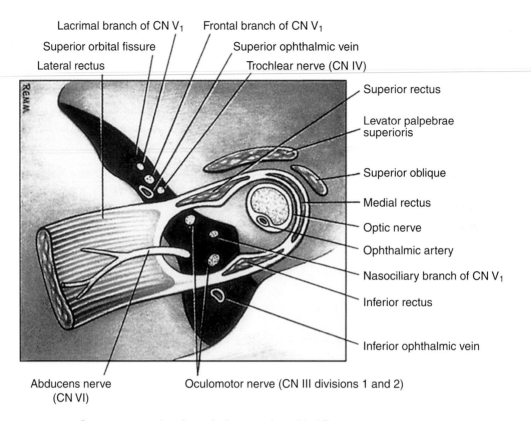

Lacrimal branch of CN V₁

Frontal branch of CN V₁

Superior orbital fissure

Superior ophthalmic vein

Lateral rectus

Trochlear nerve (CN IV)

Superior rectus

Levator palpebrae superioris

Superior oblique

Medial rectus

Optic nerve

Ophthalmic artery

Nasociliary branch of CN V₁

Inferior rectus

Inferior ophthalmic vein

Abducens nerve (CN VI)

Oculomotor nerve (CN III divisions 1 and 2)

Figure 1-8 Structures passing through the superior orbital fissure. *(From Bron AJ, Tripathi RC, Tripathi BJ. Wolff's Anatomy of the Eye and Orbit. 8th ed. London: Chapman & Hall; 1997.)*

infraorbital and zygomatic branches of CN V_2, an orbital nerve from the pterygopalatine ganglion, and the inferior ophthalmic vein. The inferior ophthalmic vein connects with the pterygoid plexus before the vein drains into the cavernous sinus.

Periorbital Sinuses

The periorbital sinuses have a close anatomical relationship with the orbits, which are located on either side of the root of the nose. The medial walls of the orbits, which border the nasal cavity anteriorly and the ethmoidal sinus (see Fig 1-3) and the sphenoid sinus posteriorly, are almost parallel. In the adult, the lateral wall of each orbit forms an angle of approximately 45° with the medial plane. The lateral walls border the middle cranial, temporal, and pterygopalatine fossae. Superior to the orbit are the anterior cranial fossa and the frontal sinus. The maxillary sinus and the palatine air cells are located inferiorly.

The periorbital sinuses offer a route for the spread of infection. Mucoceles occasionally arise from the sinuses, extend into the adjacent orbit, and may confuse the clinician in the differential diagnosis of orbital tumors. The locations of the paranasal air sinuses and their relation to anatomical features of the skull are shown in Figures 1-9 and 1-10. Figure 1-9 also shows the distribution of pain originating from sinusitis. See BCSC Section 7, *Orbit, Eyelids, and Lacrimal System,* for further discussion.

Doxanas MT, Anderson RL. *Clinical Orbital Anatomy.* Baltimore: Williams & Wilkins; 1984:232.

Zide BM. *Surgical Anatomy Around the Orbit: The System of Zones.* Philadelphia: Lippincott Williams & Wilkins; 2005.

Cranial Nerves

Six of the 12 cranial nerves (CN II–VII) directly innervate the eye and periocular tissues. Because certain tumors affecting CN I (olfactory) can give rise to important ophthalmic signs and symptoms, familiarity with the anatomy of this nerve is also important for the ophthalmologist. (Chapter 3 discusses the central and peripheral connections of CN I–VII.) See also BCSC Section 7, *Orbit, Eyelids, and Lacrimal System.*

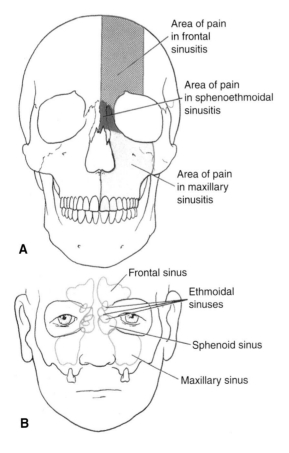

Area of pain in frontal sinusitis

Area of pain in sphenoethmoidal sinusitis

Area of pain in maxillary sinusitis

A

Frontal sinus

Ethmoidal sinuses

Sphenoid sinus

Maxillary sinus

B

Figure 1-9 **A,** Bones of the face, showing regions where pain is experienced in sinusitis. **B,** Positions of the paranasal sinuses relative to the face. *(Reproduced with permission from Snell RS, Lemp MA.* Clinical Anatomy of the Eye. *Boston: Blackwell; 1989.)*

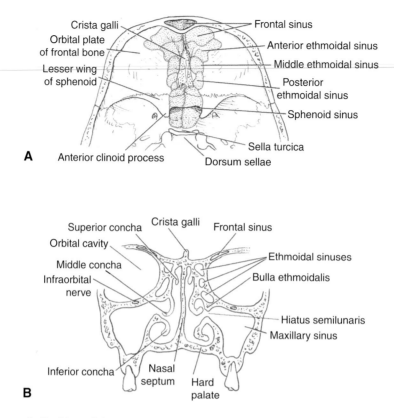

Figure 1-10 A, Position of the paranasal sinuses relative to the anterior cranial fossa, in axial view. **B,** Coronal section through the nasal cavity, showing the ethmoidal and maxillary sinuses. *(Reproduced with permission from Snell RS, Lemp MA.* Clinical Anatomy of the Eye. *Boston: Blackwell; 1989.)*

Ciliary Ganglion

The ciliary ganglion is located approximately 1 cm in front of the annulus of Zinn, on the lateral side of the ophthalmic artery between the optic nerve and the lateral rectus muscle (Figs 1-11, 1-12). It receives 3 roots:

1. A long *sensory root* arises from the nasociliary branch of CN V_1. It is 10–12 mm long and contains sensory fibers from the cornea, the iris, and the ciliary body.
2. A short *motor root* arises from the inferior division of CN III, which also supplies the inferior oblique muscle. The fibers of the motor root synapse in the ganglion, and the postganglionic fibers carry parasympathetic axons to supply the iris sphincter.
3. The *sympathetic root* comes from the plexus around the internal carotid artery. It enters the orbit through the superior orbital fissure within the tendinous ring, passes through the ciliary ganglion without synapse, and innervates ocular blood vessels and possibly the dilator muscle.

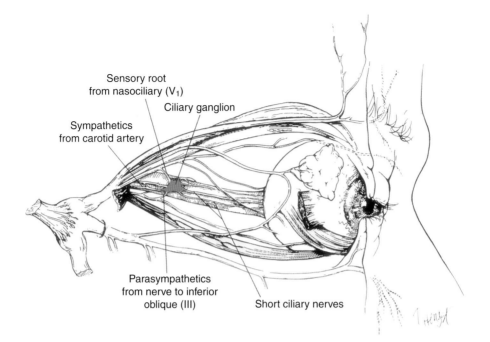

Figure 1-11 Contributions to the ciliary ganglion. *(Reproduced with permission from Doxanas MT, Anderson RL.* Clinical Orbital Anatomy. *Baltimore: Williams & Wilkins; 1984.)*

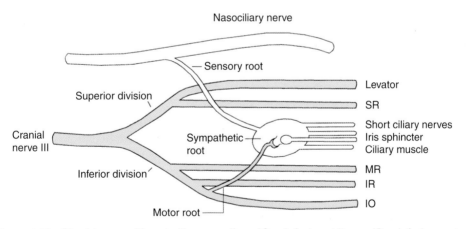

Figure 1-12 Cranial nerve III and ciliary ganglion. *IO* = inferior oblique, *IR* = inferior rectus, *MR* = medial rectus, *SR* = superior rectus. *(Illustration by Sylvia Barker.)*

Branches of the Ciliary Ganglion

Only the parasympathetic fibers synapse in the ciliary ganglion. The sympathetic fibers are postganglionic from the superior cervical ganglion and pass through it without synapse. Sensory fibers from cell bodies in the trigeminal ganglion carry sensation from the eye, orbit, and face. Together, the nonsynapsing sympathetic fibers, the sensory fibers, and the myelinated, fast-conducting postganglionic parasympathetic fibers form the short ciliary nerves.

Short Ciliary Nerves

Two groups, totaling 6–10 short ciliary nerves, arise from the ciliary ganglion (see Figs 1-11, 1-12). They travel on both sides of the optic nerve and, together with the long ciliary nerves, pierce the sclera around the optic nerve. They pass anteriorly between the choroid and the sclera into the ciliary muscle, where they form a plexus that supplies the cornea, the ciliary body, and the iris.

Extraocular Muscles

There are 7 extraocular muscles (Figs 1-13 through 1-16):

1. medial rectus
2. lateral rectus
3. superior rectus
4. inferior rectus
5. superior oblique
6. inferior oblique
7. levator palpebrae superioris

Extraocular Muscle Insertions

The 4 rectus muscles insert anteriorly on the globe. Starting at the medial rectus and then proceeding to the inferior rectus, lateral rectus, and superior rectus, the muscle insertions lie progressively farther from the limbus. An imaginary curve drawn through these insertions creates a spiral, which is called the *spiral of Tillaux* (Fig 1-17). The relationship between the muscle insertions and the ora serrata is clinically important. A misdirected suture passed through the insertion of the superior rectus muscle could perforate the retina.

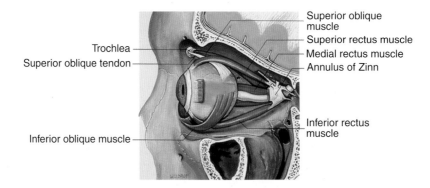

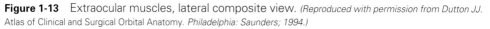
Figure 1-13 Extraocular muscles, lateral composite view. *(Reproduced with permission from Dutton JJ. Atlas of Clinical and Surgical Orbital Anatomy. Philadelphia: Saunders; 1994.)*

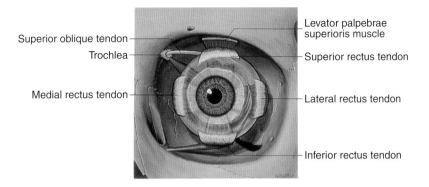

Figure 1-14 Extraocular muscles, frontal composite view. *(Reproduced with permission from Dutton JJ. Atlas of Clinical and Surgical Orbital Anatomy. Philadelphia: Saunders; 1994.)*

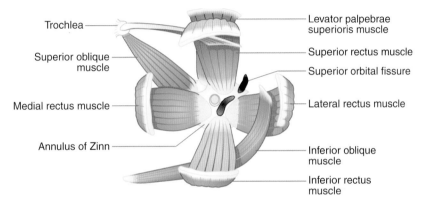

Figure 1-15 Extraocular muscles, frontal view, left eye, with globe removed. *(Reproduced with permission from Dutton JJ. Atlas of Clinical and Surgical Orbital Anatomy. Philadelphia: Saunders; 1994.)*

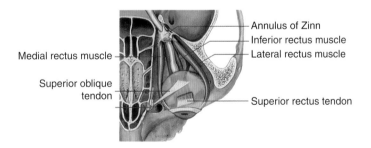

Figure 1-16 Extraocular muscles, superior composite view. *(Reproduced with permission from Dutton JJ. Atlas of Clinical and Surgical Orbital Anatomy. Philadelphia: Saunders; 1994.)*

The superior oblique muscle, after passing through the trochlea in the superior nasal orbital rim, inserts onto the sclera superiorly, under the insertion of the superior rectus. The inferior oblique muscle inserts onto the sclera in the posterior inferior temporal quadrant (see Fig 1-17; Table 1-1).

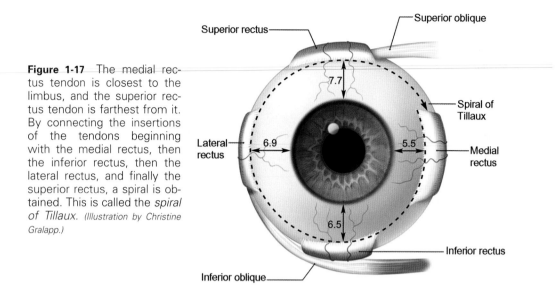

Figure 1-17 The medial rectus tendon is closest to the limbus, and the superior rectus tendon is farthest from it. By connecting the insertions of the tendons beginning with the medial rectus, then the inferior rectus, then the lateral rectus, and finally the superior rectus, a spiral is obtained. This is called the *spiral of Tillaux.* *(Illustration by Christine Gralapp.)*

Extraocular Muscle Distribution in the Orbit

Figures 1-15 and 1-16 show the arrangement of the extraocular muscles within the orbit. Note the relationship between the oblique extraocular muscles and the superior, medial, and inferior rectus muscles.

The location of the extraocular muscles within the orbit and their relationship to surrounding nerves and bone are illustrated in coronal, cross-sectional views (Figs 1-18, 1-19). Longitudinal, axial views are shown in Figures 1-20 and 1-21.

Extraocular Muscle Origins

The annulus of Zinn consists of superior and inferior orbital tendons and is the origin of the four recti muscles. The upper tendon gives rise to all of the superior rectus muscle, as well as portions of the lateral and medial rectus muscles. The inferior tendon gives rise to all of the inferior rectus muscle and portions of the medial and lateral rectus muscles. The levator palpebrae superioris muscle arises from the lesser wing of the sphenoid bone, at the apex of the orbit, just superior to the annulus of Zinn.

The superior oblique muscle originates from the periosteum of the body of the sphenoid bone, above and medial to the optic foramen. The inferior oblique muscle originates anteriorly, from a shallow depression in the orbital plate of the maxillary bone, at the anteromedial corner of the orbital floor, near the lacrimal fossa. From its origin, the inferior oblique muscle then extends posteriorly, laterally, and superiorly to insert into the globe.

Blood Supply to the Extraocular Muscles

The inferior and superior muscular branches of the ophthalmic artery, lacrimal artery, and infraorbital artery supply the extraocular muscles. The lateral rectus muscle is supplied by a single vessel derived from the lacrimal artery; the other rectus muscles receive

Table 1-1 Comparison of Extraocular Muscles

Muscle	Origin	Insertion	Blood Supply	Size
Medial rectus	Annulus of Zinn	Medially, in horizontal meridian 5.5 mm from limbus	Inferior muscular branch of ophthalmic artery	40.8 mm long; tendon: 3.7 mm long, 10.3 mm wide
Inferior rectus	Annulus of Zinn at orbital apex	Inferiorly, in vertical meridian 6.5 mm from limbus	Inferior muscular branch of ophthalmic artery and infraorbital artery	40 mm long; tendon: 5.5 mm long, 9.8 mm wide
Lateral rectus	Annulus of Zinn spanning the superior orbital fissure	Laterally, in horizontal meridian 6.9 mm from limbus	Lacrimal artery	40.6 mm long; tendon: 8 mm long, 9.2 mm wide
Superior rectus	Annulus of Zinn at orbital apex	Superiorly, in vertical meridian 7.7 mm from limbus	Superior muscular branch of ophthalmic artery	41.8 mm long; tendon: 5.8 mm long, 10.6 mm wide
Superior oblique	Medial to optic foramen, between annulus of Zinn and periorbita	To trochlea, through pulley, at orbital rim, then hooking back under superior rectus, inserting posterior to center of rotation	Superior muscular branch of ophthalmic artery	40 mm long; tendon: 20 mm long, 10.8 mm wide
Inferior oblique	From a depression on orbital floor near orbital rim (maxilla)	Posterior inferior temporal quadrant at level of macula; posterior to center of rotation	Inferior branch of ophthalmic artery and infraorbital artery	37 mm long; no tendon: 9.6 mm wide at insertion

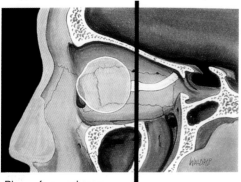

Plane of coronal scan

Figure 1-18 Location of the plane of section shown in Figure 1-19. *(Reproduced with permission from Dutton JJ. Atlas of Clinical and Surgical Orbital Anatomy. Philadelphia: Saunders; 1994.)*

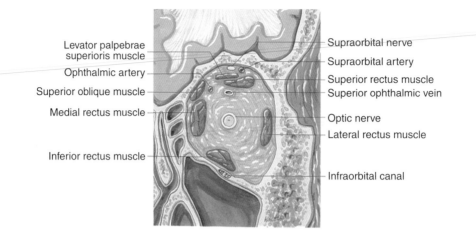

Levator palpebrae superioris muscle

Ophthalmic artery

Superior oblique muscle

Medial rectus muscle

Inferior rectus muscle

Supraorbital nerve

Supraorbital artery

Superior rectus muscle

Superior ophthalmic vein

Optic nerve

Lateral rectus muscle

Infraorbital canal

Figure 1-19 Coronal section through the central orbit just posterior to the globe. *(Reproduced with permission from Dutton JJ. Atlas of Clinical and Surgical Orbital Anatomy. Philadelphia: Saunders; 1994.)*

Figure 1-20 Location of the plane of section shown in Figure 1-21. *(Reproduced with permission from Dutton JJ. Atlas of Clinical and Surgical Orbital Anatomy. Philadelphia: Saunders; 1994.)*

Plane of axial scan

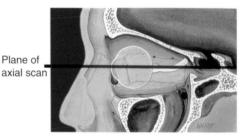

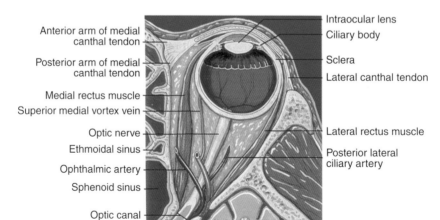

Anterior arm of medial canthal tendon

Posterior arm of medial canthal tendon

Medial rectus muscle

Superior medial vortex vein

Optic nerve

Ethmoidal sinus

Ophthalmic artery

Sphenoid sinus

Optic canal

Intraocular lens

Ciliary body

Sclera

Lateral canthal tendon

Lateral rectus muscle

Posterior lateral ciliary artery

Figure 1-21 Axial section through the midorbit at the level of the optic nerve. The third portion of the ophthalmic artery crosses the nerve in the posterior orbit. *(Reproduced with permission from Dutton JJ. Atlas of Clinical and Surgical Orbital Anatomy. Philadelphia: Saunders; 1994.)*

2 anterior ciliary arteries that communicate with the major arterial circle of the ciliary body via perforating scleral vessels. Vascular supply and venous drainage of orbital structures are discussed later in this chapter.

Innervation of the Extraocular Muscles

The lateral rectus muscle is innervated by CN VI (abducens); the superior oblique muscle is innervated by CN IV (trochlear); the levator palpebrae superioris, superior rectus, medial rectus, inferior rectus, and inferior oblique muscles are innervated by CN III. Cranial nerve III (oculomotor) has a superior and inferior division: the upper division innervates the levator palpebrae superioris and superior rectus muscles, and the lower division innervates the medial rectus, inferior rectus, and inferior oblique muscles.

Fine Structure of the Extraocular Muscles

The ratio of nerve fibers to eye muscle fibers in the extraocular muscles is very high (1:3–1:5) compared to the ratio of nerve axons to muscle fibers for skeletal muscle (1:50–1:125), thereby allowing precise control of ocular movements (Table 1-2). The fibers of the extraocular muscles are a mixture of the slow, tonic type (Felderstruktur) and the fast, twitch type (Fibrillenstruktur).

The tonic-type muscle fibers are unique to extraocular muscles. Smaller than twitch-type fibers, they have a slow, smooth contraction and tend to be located more superficially in the muscle, nearer the orbital wall. The tonic-type fibers are innervated by multiple grapelike nerve endings (en grappe) and are useful for smooth pursuit.

The twitch-type fibers are more similar to skeletal muscle fibers. Larger than tonic fibers and located deeper in the muscle, they have a fast contraction and platelike nerve endings (en plaque). Twitch fibers aid in rapid saccadic movements of the eye.

The fibers of the extraocular muscles can be classified further by contractile properties, histochemical profile, and myosin content.

Table 1-2 Extraocular Muscles

	Fast, Twitch Fibers (Fibrillenstruktur)	Slow, Tonic Fibers (Felderstruktur)
Myofibrils	Well defined	Poorly defined
Sarcoplasm	Abundant	Sparse
Sarcomere	Well developed	Poorly developed
T-system	Regular	Absent, or aberrant
Z-line	Straight	Zigzag course
M-line	Well marked	Absent
Nuclei	Located peripherally	Located centrally or eccentrically
Innervation	Thick; heavily myelinated	Thin
Neuromuscular junction	En plaque (single)	En grappe (grapelike)
Synaptic vesicles	Agranular	Granular/agranular
Acetylcholine	Twitch contraction	Tonic contraction

Porter JD, Baker RS, Ragusa RJ, Brueckner JK. Extraocular muscles: basic and clinical aspects of structure and function. *Surv Ophthalmol.* 1995;39(6):451–484.

Spencer FR, Porter JD. Structural organization of the extraocular muscles. In: Buttner-Ennever JA, ed. *Neuroanatomy of the Oculomotor System.* Amsterdam: Elsevier; 1988.

Eyelids

The *palpebral fissure* is the exposed zone between the upper and lower eyelids (Fig 1-22). Normally, the adult fissure is 27–30 mm long and 8–11 mm wide. The upper eyelid, more mobile than the lower, can be raised 15 mm by the action of the levator muscle alone. If the frontalis muscle of the brow is used, the palpebral fissure can be widened an additional 2 mm. The levator muscle is innervated by CN III. See also BCSC Section 7, *Orbit, Eyelids, and Lacrimal System.*

Anatomy

Although small in surface area, the eyelid is complex in its structure and function. When describing the anatomy of the upper eyelid, it is helpful to divide it into distinct segments from the dermal surface inward. These segments are the skin, the eyelid margin, the sub-cutaneous tissue, the orbicularis muscle, orbital septum, levator muscle, Müller muscle, tarsus, and conjunctiva (Figs 1-23 through 1-26).

Skin

The eyelid skin, the thinnest in the body, contains fine hairs, sebaceous glands, and sweat glands. A superior eyelid fold is present near the upper border of the tarsus, where the

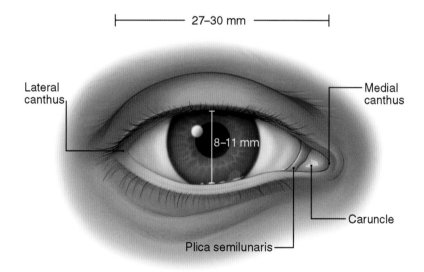

Figure 1-22 Landmarks of the external eye. *(Illustration by Christine Gralapp.)*

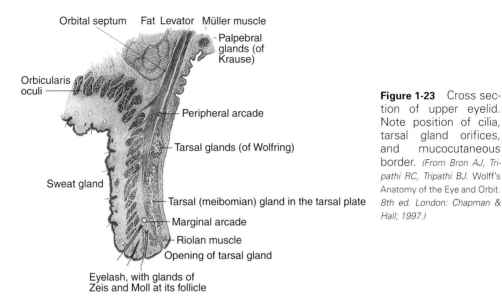

Orbital septum   Fat Levator Müller muscle

Palpebral glands (of Krause)

Orbicularis oculi

Peripheral arcade

Tarsal glands (of Wolfring)

Sweat gland

Tarsal (meibomian) gland in the tarsal plate

Marginal arcade

Riolan muscle

Opening of tarsal gland

Eyelash, with glands of Zeis and Moll at its follicle

Figure 1-23   Cross section of upper eyelid. Note position of cilia, tarsal gland orifices, and mucocutaneous border. *(From Bron AJ, Tripathi RC, Tripathi BJ. Wolff's Anatomy of the Eye and Orbit. 8th ed. London: Chapman & Hall; 1997.)*

levator aponeurosis establishes its first insertional attachments. (In many individuals of Asian descent, there are few attachments of the levator aponeurosis to the skin near the upper tarsal border, and the superior eyelid fold is minimal or absent.) The aponeurosis forms its firmest attachments on the anterior aspect of the tarsus about 3 mm superior to the eyelid margin.

Margin

The eyelid margin contains several important landmarks (Fig 1-27). A small opening, the punctum of the canaliculus, presents medially at the summit of each lacrimal papilla. The superior punctum, normally hidden by slight internal rotation, is located more medially. The inferior punctum is usually apposed to the globe and is not normally visible without eversion.

Along the entire length of the free margin of the eyelid is the delicate *gray line* (or *intermarginal sulcus*), corresponding histologically to the most superficial portion of the orbicularis muscle, the muscle of Riolan, and to the avascular plane of the lid. Anterior to this line, the eyelashes (or cilia) arise, and behind it are the openings of the tarsal (or meibomian) glands just anterior to the mucocutaneous junction.

The eyelashes are arranged in 2 or 3 irregular rows along the anterior dermal edge of the eyelid margin. They are usually longer and more numerous on the upper eyelid than on the lower one. The margins contain the *glands of Zeis,* which are modified sebaceous glands associated with the cilia, and the *glands of Moll,* apocrine sweat glands of skin (Table 1-3).

Subcutaneous connective tissue

The loose connective tissue of the eyelid contains no fat. Blood or other fluids can accumulate beneath the skin and result in rapid and dramatic swelling of the lids.

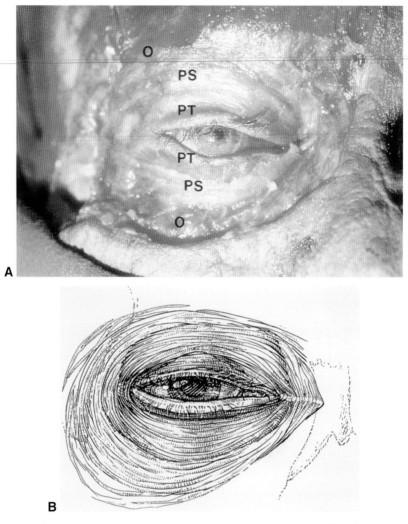

Figure 1-24 **A,** Photo shows the eye with the periorbital skin removed and orbicularis oculi muscle, which is innervated by CN VII, exposed. This muscle acts as an antagonist to the levator palpebrae superioris muscle, which is innervated by CN III. The orbicularis muscle is divided into the palpebral and orbital *(O)* portions. The palpebral portion is further divided into pretarsal *(PT)* and preseptal *(PS)* portions. **B,** Diagram depicts the arrangement of muscle fibers of the orbicularis muscle. *(Reproduced with permission from Zide BM, Jelks GW. Surgical Anatomy of the Orbit. New York: Raven; 1985.)*

Orbicularis oculi muscle

The *orbicularis oculi muscle* is arranged in several concentric bands around the palpebral fissure and can be subdivided into orbital and palpebral parts (see Fig 1-24). The muscle fibers are short and are connected by myomyous junctions. Of all the facial muscles, the orbicularis muscle has fibers with the smallest diameter. Innervation is by the facial nerve (CN VII), and end plates are arranged in clusters over the entire length of the muscle. This

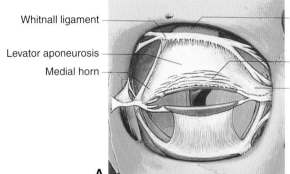

Whitnall ligament

Levator aponeurosis

Medial horn

Levator palpebrae superioris muscle

Fascial slips to orbicularis muscle

Lateral horn

A

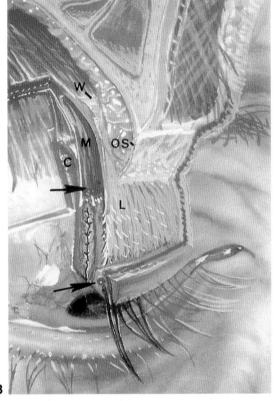

W

M OS

C

L

B

Figure 1-25 A, The upper and lower tarsal plates and their attachments to the levator aponeurosis and to the Whitnall ligament. **B,** The 3-dimensional organization of the upper eyelid. For convenience, the upper eyelid may be divided into anterior and posterior lamellae. The *anterior lamella* consists of the skin and orbicularis muscle and its associated fascial and vascular structures. Note the marginal artery *(lower arrow)* approximately 3.0–3.5 mm above the eyelid margin. The *posterior lamella* consists of the levator aponeurosis *(L),* tarsus *(blue),* Müller muscle *(M),* and conjunctival lining *(C).* At a variable height above the superior edge of the tarsus, the orbital septum *(OS)* forms the anterior border of the preaponeurotic fat space. The peripheral arterial arcade is situated *(upper arrow)* at the level of the superior edge of the tarsus, posterior to the levator aponeurosis within the so-called *pretarsal space.* The levator muscle usually becomes aponeurotic at the equator of the globe in the superior orbit. The aponeurosis courses anteriorly to insert onto the lower two thirds of the anterior tarsal plate. The levator muscle provides origin to the Müller muscle, the nonstriated, sympathetically innervated elevator of the upper eyelid, which inserts into the superior edge of the tarsus and into the conjunctiva of the superior fornix. The superior transverse ligament of Whitnall *(W)* is noted as a fascial condensation along the upper aspect of the levator muscle. This ligament attaches to the trochlear fascia medially and the fascia of the orbital lobe of the lacrimal gland laterally. *(Part A reproduced with permission from Dutton JJ.* Atlas of Clinical and Surgical Orbital Anatomy. *Philadelphia: Saunders; 1994; part B reproduced with permission from Zide BM, Jelks GW.* Surgical Anatomy of the Orbit. *New York: Raven; 1985.)*

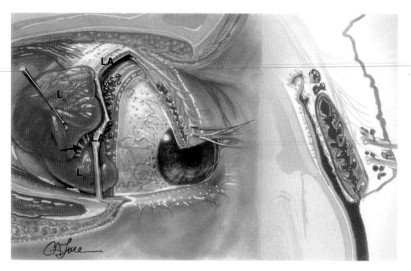

Figure 1-26 The lacrimal secretory system: (1) The conjunctival and tarsal mucin-secreting goblet cells *(green)* produce a mucoprotein layer covering the epithelial surface of the cornea and conjunctiva. (2) The accessory lacrimal exocrine glands of Krause and Wolfring are present in the subconjunctival tissues *(blue)* and contribute to the aqueous layer of the precorneal tear film. (3) Oil-producing meibomian glands and palpebral glands of Zeis and Moll *(pink)*. The orbital lobe of the lacrimal gland *(L$_o$)* and the palpebral lobe of the lacrimal gland *(L$_p$)* are separated by the lateral horn of the levator palpebrae superioris *(LA)*. The tear ducts *(arrow)* from the orbital portion traverse the palpebral portion. *(Reproduced with permission from Zide BM, Jelks GW. Surgical Anatomy of the Orbit. New York: Raven; 1985.)*

Figure 1-27 Anatomical landmarks of the lower eyelid margin. The gray line, or inter-marginal sulcus, is seen between the bases of the cilia and the orifices of the meibomian glands. The lower eyelid has been slightly everted in this view to clearly expose the inferior lacrimal puncta. *(Illustration by Christine Gralapp.)*

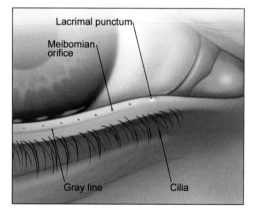

arrangement may influence the action of botulinum A toxin, which is used in the treatment of blepharospasm.

Lander T, Wirtschafter JD, McLoon LK. Orbicularis oculi muscle fibers are relatively short and heterogeneous in length. *Invest Ophthalmol Vis Sci.* 1996;37(9):1732–1739.

The orbital part inserts in a complex way into the medial canthal tendon and into other portions of the orbital rim and the corrugator supercilii muscle. The orbital part acts like a sphincter and functions solely as a voluntary muscle.

Table 1-3 Glands of the Eye and Adnexa

Glands	Location	Secretion	Content
Lacrimal	Orbital gland	Exocrine	Aqueous
	Palpebral gland	Exocrine	Aqueous
Accessory lacrimal	Plica, caruncle	Exocrine	Aqueous
Krause	Eyelid	Exocrine	Aqueous
Wolfring	Eyelid	Exocrine	Aqueous
Meibomian	Tarsus	Holocrine	Oily
Zeis	Follicles of cilia	Holocrine	Oily
	Eyelid, caruncle	Holocrine	Oily
Moll	Eyelid	Eccrine	Sweat
Goblet cell	Conjunctiva	Holocrine	Mucus
	Plica, caruncle	Holocrine	Mucus

The palpebral part of the orbicularis functions both voluntarily and involuntarily in spontaneous and reflex blinking. The preseptal and pretarsal portions unite along the superior palpebral furrow. The pretarsal orbicularis muscle is firmly adherent to the tarsus, with a portion of it attaching to the anterior lacrimal crest and the posterior lacrimal crest (sometimes called the Horner muscle), and plays a role in the drainage of tears (Fig 1-28).

Orbicularis fibers extend to the eyelid margin, where there is a small bundle of striated muscle fibers called the *muscle of Riolan*. Disinsertion of the lower eyelid retractors from the tarsus may result in laxity of the lower eyelid, followed by spastic entropion, an inward turning of the eyelid margin.

Orbital septum

A thin sheet of connective tissue called the *orbital septum* encircles the orbit as an extension of the periosteum of the roof and the floor of the orbit (see Fig 1-23). It also attaches to the anterior surface of the levator muscle. Posterior to the orbital septum is the orbital fat. In both the upper and lower eyelids, the orbital septum attaches to the aponeurosis. The orbital septum thus provides a barrier to anterior or posterior extravasation of blood

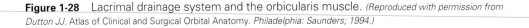

Figure 1-28 Lacrimal drainage system and the orbicularis muscle. *(Reproduced with permission from Dutton JJ. Atlas of Clinical and Surgical Orbital Anatomy. Philadelphia: Saunders; 1994.)*

or the spread of inflammation. The intermuscular orbital septa can be identified in coronal MRI studies with fat suppression and gadolinium enhancement.

Superiorly, the septum is attached firmly to the periosteum of the superior half of the orbital margin. It passes medially in front of the trochlea and continues along the medial margin of the orbit, along the margin of the frontal process of the maxillary bone, and on to the inferior margin of the orbit. Here, the septum also delimits the lateral spread of edema, inflammation, or blood trapped anterior to it and appears clinically as a dramatic barrier to these processes.

Levator muscle

The *levator palpebrae superioris muscle* originates from the lesser wing of the sphenoid bone (see Fig 1-25). The body of the levator muscle overlies the superior rectus as it travels anteriorly toward the eyelid. The Whitnall ligament results from a condensation of tissue surrounding the superior rectus and levator muscles. Near the Whitnall ligament, the levator muscle changes direction from horizontal to more vertical, and it divides anteriorly into the aponeurosis and posteriorly into the superior tarsal (Müller's) muscle.

The aponeurosis inserts into the anterior surface of the tarsus and passes by the medial and lateral horns into the canthal tendons. The fibrous elements of the aponeurosis pass through the orbicularis muscle and insert subcutaneously to produce the superior eyelid fold. The aponeurosis also inserts into the trochlea of the superior oblique muscle and into the fibrous tissue bridging the supraorbital notch. Attachments also exist with the conjunctiva of the upper fornix and with the orbital septum.

The levator muscle and tendon are 50–55 mm long. The muscle, which elevates the upper eyelid, is 40 mm long and is innervated by the superior division of CN III.

Müller muscle

The *Müller muscle* is a smooth (nonstriated), sympathetically innervated muscle that originates from the undersurface of the levator muscle in the upper eyelid. A similar smooth muscle arises from the capsulopalpebral head of the inferior rectus in the lower eyelid. The Müller muscle attaches to the upper border of the upper tarsus and to the conjunctiva of the upper fornix. The capsulopalpebral muscle, which is much weaker than the Müller muscle, attaches to the lower border of the lower tarsus.

Tarsus

The *tarsal plates* consist of dense connective tissue, not cartilage. They are attached to the orbital margin by the medial and lateral palpebral ligaments. Although the upper and lower tarsal plates are similar in length (29 mm) and in thickness (1 mm), the upper tarsus is almost 3 times as wide vertically (11 mm) as the lower tarsus (4 mm).

The *tarsal (meibomian) glands* are modified holocrine sebaceous glands that are oriented vertically in parallel rows through the tarsus (Fig 1-29). Their distribution and number within the eyelid can be observed by infrared transillumination (Fig 1-30) of the eyelid. A single row of 30–40 meibomian orifices is present in the upper eyelid, but there are only 20–30 orifices in the lower lid. Oil from these orifices forms a reservoir on the skin of the lid margin and is spread onto the tear film with each blink.

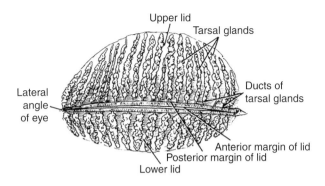

Upper lid
Tarsal glands
Lateral angle of eye
Ducts of tarsal glands
Anterior margin of lid
Posterior margin of lid
Lower lid

Figure 1-29 Posterior view of the eyelids with the palpebral fissure nearly closed. Note the tarsal glands with their short ducts and orifices. The palpebral conjunctiva has been removed to show the tarsal glands in situ. *(Reproduced with permission from Snell RS, Lemp MA.* Clinical Anatomy of the Eye. *Boston: Blackwell; 1989.)*

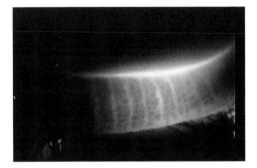

Figure 1-30 Distribution of the meibomian glands in the lower eyelid, as revealed by infrared transillumination of the eyelid. The glands appear as dark gray linear structures. *(Courtesy of William Mathers, MD.)*

The hair bulbs of the cilia are located anterior to the tarsus and the meibomian gland orifices. Misdirection in the orientation of the eyelashes (trichiasis) or aberrant growth through the orifices of the meibomian glands (distichiasis) may occur as either a congenital or an acquired defect; occasionally these defects are hereditary.

Conjunctiva

The palpebral conjunctiva is a transparent vascularized membrane covered by a nonkeratinized epithelium that lines the inner surface of the eyelids. Continuous with the conjunctival fornices (cul-de-sacs), it merges with the bulbar conjunctiva before terminating at the limbus (Fig 1-31). The conjunctiva is discussed in more detail later in this chapter.

Vascular Supply of the Eyelids

The blood supply of the eyelids is derived from the facial system, which arises from the external carotid artery, and the orbital system, which originates from the internal carotid artery along branches of the ophthalmic artery (Fig 1-32). The superficial and deep plexuses of arteries provide a vast blood supply to the upper and lower eyelids. The facial artery becomes the angular artery as it passes upward, forward, and lateral to the nose, where it serves as an important landmark in dacryocystorhinostomy (DCR).

The *marginal arterial arcade* is located 3 mm from the free border of the eyelid, just above the ciliary follicles. It is either between the tarsal plate and the orbicularis or within

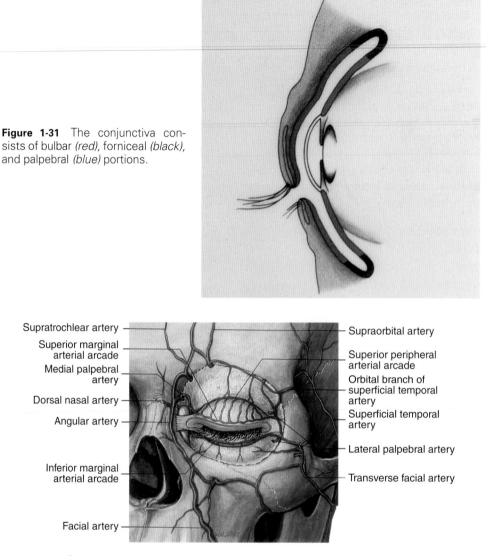

Figure 1-31 The conjunctiva consists of bulbar *(red)*, forniceal *(black)*, and palpebral *(blue)* portions.

Supratrochlear artery

Superior marginal arterial arcade

Medial palpebral artery

Dorsal nasal artery

Angular artery

Inferior marginal arterial arcade

Facial artery

Supraorbital artery

Superior peripheral arterial arcade

Orbital branch of superficial temporal artery

Superficial temporal artery

Lateral palpebral artery

Transverse facial artery

Figure 1-32 Periorbital and eyelid arteries, frontal view. *(Reproduced with permission from Dutton JJ. Atlas of Clinical and Surgical Orbital Anatomy. Philadelphia: Saunders; 1994.)*

the tarsus. A smaller peripheral arcade runs along the upper margin of the tarsal plate within the Müller muscle.

The venous drainage of the eyelids can be divided into 2 portions: a superficial, or pretarsal, system, which drains into the internal and external jugular veins; and a deep, or posttarsal, system, which flows into the cavernous sinus.

Lymphatics of the Eyelids

Lymphatic vessels are found in the eyelids and conjunctiva, but neither lymphatic vessels nor nodes are present in the orbit. Lymphatic drainage from the eyelids parallels the course of the veins (Fig 1-33). Two groups of lymphatics exist: (1) a medial group that drains into the submandibular lymph nodes and (2) a lateral group that drains into the superficial preauricular lymph nodes.

Clinically, swelling of the lymph nodes is a diagnostic sign of several external eye infections, including adenoviral conjunctivitis and Parinaud oculoglandular syndrome.

Accessory Eyelid Structures

Caruncle

The caruncle is a small, fleshy, ovoid structure attached to the inferomedial side of the plica semilunaris (see Fig 1-22). As a piece of modified skin, it contains sebaceous glands and fine, colorless hairs. The surface is covered by nonkeratinized, stratified squamous epithelium.

Plica semilunaris

The plica semilunaris is a narrow, highly vascular, crescent-shaped fold of the conjunctiva located lateral to and partly under the caruncle (see Fig 1-22). Its lateral border is free and separated from the bulbar conjunctiva, which it resembles histologically. The epithelium of the plica is rich in goblet cells. The plica's stroma contains fat and some nonstriated muscle. The plica is a vestigial structure analogous to the nictitating membrane, or third eyelid, of dogs and other animals.

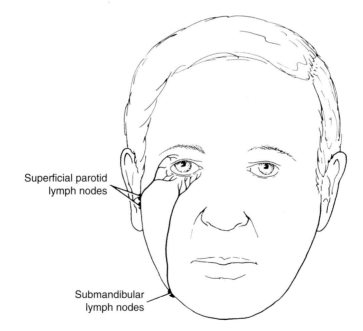

Superficial parotid
lymph nodes

Submandibular
lymph nodes

Figure 1-33 The lymphatic drainage of the eyelids. *(Reproduced with permission from Snell RS, Lemp MA. Clinical Anatomy of the Eye. Boston: Blackwell; 1989.)*

Lacrimal Gland and Excretory System

For further discussion of the lacrimal system, see BCSC Section 7, *Orbit, Eyelids, and Lacrimal System.*

Lacrimal Gland

The main lacrimal gland is located in a shallow depression within the orbital part of the frontal bone. The gland is separated from the orbit by fibroadipose tissue and divided into 2 parts by a lateral expansion of the levator aponeurosis (Fig 1-34). When the upper eyelid is everted, the smaller, palpebral part can be seen in the superolateral conjunctival fornix. An isthmus of glandular tissue occasionally exists between the palpebral lobe and the main orbital gland.

A variable number of thin-walled excretory ducts, blood vessels, lymphatics, and nerves pass from the main orbital gland into the palpebral lacrimal gland. The ducts continue downward, and about 12 of them empty into the conjunctival fornix approximately 5 mm above the superior margin of the upper tarsus. Because the lacrimal excretory ducts pass through the palpebral portion of the gland, biopsy of the lacrimal gland is usually performed on the main part to avoid sacrificing the ducts.

The lacrimal glands are exocrine glands that produce a serous secretion. The body of each gland contains 2 cell types (Fig 1-35):

1. acinar cells, which line the lumen of the gland
2. myoepithelial cells, which surround the parenchyma and are covered by a basement membrane

The lacrimal artery, a branch of the ophthalmic artery, supplies the gland. The lacrimal gland receives secretomotor cholinergic, vasoactive intestinal polypeptide (VIP)-

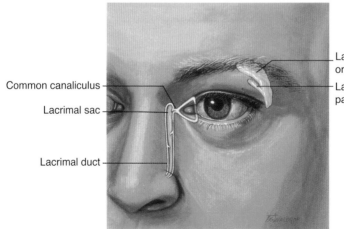

Figure 1-34   Lacrimal system. *(Reproduced with permission from Dutton JJ.* Atlas of Clinical and Surgical Orbital Anatomy. *Philadelphia: Saunders; 1994.)*

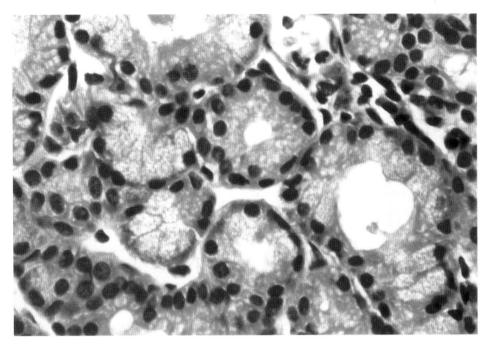

Figure 1-35 Higher magnification of lacrimal gland lobules. Note that the acinar cells forming the lobules are surrounded by myoepithelial cells that contain flattened nuclei (H&E×64). *(Courtesy of Thomas A. Weingeist, PhD, MD.)*

ergic, and sympathetic nerve fibers in addition to a sensory innervation via the lacrimal nerve (CN V$_1$). Cyclic adenosine monophosphate is the second messenger for VIP and β-adrenergic stimulation of the gland; cholinergic stimulation acts through an inositol 1,4,5-triphosphate–activated protein kinase C. The gland also contains α$_1$-adrenergic receptors. Extremely complex, the gland's neuroanatomy governs both reflex and psychogenic stimulation. See BCSC Section 5, *Neuro-Ophthalmology.*

Accessory Glands

The accessory lacrimal *glands of Krause* and *Wolfring* are located at the proximal lid borders or in the fornices and are cytologically identical to the main lacrimal gland, receiving a similar innervation. They account for about 10% of the total lacrimal secretory mass.

Lacrimal Excretory System

The lacrimal drainage system includes the upper and lower puncta, the lacrimal canaliculi, the lacrimal sac, and the nasolacrimal duct (see Fig 1-28; Fig 1-36). The lacrimal papillae are located at the extreme nasal border of the eyelids at their junction with the inner canthus. The puncta are directed posteriorly into the tear lake at the inner canthus. Each tiny opening, or *lacrimal punctum,* is about 0.3 mm in diameter. The inferior punctum is 6.5 mm from the medial canthus; the superior punctum is 6.0 mm from it. These openings lead to the *lacrimal canaliculi,* the *lacrimal sac,* and finally the *nasolacrimal duct* to the

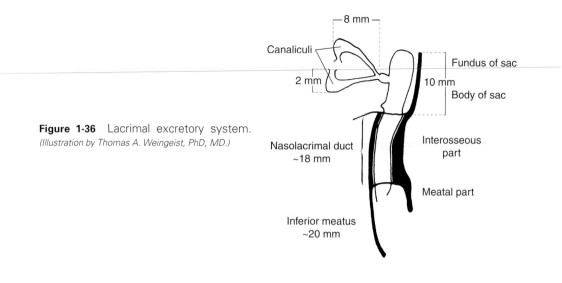

Figure 1-36 Lacrimal excretory system.
(Illustration by Thomas A. Weingeist, PhD, MD.)

nose. In 90% of people, the canaliculi join to form a common canaliculus. In about 30% of full-term neonates, the outlet of the nasolacrimal duct is closed and may remain so for up to 6 months. Occasionally, probing may be necessary to achieve patency.

The lacrimal puncta and the canaliculi are lined with stratified squamous nonkeratinized epithelium that merges with the epithelium of the eyelid margins. Near the lacrimal sac, the epithelium changes into 2 layers: (1) a superficial columnar layer and (2) a deep, flattened cell layer. Goblet cells and occasional cilia are present. In the canaliculi, the substantia propria consists of collagenous connective tissue and elastic fibers. The wall of the lacrimal sac resembles adenoid tissue and has a rich venous plexus and many elastic fibers.

Conjunctiva

The conjunctiva can be divided into 3 geographic zones: palpebral, fornical, and bulbar. The *palpebral conjunctiva* begins at the mucocutaneous junction of the eyelid and covers the lid's inner surface. This part adheres firmly to the tarsus. The tissue becomes redundant and freely movable in the fornices *(forniceal conjunctiva),* where it becomes enmeshed with fibrous elements of the levator aponeurosis and Müller muscle in the upper eyelid. In the lower eyelid, fibrous expansions of the inferior rectus muscle sheath fuse with the inferior tarsal muscle, the equivalent of the Müller muscle. The conjunctiva is reflected at the cul-de-sac and attaches to the globe. The delicate *bulbar conjunctiva* is freely movable but fuses with the Tenon capsule and inserts into the limbus.

Anterior ciliary arteries supply blood to the bulbar conjunctiva. The tarsal conjunctiva is supplied by branches of the marginal arcades of the lids. The proximal arcade, running along the upper border of the lid, sends branches proximally to supply the fornical and then the bulbar conjunctiva as the posterior conjunctival arteries. The limbal blood supply derives from the ciliary arteries through the anterior conjunctival arteries. The vascular watershed between the anterior and posterior territories lies approximately 3 or 4 mm from the limbus. The innervation of the conjunctiva is derived from the ophthalmic division of CN V.

The conjunctiva is a mucous membrane consisting of a nonkeratinizing squamous epithelium with numerous goblet cells and a thin, richly vascularized substantia propria containing lymphatic vessels, plasma cells, macrophages, and mast cells. A lymphoid layer extends from the bulbar conjunctiva to the subtarsal folds of the lids. In places, specialized aggregations of *conjunctiva-associated lymphoid tissue (CALT)* correspond to *mucosa-associated lymphoid tissue (MALT)* elsewhere and comprise collections of T and B lymphocytes underlying a modified epithelium. These regions are concerned with antigen processing.

The conjunctival epithelium varies from 2 to 5 cells in thickness. The basal cells are cuboidal and evolve into flattened polyhedral cells as they reach the surface. The goblet cells (unicellular mucous glands) are concentrated in the inferior and medial portion of the conjunctiva, especially in the region of the caruncle and plica semilunaris. They are sparsely distributed throughout the remainder of the conjunctiva and are absent in the limbal region.

Knop N, Knop E. Conjunctiva-associated lymphoid tissue in the human eye. *Invest Ophthalmol Vis Sci.* 2000;41(6):1270–1279.

Tenon Capsule

The Tenon capsule (the *fascia bulbi*) is an envelope of elastic connective tissue that fuses posteriorly with the optic nerve sheath and anteriorly with a thin layer of tissue called the *intermuscular septum,* 3 mm posterior to the limbus. The Tenon capsule is the cavity within which the globe moves. It is composed of compactly arranged collagen fibers and a few fibroblasts.

The Tenon capsule is thickest in the area of the equator of the globe. Connections between the Tenon capsule and the periorbital tissues help suspend the globe in the orbit. The extraocular muscles penetrate this connective tissue about 10 mm posterior to their insertions. The connective tissues form sleeves around the penetrating extraocular muscles, creating pulleys suspended from the periorbita. These pulleys stabilize the position of the muscles relative to the orbit during eye movements. The pulleys are connected to one another and to the Tenon fascia by connective tissue bands containing collagen, elastin, and smooth muscle (Fig 1-37).

Demer JL. Mechanics of the orbita. *Dev Ophthalmol.* 2007;40:132–157.

The suspensory ligament of Lockwood (Fig 1-38) is a fusion of the sheath of the inferior rectus muscle, the inferior tarsal muscle, and the check ligaments of the medial and lateral rectus muscles. It provides support for the globe and the anterioinferior orbit. The fusion of the sheath of the inferior rectus muscles, the Lockwood ligament, and the inferior tarsal muscle is an important consideration in surgery, because an operation on the inferior rectus muscle may be associated with palpebral fissure changes.

Figure 1-37 Diagram of the orbital connective tissues. *IR* = inferior rectus, *LPS* = levator palpebrae superioris, *LR* = lateral rectus, *MR* = medial rectus, *SO* = superior oblique, *SR* = superior rectus. *(From Demer JL, Miller JM, Pouken V, Vinters HV, Glasgow BJ. Evidence for fibromuscular pulleys of the recti extraocular muscles. Invest Ophthalmol Vis Sci. 1995;36(6):1125. © Association for Research in Vision and Ophthalmology.)*

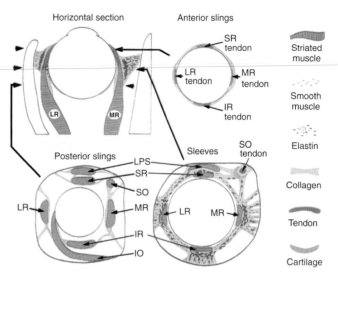

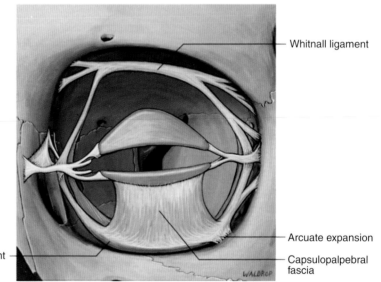

Figure 1-38 Eyelids, anterior fascial support system. *(Reproduced with permission from Dutton JJ. Atlas of Clinical and Surgical Orbital Anatomy. Philadelphia: Saunders; 1994.)*

Vascular Supply and Drainage of the Orbit

Posterior and Anterior Ciliary Arteries

Approximately 20 short posterior ciliary arteries and 10 short posterior ciliary nerves enter the globe in a ring around the optic nerve (Figs 1-39 through 1-41). Usually, 2 long ciliary arteries and nerves enter the sclera on either side of the optic nerve close to the horizontal

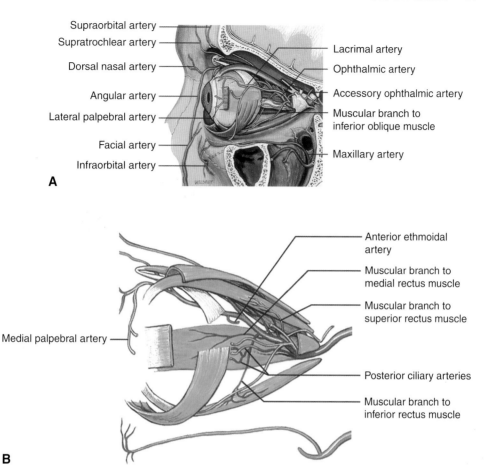

Supraorbital artery

Supratrochlear artery

Dorsal nasal artery

Angular artery

Lateral palpebral artery

Facial artery

Infraorbital artery

A

Lacrimal artery

Ophthalmic artery

Accessory ophthalmic artery

Muscular branch to inferior oblique muscle

Maxillary artery

Anterior ethmoidal artery

Muscular branch to medial rectus muscle

Muscular branch to superior rectus muscle

Medial palpebral artery

Posterior ciliary arteries

Muscular branch to inferior rectus muscle

B

Figure 1-39 Orbital arteries. **A,** Lateral view with extraocular muscles, composite view. **B,** Central dissection. *(Reproduced with permission from Dutton JJ.* Atlas of Clinical and Surgical Orbital Anatomy. *Philadelphia: Saunders; 1994.)*

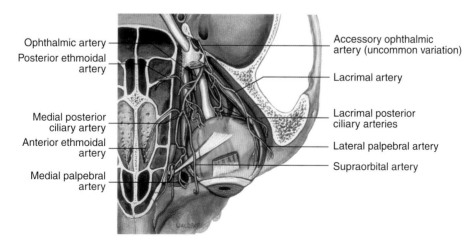

Ophthalmic artery

Posterior ethmoidal artery

Medial posterior ciliary artery

Anterior ethmoidal artery

Medial palpebral artery

Accessory ophthalmic artery (uncommon variation)

Lacrimal artery

Lacrimal posterior ciliary arteries

Lateral palpebral artery

Supraorbital artery

Figure 1-40 Orbital arteries, superior composite view. *(Reproduced with permission from Dutton JJ.* Atlas of Clinical and Surgical Orbital Anatomy. *Philadelphia: Saunders; 1994.)*

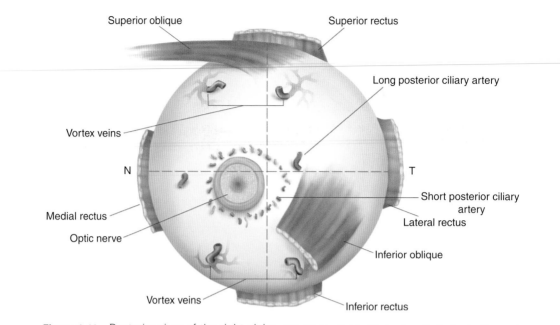

Figure 1-41 Posterior view of the right globe. *(Modified by Cyndie Wooley from illustration by Thomas A. Weingeist, PhD, MD.)*

meridian. The course of these vessels can usually be followed for a short distance in the suprachoroidal space. The posterior ciliary vessels originate from the ophthalmic artery and supply the whole uveal tract, the cilioretinal arteries, the sclera, the margin of the cornea, and the adjacent conjunctiva. Occlusion of the posterior ciliary vessels (as in giant cell arteritis) may have profound consequences for the eye, such as anterior ischemic optic neuropathy.

The anterior ciliary arteries also arise from the ophthalmic artery and usually supply (in pairs) the superior, medial, and inferior rectus muscles (Figs 1-42, 1-43). A single anterior ciliary vessel enters the lateral rectus muscle from the lacrimal artery. The anterior and posterior ciliary vessels usually anastomose with the long posterior ciliary vessels via anastomoses that perforate the sclera anterior to the rectus muscle insertions. Within the eye, the posterior ciliary vessel forms the intramuscular circle of the iris, from which branches supply the major arterial circle (which is usually discontinuous). This circle lies within the apex of the ciliary muscle, which it supplies together with the iris. The iris vessels have a radial arrangement that is visible upon slit-lamp examination in lightly pigmented blue irises. This can be distinguished from the irregular new iris vessels formed in rubeosis iridis.

Vortex Veins

The vortex veins drain the venous system of the choroid, ciliary body, and iris (see Fig 1-41; Fig 1-44). Each eye contains 4 to 7 (or more) veins. One or more veins are usually located

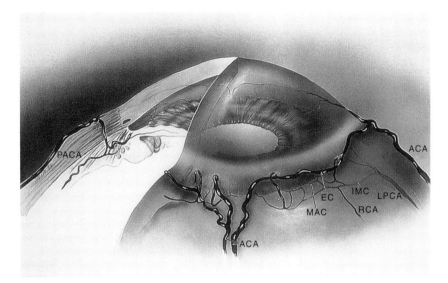

Figure 1-42 Three-dimensional representation of the multilevel collateral circulation in the primate anterior uvea in both surface and cutaway views. To the left, in cross section, perforating branches of the anterior ciliary artery are shown as they pass through the sclera to supply the intramuscular circle and major arterial circle. *ACA* = anterior ciliary artery, *EC* = episcleral circle, *IMC* = intramuscular circle, *LPCA* = long posterior ciliary artery, *MAC* = major arterial circle, *PACA* = posterior perforating anterior ciliary artery, *RCA* = recurrent ciliary artery. *(Reproduced with permission from Morrison JC, Van Buskirk EM. Anterior collateral circulation in the primate eye.* Ophthalmology. *1983;90:707.)*

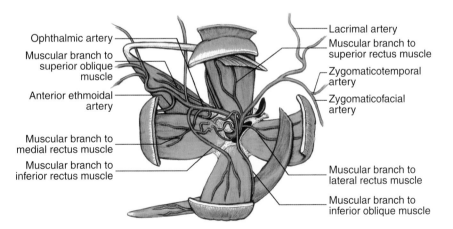

Figure 1-43 Orbital arteries, frontal view with extraocular muscles. *(Reproduced with permission from Dutton JJ.* Atlas of Clinical and Surgical Orbital Anatomy. *Philadelphia: Saunders; 1994.)*

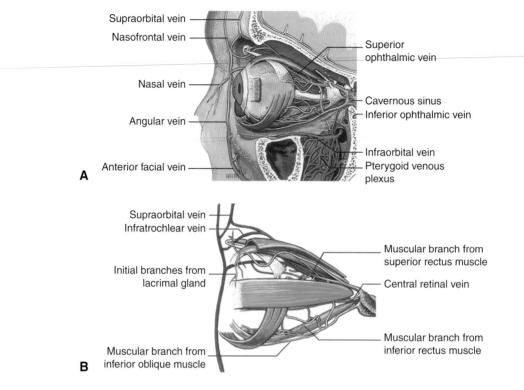

Supraorbital vein
Nasofrontal vein
Superior ophthalmic vein
Nasal vein
Cavernous sinus
Inferior ophthalmic vein
Angular vein
Infraorbital vein
Pterygoid venous plexus
Anterior facial vein
A

Supraorbital vein
Infratrochlear vein
Muscular branch from superior rectus muscle
Initial branches from lacrimal gland
Central retinal vein
Muscular branch from inferior rectus muscle
Muscular branch from inferior oblique muscle
B

Figure 1-44 Orbital veins, lateral view. **A,** Composite view. **B,** Central dissection. *(Reproduced with permission from Dutton JJ. Atlas of Clinical and Surgical Orbital Anatomy. Philadelphia: Saunders; 1994.)*

in each quadrant and exit 14–25 mm from the limbus between the rectus muscles. The ampullae of the vortex veins are 8–9 mm from the ora serrata and are visible by indirect ophthalmoscopy. A circle connecting these ampullae corresponds roughly to the equator and divides the central or posterior fundus from the peripheral portion.

CHAPTER 2

The Eye

Topographic Features of the Globe

The eyeball, or globe, is not a true sphere. The radius of curvature of the cornea (8 mm) is smaller than that of the sclera (12 mm), making the shape of the globe an oblate spheroid (Fig 2-1). The anteroposterior diameter of the adult eye is approximately 23–25 mm. Myopic eyes tend to be longer, and hyperopic eyes tend to be shorter. The average transverse diameter of the adult eye is 24 mm.

The eye contains 3 compartments: the anterior chamber, the posterior chamber, and the vitreous cavity. The anterior chamber, the space between the iris and the

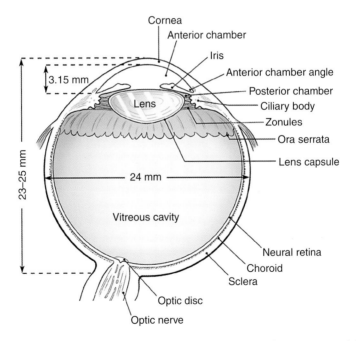

Figure 2-1 Sagittal section of eye with absent vitreous and major structures identified. Dimensions are approximate and are the average dimension in the normal adult eye. *(Illustration by Christine Gralapp.)*

cornea, is filled with aqueous fluid. It is about 3 mm deep, with an average volume of 200 μL. The posterior chamber is the anatomical portion of the eye posterior to the iris and anterior to the lens and vitreous face. It is also filled with aqueous fluid and has an average volume of 60 μL. The largest compartment of the eye is the vitreous cavity, which makes up more than two thirds of the volume of the eye (5–6 mL) and contains the vitreous gel. The total volume of the average adult eye is approximately 6.5–7 mL.

The eyeball is composed of 3 concentric layers. The outermost layer consists of the clear *cornea* anteriorly and the opaque white *sclera* posteriorly. The outermost corneo-scleral layer is composed of tough and protective tissues.

The cornea occupies the center of the anterior pole of the globe. Because the sclera and conjunctiva overlap the cornea anteriorly, slightly more above and below than medi-ally and laterally, the cornea appears elliptical when viewed from the front. In the adult, it measures about 12 mm in the horizontal meridian and about 11 mm in the vertical. From behind, when the cornea is viewed at its posterior landmark (the Schwalbe line—the termination of Descemet's membrane), its circumference appears circular. The cornea is about 1 mm thick at its periphery and is 0.5 mm thick centrally. The limbus, which bor-ders the cornea and the sclera, is gray and translucent.

In contrast to the transparent cornea, the sclera is opaque and white. Thinnest just be-hind the insertions of the rectus muscles (0.3 mm), the sclera increases to approximately 1 mm thick posteriorly but becomes thin and sievelike at the lamina cribrosa, where the axons of the ganglion cells exit to form the optic nerve.

The middle layer of the globe is the *uvea,* which consists of the choroid, ciliary body, and iris. Highly vascular, it serves a nutritive and supportive function.

The innermost layer of the globe is the *retina.* This photosensitive layer contains the photoreceptors and neural elements that initiate the processing of visual information.

Other important surface features of the globe, such as the vortex veins, the posterior ciliary artery and nerves, extraocular muscle insertions, and the optic nerve and its sur-rounding meningeal sheaths, are discussed in Chapter 1.

Precorneal Tear Film

The exposed surfaces of the cornea and globe are covered by the precorneal tear film, which is composed of 3 layers: a *superficial oily layer* produced predominantly by the meibomian glands; a *middle aqueous layer* produced by the main and accessory lacrimal glands; and a *deep mucin layer* derived from the conjunctival goblet cells. The surface cells of the cornea and conjunctiva also express a mucinous glycocalyx.

Maintenance of the precorneal tear film is vital for normal corneal function. In addi-tion to lubricating the surface of the cornea and conjunctiva, tears produce a smooth opti-cal surface, provide oxygen and other nutrients, and contain immunoglobulins, lysozyme, and lactoferrin. Aberrations in the tear film result from a variety of diseases (eg, dry eye) that profoundly affect the integrity of the surface.

Cornea

Characteristics of the Central and Peripheral Cornea

The air–tear interface at the surface of the cornea forms a positive lens of approximately 43 diopters (D) in air and constitutes the main refractive element of the eye (Fig 2-2). The central third of the cornea is nearly spherical and measures about 4 mm in diameter in the normal eye. Because the posterior surface of the cornea is more curved than the anterior surface, the central cornea is thinner (0.5 mm) than the peripheral cornea (1.0 mm). The cornea becomes flatter in the periphery, but the rate of flattening is not symmetric. Flattening is more extensive nasally and superiorly than temporally and inferiorly. This topography is important in contact lens fitting. BCSC Section 8, *External Disease and Cornea*, discusses the cornea in detail.

Epithelium and Basal Lamina

The anterior surface of the cornea is derived from surface ectoderm and is covered by a nonkeratinized, stratified squamous epithelium whose basal columnar layer is attached to a basal lamina by hemidesmosomes (Fig 2-3). The basal cells have a width of 12 μm and a density of approximately 6000 cells/mm². The occasional recurrence of corneal erosion following a traumatic corneal abrasion may be due to improper formation of hemidesmosomes after an epithelial abrasion.

Overlying the basal cell layer are 2 or 3 layers of polygonal "wing" cells. The superficial corneal epithelial cells are extremely thin (30 μm) and are attached to one another by occluding zonules. These zonules confer the properties of a semipermeable membrane to the epithelium. Microplicae and microvilli make the apical surfaces of the wing cells highly irregular; however, the precorneal tear film renders the surfaces optically smooth. Although the deeper epithelial cells are firmly attached to one another by desmosomes, they migrate continuously from the basal region toward the tear film, into which they are shed. They also migrate centripetally from their stem cell source at the limbus. Division of the slow-cycling stem cells gives rise to a progeny of daughter cells (transient amplifying cells), whose division serves to maintain the corneal epithelium. Diffuse damage to the limbal stem cells (eg, by chemical burns, trachoma) leads to chronic epithelial surface defects.

Fine BS, Yanoff M. *Ocular Histology: A Text and Atlas.* 2nd ed. Hagerstown, MD: Harper & Row; 1979:163–168.

Nonepithelial Cells

Nonepithelial cells may appear within the corneal epithelial layer. Wandering histiocytes, macrophages, lymphocytes, and pigmented melanocytes are frequent components of the peripheral cornea. Antigen-presenting Langerhans cells are found peripherally and move centrally with age or in response to keratitis.

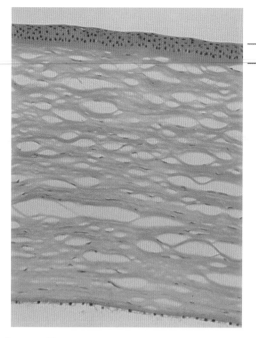

See Figure 2-3 below for diagram of this portion

Figure 2-2 Cornea. The empty spaces in the stroma are artifactitious (H&E ×32). *(Courtesy of Thomas A. Weingeist, PhD, MD.)*

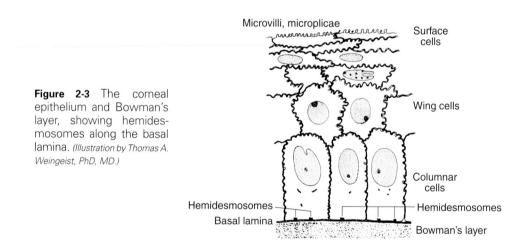

Figure 2-3 The corneal epithelium and Bowman's layer, showing hemides- mosomes along the basal lamina. *(Illustration by Thomas A. Weingeist, PhD, MD.)*

Microvilli, microplicae

Surface cells

Wing cells

Columnar cells

Hemidesmosomes

Basal lamina

Hemidesmosomes

Bowman's layer

Bowman's Layer

Beneath the basal lamina is Bowman's layer, or Bowman's membrane, a tough layer consisting of randomly dispersed collagen fibrils. It is a modified region of the anterior stroma 8–14 µm thick. Unlike Descemet's membrane, it is not restored after injury but is replaced by scar tissue.

Stroma

The stroma constitutes approximately 90% of the total corneal thickness in humans (see Fig 2-5). It is composed of collagen-producing keratocytes, ground substance, and collagen lamellae. The collagen fibrils form obliquely oriented lamellae in the anterior third of the stroma (with some interlacing) and parallel lamellae in the posterior two thirds. The corneal collagen fibrils extend across the entire diameter of the cornea, finally winding circumferentially around the limbus. The fibrils are remarkably uniform in size and separation, and this regularity helps determine the transparency of the cornea. Separation of the collagen fibrils by edema fluid leads to stromal clouding. The macroperiodicity of the fibrils (640 Å) is typical of collagen. The stroma's collagen types are I, III, V, and VI. Type VII forms the anchoring fibril of the epithelium.

The ground substance of the cornea consists of proteoglycans that run along and between the collagen fibrils. Their glycosaminoglycan components (eg, keratan sulfate) are highly charged and account for the swelling property of the stroma. The keratocytes lie between the corneal lamellae and synthesize both collagen and proteoglycans. Ultrastructurally, they resemble fibrocytes.

The cornea has approximately 2.4 million keratocytes, which occupy about 5% of the stromal volume; the density is higher anteriorly (1058 cells/mm^2) than posteriorly (771 cells/mm^2). Keratocytes are highly active cells, rich in mitochondria, rough endoplasmic reticula, and Golgi apparatuses. They have attachment structures, communicate by gap junctions, and have unusual fenestrations in their plasma membranes. Their flat profile and even distribution in the coronal plane ensure a minimum disturbance of light transmission. Studies with vital dyes suggest that there may be at least 3 different types of keratocytes.

Müller LJ, Pels L, Vrensen GF. Novel aspects of the ultrastructural organization of human corneal keratocytes. *Invest Ophthalmol Vis Sci.* 1995;36(13):2557–2567.

Mustonen RK, McDonald MB, Srivannaboon S, Tan AL, Doubrava MW, Kim CK. Normal human corneal cell populations evaluated by in vivo scanning slit confocal microscopy. *Cornea.* 1998;17(5):485–492.

Descemet's Membrane

The basal lamina of the corneal endothelium, Descemet's membrane, is periodic acid–Schiff (PAS)-positive (Fig 2-4). It is a true basement membrane, and its thickness increases with age. At birth, it is 3–4 μm thick; thickness increases throughout life to an adult level of 10–12 μm. It is composed of an anterior banded zone that develops in utero and a posterior nonbanded zone that is laid down by the corneal endothelium throughout life (Fig 2-5). These zones provide a historical record of the synthetic function of the endothelium. Like other basal laminae, Descemet's membrane is rich in type IV collagen.

Peripheral excrescences of Descemet's membrane, known as *Hassall-Henle warts,* are common, especially among elderly people. Central excrescences (cornea guttae) also appear with increasing age.

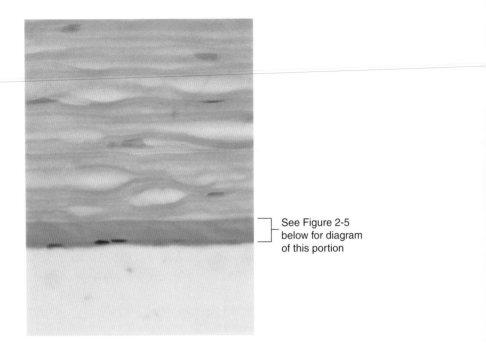

See Figure 2-5 below for diagram of this portion

Figure 2-4 Posterior cornea. Note the appearance of Descemet's membrane and the corneal endothelium (H&E ×64). *(Courtesy of Thomas A. Weingeist, PhD, MD.)*

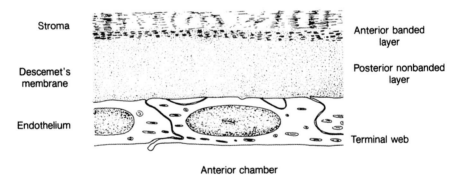

Stroma

Descemet's membrane

Endothelium

Anterior banded layer

Posterior nonbanded layer

Terminal web

Anterior chamber

Figure 2-5 Corneal endothelium and Descemet's membrane. *(Illustration by Thomas A. Weingeist, PhD, MD.)*

Endothelium

The corneal endothelium is composed of a single layer of mostly hexagonal cells derived from the neural crest (Fig 2-6). The corneal endothelium is therefore of neuroectodermal origin. Approximately 500,000 cells are present, with a density of about 3000 cells/mm^2.

The size, shape, and morphology of the endothelial cells can be observed by specular microscopy at the slit lamp. The apical surfaces of these cells face the anterior chamber; their basal surfaces abut Descemet's membrane. Typically, young endothelial cells have a large nucleus and abundant mitochondria. The active transport of ions by these cells leads

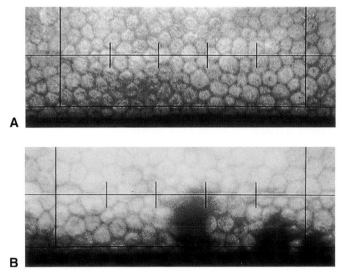

Figure 2-6 Specular micrographs of the corneal endothelium. **A,** Normal patient. **B,** Patient with Fuchs endothelial dystrophy. Both were taken at the same magnification. Bottom micrograph shows larger, more irregular cells (polymegethism); the 3 dark areas toward the bottom are cornea guttae. *(Courtesy of David Palay, MD, and David Litoff, MD.)*

to the transfer of water from the corneal stroma and the maintenance of stromal deturgescence and transparency. Mitosis of the endothelium is rare in humans, and the overall number of endothelial cells decreases with age.

Adjacent endothelial cells interdigitate in a complex way and form a variety of adherent junctions, but desmosomes are never seen between normal cells. In cross section, pinocytotic vesicles and a terminal web (a meshwork of fine fibrils that increases the density of the cytoplasm) can be seen toward the apical surface of the cells. Junctional complexes are present at the overlapping apicolateral boundaries of contiguous cells. They form a significant but lesser barrier to ion and water flow than the tight junctions of the epithelium.

Endothelial cell dysfunction and loss—through surgical injury, inflammation, or inherited disease (eg, Fuchs endothelial dystrophy)—may cause endothelial decompensation, stromal edema, and visual failure. In humans, endothelial mitosis is limited, and destruction of cells causes cell density to decrease and residual cells to spread and enlarge.

Foster CS, Azar DT, Dohlman CH. *Smolin and Thoft's The Cornea: Scientific Foundations and Clinical Practice.* 4th ed. Philadelphia: Lippincott Williams & Wilkins; 2004.

Sclera

The sclera covers the posterior four fifths of the surface of the globe, with an anterior opening for the cornea and a posterior opening for the optic nerve. The tendons of the rectus muscles insert into the superficial scleral collagen. The Tenon capsule covers the sclera and rectus muscles anteriorly, and both are overlain by the bulbar conjunctiva. The capsule and conjunctiva fuse near the limbus.

The sclera is thinnest (0.3 mm) just behind the insertions of the rectus muscles and thickest (1.0 mm) at the posterior pole around the optic nerve head. It is 0.4–0.5 mm thick at the equator and 0.6 mm thick anterior to the muscle insertions. Because of the thinness of the sclera, strabismus and retinal detachment surgery require careful placement of sutures. Scleral rupture following blunt trauma can occur at a number of sites: in a circumferential arc parallel to the corneal limbus opposite the site of impact, at the insertion of the rectus muscles, or at the equator of the globe. The most common site is the superonasal quadrant near the limbus.

The sclera, like the cornea, is essentially avascular except for the superficial vessels of the episclera and the intrascleral vascular plexus located just posterior to the limbus. A number of channels, or *emissaria,* penetrate the sclera, allowing for the passage of arteries, veins, and nerves. Extraocular extension of malignant melanoma of the choroid often occurs by way of the emissaria.

Branches of the ciliary nerves that supply the cornea sometimes leave the sclera to form loops posterior to the nasal and temporal limbus. These nerve loops, called *Axenfeld loops,* are sometimes pigmented and, consequently, have been mistaken for uveal tissue or malignant melanoma.

Anteriorly, the episclera consists of a dense vascular connective tissue that merges deeply with the superficial sclera and superficially with the Tenon capsule and the conjunctiva. The scleral stroma is composed of bundles of collagen, fibroblasts, and a moderate amount of ground substance. Collagen fibrils of the sclera vary in size and shape and have been shown to taper at their ends, indicating that they are not continuous fibers as in the cornea. In general, the outer scleral collagen fibers have a larger diameter (1600 Å) than the inner collagen fibers have (1000 Å). The inner layer of the sclera *(lamina fusca)* blends imperceptibly with the suprachoroidal and supraciliary lamellae of the uveal tract. The collagen fibers in this portion of the sclera branch and intermingle with the outer ciliary body and choroid. The bundles of collagen fibers contain electron-dense bodies, fibroblasts, and melanocytes. The opaque, porcelain-white appearance of the sclera contrasts markedly with the transparency of the cornea and is primarily due to 2 things: (1) the greater variation in fibril separation and diameter and (2) the greater degree of fibril interweave in the sclera. In addition, the lack of vascular elements such as the scleral emissaria contributes to corneal clarity.

Limbus

The transition zone between the peripheral cornea and the anterior sclera, known as the *limbus,* is defined differently by anatomists, pathologists, and clinicians. Although not a distinct anatomical structure, the limbus is important for 2 reasons: (1) its relationship to the chamber angle and (2) its use as a surgical landmark. The following structures are included in the limbus:

- conjunctiva and limbal palisades
- Tenon capsule

- episclera
- corneoscleral stroma
- aqueous outflow apparatus

The transition from opaque sclera to clear cornea occurs gradually over 1.0–1.5 mm and is difficult to define histologically. The corneoscleral junction begins centrally in a plane connecting the end of Bowman's layer and the Schwalbe line, the termination of Descemet's membrane. Internally, its posterior limit is the anterior tip of the scleral spur. Pathologists consider the posterior limit of the limbus to be formed by another plane perpendicular to the surface of the eye, approximately 1.5 mm posterior to the termination of Bowman's layer in the horizontal meridian and 2.0 mm posterior in the vertical meridian, where there is greater scleral overlap (Fig 2-7).

The surgical limbus can be divided conceptually into 2 equal zones: (1) an anterior bluish gray zone overlying clear cornea and extending from Bowman's layer to the Schwalbe line and (2) a posterior white zone overlying the trabecular meshwork and extending from the Schwalbe line to the scleral spur, or iris root. Familiarity with these landmarks is essential to the surgeon performing a cataract extraction or a glaucoma-filtering procedure.

Jaffe NS, Jaffe MS, Jaffe GF. *Cataract Surgery and Its Complications.* 6th ed. Philadelphia: Elsevier/Mosby; 1997.

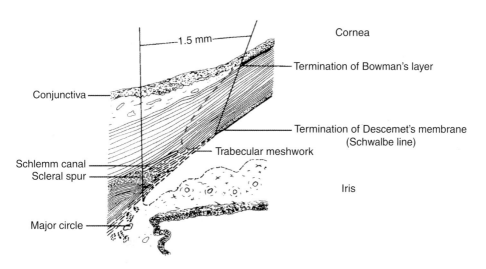

Figure 2-7 Anterior chamber angle and limbus, depicting the concept of the limbus. *Solid lines* represent the limbus as seen by pathologists; the *green dotted line* represents the limbus as seen by anatomists. *(Illustration by Thomas A. Weingeist, PhD, MD.)*

Anterior Chamber

The anterior chamber is bordered anteriorly by the cornea and posteriorly by the iris diaphragm and the pupil. The anterior chamber angle, which lies at the junction of the cornea and the iris, consists of the following structures (Fig 2-8):

- Schwalbe line
- the Schlemm canal and trabecular meshwork
- scleral spur
- anterior border of the ciliary body (where its longitudinal fibers insert into the scleral spur)
- iris

The depth of the anterior chamber varies. It is deeper in aphakia, pseudophakia, and myopia and shallower in hyperopia. In the normal adult emmetropic eye, the anterior chamber is approximately 3 mm deep at its center and reaches its narrowest point slightly central to the angle recess. The volume of the anterior chamber is about 200 μL in the emmetropic eye.

The anterior chamber is filled with *aqueous humor*, which is produced by the ciliary epithelium in the posterior chamber. The fluid passes through the pupil aperture and drains chiefly by the conventional pathway through the trabecular meshwork into the Schlemm canal and partly by the nontrabecular uveoscleral drainage pathway, across the ciliary body into the supraciliary space. The uveoscleral pathway, thought to be influenced by age, accounts for up to 50% of aqueous outflow in young people. BCSC Section 10, *Glaucoma*, discusses the anterior chamber and aqueous humor in detail.

High-resolution ultrasound biomicroscopy provides detailed 2-dimensional views of the anterior segment of the eye and is performed in vivo (Fig 2-9), allowing the clinician to view the relationship of the structures in the anterior segment under different pathologic conditions.

The internal scleral sulcus accommodates the Schlemm canal externally and the trabecular meshwork internally. The Schwalbe line, the periphery of Descemet's membrane, forms the anterior margin of the sulcus; the scleral spur is its posterior landmark. The scleral spur receives the insertion of the longitudinal ciliary muscle, and contraction opens up the trabecular spaces. Contractile cells are found within the scleral spur, as are structures resembling mechanoreceptors, which receive a sensory innervation.

Myofibroblast-like scleral spur cells with contractile properties are disposed circumferentially within the scleral spur. They are connected by elastic tissue to the trabecular meshwork; in experiments, stimulation with vasoactive intestinal polypeptide (VIP) or calcitonin gene–related peptide (CGRP) causes an increase in outflow facility. Individual scleral spur cells are innervated by unmyelinated axons, the terminals of which contact the cell membranes of the spur cells without an intervening basal lamina. The nerve fibers in this region are immunoreactive for neuropeptide Y, substance P, CGRP, VIP, and nitrous oxide and therefore are mediated by sympathetic, sensory, and pterygopalatine nerve pathways. There are no cholinergic fibers in this region.

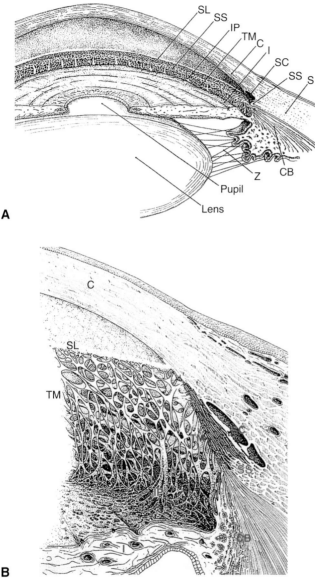

Figure 2-8 Semidiagrammatic representation of the structures of the angle of the anterior chamber and ciliary body. **A,** Composite gonioscopic and cross-sectional view of the anterior segment of the eye. **B,** Enlarged view. Note the superimposed trabecular sheets with intratrabecular spaces through which aqueous humor percolates to reach the Schlemm canal. *C* = cornea, *CB* = ciliary body, *I* = iris, *IP* = iris process, *S* = sclera, *SC* = Schlemm canal, *SL* = Schwalbe line, *SS* = scleral spur, *TM* = trabecular meshwork, *Z* = zonular fibers. *(Reproduced with permission from Tripathi RC, Tripathi BJ. Functional anatomy of the anterior chamber angle. In: Jakobiec FA, ed.* Ocular Anatomy, Embryology, and Teratology. *Philadelphia: Harper & Row; 1982.)*

Tamm ER, Koch TA, Mayer B, Stefani FH, Lütjen-Drecoll E. Innervation of myofibroblast-like scleral spur cells in human and monkey eyes. *Invest Ophthalmol Vis Sci.* 1995;36(8): 1633–1644.

Myelinated nerve fibers extending forward from the ciliary region to the inner aspect of the scleral spur give branches to the meshwork and to club-shaped endings in the scleral spur. These endings have the morphologic features of mechanoreceptors found elsewhere in the body, such as in the carotid. The endings are incompletely covered by a Schwann cell sheath and make contact with extracellular matrix materials such as elastin.

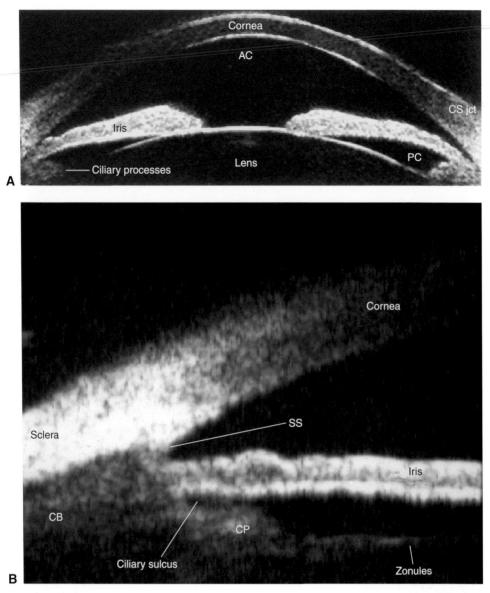

Figure 2-9 **A,** Ultrasound biomicroscopic composite image of the anterior segment, including the anterior chamber *(AC)*. The iris is slightly convex, indicating mild pupillary block. The corneoscleral junction *(CS jct)*, ciliary processes, and posterior chamber *(PC)* region are clearly imaged. The angle is narrow but open. Iris–lens contact is small. **B,** High-resolution ultrasound image of the anterior segment. Note the location of the ciliary sulcus. *CB* = ciliary body, *CP* = ciliary process, *SS* = scleral spur. *(Part A courtesy of Charles Pavlin, MD; part B courtesy of K. Nischal, MD.)*

Various functions have been proposed for these endings, including (1) proprioception to the ciliary muscle, which inserts into the scleral spur, signaling contraction of the scleral spur cells, and (2) baroreception in response to changes in intraocular pressure.

Trabecular Meshwork

The relationship of the trabecular meshwork (see Figs 2-7, 2-8) and the Schlemm canal to other structures is complex because the outflow apparatus is composed of tissue derived from the cornea, sclera, iris, and ciliary body (Fig 2-10).

The *trabecular meshwork* is a circular spongework of connective tissue lined by trabeculocytes. These cells have contractile properties, which may influence outflow resistance. They also have phagocytic properties. The meshwork is roughly triangular in cross section, with the apex at the Schwalbe line and the base formed by the scleral spur and the ciliary body. Some trabecular tissue passes posterior to the spur. The trabecular meshwork can be divided into 3 layers (see Fig 2-2 in BCSC Section 10, *Glaucoma*, Chapter 2):

1. uveal portion
2. corneoscleral meshwork
3. juxtacanalicular tissue, which is directly adjacent to the Schlemm canal

The uveal and corneoscleral meshwork can be divided by an imaginary line drawn from the Schwalbe line to the scleral spur. The uveal meshwork lies internal and the corneoscleral meshwork lies external to this line.

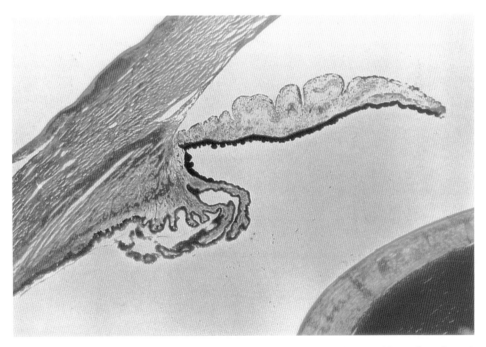

Figure 2-10 Anterior chamber angle, ciliary body, and peripheral lens. Note the triangular shape of the ciliary body. The muscle fibers appear red in contrast with the connective tissue. The scleral spur is clearly delineated from the ciliary muscle in the region of the trabecular meshwork. The lens is artifactually displaced posteriorly. (Masson trichrome ×8). *(Courtesy of Thomas A. Weingeist, PhD, MD.)*

Uveal Trabecular Meshwork

The *uveal meshwork* is composed of cordlike trabeculae, with fewer elastic fibers than in the corneoscleral meshwork. The trabeculocytes usually contain pigment granules, and the trabecular apertures are less circular and larger than those of the corneoscleral meshwork.

Corneoscleral Meshwork

The *corneoscleral meshwork* consists of a series of thin, flat, perforated connective tissue sheets arranged in a laminar pattern. Each trabecular beam is covered by a monolayer of thin trabecular cells exhibiting multiple pinocytotic vesicles. The basal lamina of these cells forms the outer cortex of the trabecular beam; the inner core is of collagen and elastic fibers.

Pericanalicular Connective Tissue

Pericanalicular connective tissue invests the entire extent of the Schlemm canal. On its trabecular aspect, between the outermost layers of the corneoscleral meshwork and the endothelial lining of the Schlemm canal, lies the *endothelial meshwork,* a multilayered collection of cells forming a loose network. Spaces exist between these cells, up to 10 μm in width, through which aqueous humor can percolate to reach the endothelial lining of the Schlemm canal. This region of the drainage system makes the greatest contribution to outflow resistance, partly because the pathway is narrow and tortuous and partly because of the resistance offered by extracellular proteoglycans and glycoproteins.

Schlemm Canal

The Schlemm canal is a circular tube closely resembling a lymphatic vessel. It is formed by a continuous monolayer of nonfenestrated endothelium and a thin connective tissue wall. The basement membrane of the endothelium is poorly defined. The lateral walls of the endothelial cells are joined by tight junctions. Micropinocytotic vesicles are present at both the apical and the basal surfaces of the cells. Larger vesicles (so-called giant vacuoles) have been observed along the internal canal wall (Figs 2-11, 2-12). These vacuoles are lined by a single membrane, and their size and number are increased by increasing intraocular pressure. They are thought to contribute to the pressure-dependent outflow of aqueous.

Collector Channels

Approximately 25–30 collector channels arise from the Schlemm canal (Fig 2-13) and drain into the deep and midscleral venous plexuses. Up to 8 of these channels drain directly into the episcleral venous plexus as aqueous veins (Fig 2-14), which are visible in the conjunctiva by biomicroscopy.

Aging brings about a twofold to threefold thickening of trabecular sheets; the cortex thickens and the core thins. There is loss of endothelial cellularity, an increase in

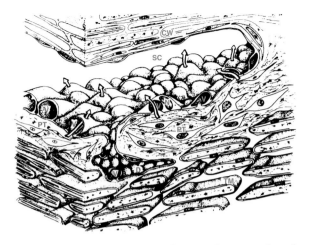

Figure 2-11 The walls of the Schlemm canal *(SC)* and adjacent trabecular meshwork *(TM)*. The endothelial lining of the trabecular wall of the Schlemm canal is very irregular; normally, the cells show luminal bulges corresponding to cell nuclei *(N)* and macrovacuolar configurations *(V)*. The latter represent cellular invaginations from the basal aspect that eventually open on the apical aspect of the cell to form transcellular channels *(arrows)* through which aqueous humor flows down a pressure gradient. A diverticulum *(D)*—its endothelial lining continuous with that of the canal—is shown on the inner wall of the Schlemm canal next to macrovacuolar configurations. Such blind, tortuous diverticula course for a variable distance into the trabecular meshwork but remain separated from the open spaces of the meshwork by their continuous endothelial lining. The endothelial lining of the trabecular wall is supported by interrupted, irregular basement membrane and a zone of pericanalicular connective tissue *(PT)* of variable thickness. The cellular element predominates in this zone, and the fibrous elements, especially elastic fibers, are irregularly arranged in a netlike fashion. Here, the open spaces are narrower than those of the trabecular meshwork. The corneoscleral trabecular sheets show frequent branching, and the endothelial covering may be shared between adjacent sheets. The corneoscleral wall *(CW)* of the Schlemm canal is more compact than the trabecular wall, with a lamellar arrangement of collagen and elastic tissue predominating. *(Reproduced with permission from Tripathi RC, Tripathi BJ. Functional anatomy of the anterior chamber angle. In: Jakobiec FA, ed. Ocular Anatomy, Embryology, and Teratology. Philadelphia: Harper & Row; 1982.)*

connective tissue (eg, in the endothelial meshwork), and an accumulation of debris in the meshwork and of glycosaminoglycans in the extracellular space. Such changes are exaggerated in chronic open-angle glaucoma.

Uveal Tract

The uveal tract is the main vascular compartment of the eye. It consists of 3 parts:

1. iris
2. ciliary body (located in the anterior uvea)
3. choroid (located in the posterior uvea)

The uveal tract is firmly attached to the sclera at only 3 sites: the scleral spur, the exit points of the vortex veins, and the optic nerve. These attachments account for the characteristic anterior balloons formed in choroidal detachment.

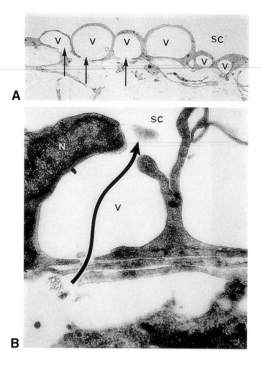

Figure 2-12 A, Low-magnification electron micrograph of the endothelial lining of the Schlemm canal *(SC)* shows that the majority of the vacuolar configurations *(V)* at this level have direct communication *(arrows)* with the subendothelial extracellular spaces, which contain aqueous humor (×3970). **B,** Electron micrograph of a vacuolar structure that shows both basal and apical openings, thus constituting a vacuolar transcellular channel *(arrow)*. Through this channel, the fluid-containing extracellular space on the basal aspect of the cell is temporarily connected with the lumen of the Schlemm canal, allowing bulk outflow of aqueous humor. *N* = indented nucleus of the cell (×23,825). *(Reproduced with permission from Tripathi RC, Tripathi BJ. Functional anatomy of the anterior chamber angle. In: Jakobiec FA, ed. Ocular Anatomy, Embryology, and Teratology. Philadelphia: Harper & Row; 1982.)*

Iris

The iris is the most anterior extension of the uveal tract (Figs 2-15, 2-16). It is made up of blood vessels and connective tissue, in addition to the melanocytes and pigment cells that are responsible for its distinctive color. The mobility of the iris allows the pupil to change size. During mydriasis, the iris is thrown into a number of ridges and folds; during miosis, its anterior surface appears relatively smooth. The iris diaphragm subdivides the anterior segment into the anterior and posterior chambers.

Stroma

The iris stroma is composed of pigmented cells (melanocytes) and nonpigmented cells, collagen fibrils, and a matrix containing hyaluronic acid. The aqueous humor flows freely through the loose stroma along the anterior border of the iris, which contains multiple crypts and crevices that vary in size, shape, and depth. This surface is covered by an interrupted layer of connective tissue cells that merges with the ciliary body.

The overall structure of the iris stroma remains similar in irides of all colors. Differences in color are related to the amount of pigmentation in the anterior border layer and the deep stroma. The stroma of blue irides is lightly pigmented, and brown irides have a densely pigmented stroma that absorbs light.

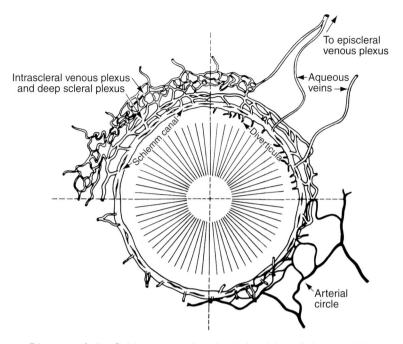

Figure 2-13 Diagram of the Schlemm canal and relationships of the arteriolar and venous vascular supply. For clarity, the various systems have been limited to only parts of the circumference of the canal. Small, tortuous, blind diverticula (so-called Sondermann channels) extend from the canal into the trabecular meshwork. Externally, the collector channels arising from the Schlemm canal anastomose to form the intrascleral and deep scleral venous plexuses. At irregular intervals around the circumference, aqueous veins arise from the intrascleral plexus and connect directly to the episcleral veins. The arteriolar supply closely approximates the canal, but no direct communication occurs between the two. *(Reproduced with permission from Tripathi RC, Tripathi BJ. Functional anatomy of the anterior chamber angle. In: Jakobiec FA, ed.* Ocular Anatomy, Embryology, and Teratology. *Philadelphia: Harper & Row; 1982:276.)*

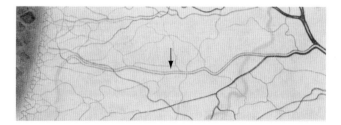

Figure 2-14 Aqueous vein *(arrow)*. Collector channels from the Schlemm canal drain into the episcleral venous plexus. With high magnification of the slit-lamp biomicroscope, they are visible near the limbus. Laminar flow and the mixing of aqueous and blood are visible. *(Reproduced with permission from Thiel R. Atlas of Diseases of the Eye. Amsterdam: Elsevier; 1963.)*

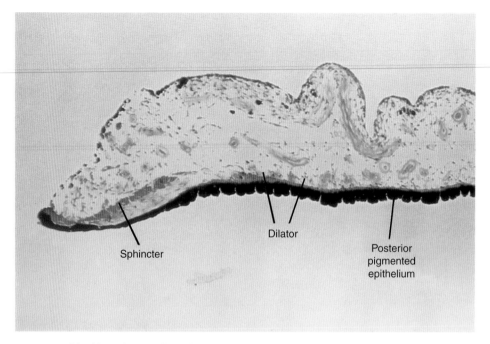

Figure 2-15 Iris. Note the relationship between the sphincter and dilator muscles (H&E ×20). *(Courtesy of Thomas A. Weingeist, PhD, MD.)*

Vessels and Nerves

Blood vessels form the bulk of the iris stroma. Most follow a radial course, arising from the major arterial circle and passing to the center of the pupil. In the region of the *collarette* (the thickest portion of the iris), anastomoses occur between the arterial and venous arcades to form the minor vascular circle of the iris, which is often incomplete. The major arterial circle is located at the apex of the ciliary body, not the iris. In humans, the anterior border layer is normally avascular. The diameter of the capillaries is relatively large. Their endothelium is nonfenestrated and is surrounded by a basement membrane, associated pericytes, and a zone of collagenous filaments. The intima has no internal elastic lamina.

Myelinated and nonmyelinated nerve fibers serve sensory, vasomotor, and muscular functions throughout the stroma.

Posterior Pigmented Layer

The posterior surface of the iris is densely pigmented and appears velvety smooth and uniform. It is continuous with the nonpigmented epithelium of the ciliary body and thence with the neurosensory portion of the retina. The polarity of its cells is maintained from embryogenesis. The basal surface of the pigmented layer borders the posterior chamber. The apical surface faces the stroma and adheres to the anterior pigmented layer, which gives rise to the dilator muscle (Fig 2-17).

The posterior pigmented layer of the iris curves around the pupillary margin and extends for a short distance onto the anterior border layer of the iris stroma as the pigment

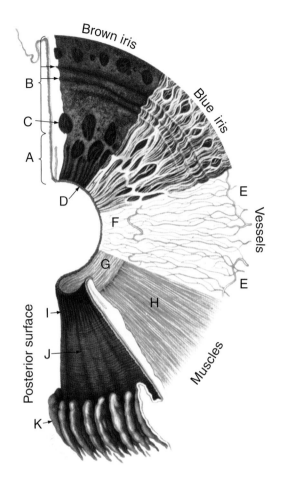

Figure 2-16 Composite drawing of the surfaces and layers of the iris, beginning at the upper left and proceeding clockwise. The iris cross section shows the pupillary *(A)* and ciliary *(B)* portions; the surface view shows a brown iris with its dense, matted anterior border layer. Circular contraction furrows are shown *(arrows)* in the ciliary portion of the iris. Fuchs crypts *(C)* are seen at either side of the collarette in the pupillary and ciliary portions and peripherally near the iris root. The pigment ruff is seen at the pupillary edge *(D)*. The blue iris surface shows a less dense anterior border layer and more prominent trabeculae. The iris vessels are shown beginning at the major arterial circle in the ciliary body *(E)*. Radial branches of the arteries and veins extend toward the pupillary region. The arteries form the incomplete minor arterial circle *(F)*, from which branches extend toward the pupil, forming capillary arcades. The sector below demonstrates the circular arrangement of the sphincter muscle *(G)* and the radial processes of the dilator muscle *(H)*. The posterior surface of the iris shows the radial contraction furrows *(I)* and the structural folds *(J)* of Schwalbe. Circular contraction folds are also present in the ciliary portion. The pars plicata of the ciliary body is at *(K)*. *(Reproduced with permission from Bron AJ, Tripathi RC, Tripathi BJ. Wolff's Anatomy of the Eye and Orbit. 8th ed. London: Chapman & Hall; 1997. Originally from Hogan MJ, Alvarado JA, and Weddell JE. Histology of the Human Eye. Philadelphia: WB Saunders; 1971.)*

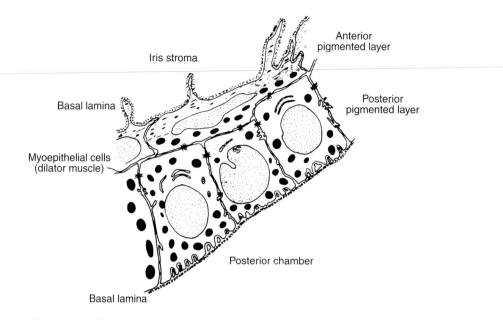

Figure 2-17 Posterior layer of the iris. *(Illustration by Thomas A. Weingeist, PhD, MD.)*

ruff. In rubeosis iridis, the pigmented layer extends farther onto the anterior surface of the iris, a condition called *ectropion*. The term *ectropion uveae* is a misnomer, because all of these layers are derived from neuroectoderm.

Dilator Muscle

The dilator muscle is derived embryologically from the outer layer of the optic cup, which is neuroectoderm. It lies parallel and anterior to the posterior pigmented epithelium. The smooth muscle cells contain fine myofilaments and melanosomes. The myofibrils are confined mainly to the basal portion of the cells and extend anteriorly into the iris stroma. The melanosomes and the nucleus are in the apical region of each myoepithelial cell.

There is dual sympathetic and parasympathetic innervation. The dilator muscle contracts in response to sympathetic α_1-adrenergic stimulation; cholinergic parasympathetic stimulation may have an inhibitory role.

The *first-order neuron* of the sympathetic chain begins in the ipsilateral posterolateral hypothalamus and passes through the brainstem to synapse in the intermediolateral gray matter of the spinal cord, chiefly at thoracic level 1. The *second-order preganglionic neuron* exits the spinal cord, passes over the pulmonary apex and through the stellate ganglion without synapsing, and synapses in the superior cervical ganglion. The *third-order postganglionic neuron* originates here, joins the internal carotid plexus, enters the cavernous sinus, and travels with the ophthalmic division of CN V to the orbit and then to the dilator muscle. Interruption of the sympathetic nerve supply results in Horner syndrome, with miosis, in addition to ptosis and anhydrosis.

Sphincter Muscle

Like the dilator muscle, the sphincter muscle is derived from neuroectoderm. It is composed of a circular band of smooth muscle fibers and is located near the pupillary margin in the deep stroma, anterior to the pigment epithelium of the iris. Although dual innervation has been demonstrated morphologically, the sphincter muscle receives its primary innervation from parasympathetic nerve fibers that originate in the CN III nucleus, and it responds pharmacologically to muscarinic stimulation. The reciprocal sympathetic innervation to the sphincter appears to serve an inhibitory role, helping to relax the sphincter in darkness.

The fibers subserving the sphincter muscle leave the Edinger-Westphal subnucleus and follow the inferior division of CN III after it bifurcates in the cavernous sinus. The fibers continue in the branch supplying the inferior oblique muscle, exit, and synapse with postganglionic fibers in the ciliary ganglion. The postganglionic fibers travel with the short ciliary nerves to the iris sphincter. They are unusual in that they are myelinated, presumably reflecting a need for fast conduction.

Ciliary Body

The ciliary body, which is triangular in cross section, bridges the anterior and posterior segments (see Fig 2-10). The apex of the ciliary body is directed posteriorly toward the ora serrata. The base of the ciliary body gives rise to the iris. The only attachment of the ciliary body to the sclera is at its base, via its longitudinal muscle fibers, where they insert into the scleral spur.

The ciliary body has 2 principal functions: aqueous humor formation and lens accommodation. It also plays a role in the trabecular and uveoscleral outflow of aqueous humor.

Ciliary Epithelium and Stroma

The ciliary body is 6–7 mm wide and consists of 2 parts: the pars plana and the pars plicata. The *pars plana* is a relatively avascular, smooth pigmented zone; it is 4 mm wide and extends from the ora serrata to the ciliary processes. The safest posterior surgical approach to the vitreous cavity is through the pars plana, located 3–4 mm from the corneal limbus. The *pars plicata* is richly vascularized and consists of approximately 70 radial folds, or ciliary processes. The zonular fibers of the lens attach primarily in the valleys of the ciliary processes but also along the pars plana.

The capillary plexus of each ciliary process is supplied by arterioles as they pass anteriorly and posteriorly from the major arterial circle; each plexus is drained by 1 or 2 large venules located at the crest of each process. Sphincter tone within the arteriolar smooth muscle affects the capillary hydrostatic pressure gradient. In addition, it influences whether blood flows into the capillary plexus or directly to the draining choroidal vein, bypassing the plexus completely. Neuronal innervation of the vascular smooth muscle and humoral vasoactive substances may be important in determining regional blood flow, capillary surface area available for exchange of fluid, and hydrostatic capillary pressure. All of these affect the rate of aqueous humor formation.

The ciliary body is lined by a double layer of epithelial cells, the nonpigmented and the pigmented epithelium (Fig 2-18). The inner, nonpigmented, epithelium is located between the aqueous humor of the posterior chamber and the outer pigmented epithelium. The apices of the nonpigmented and pigmented cell layers are fused by a complex system of junctions and cellular interdigitations. Along the lateral intercellular spaces, near the apical border of the nonpigmented epithelium, are tight junctions (*zonulae occludentes*) that maintain the blood–aqueous barrier. The basal surface of the nonpigmented epithelium, which borders the posterior chamber, is covered by the basal lamina, which is multilaminar in the valleys of the processes. The basal lamina of the pigmented epithelium, which faces the iris stroma, is thick and more homogeneous than that of the nonpigmented epithelium.

The pigmented epithelium is relatively uniform throughout the ciliary body. Its cuboidal cells are characterized by multiple basal infoldings, a large nucleus, mitochondria, extensive endoplasmic reticulum, and many melanosomes. The nonpigmented epithelium tends to be cuboidal in the pars plana region but columnar in the pars plicata. It also has multiple basal infoldings, abundant mitochondria, and large nuclei. The endoplasmic reticulum and Golgi complex in these cells are important to aqueous humor formation. Sometimes melanosomes are present, especially anteriorly, near the iris.

The uveal portion of the ciliary body consists of comparatively large fenestrated capillaries, collagen fibrils, and fibroblasts. The main arterial supply to the ciliary body comes from the anterior and the long posterior ciliary arteries, which join together to form a multilayered arterial plexus consisting of a superficial episcleral plexus, a deeper intramuscular plexus, and an incomplete major arterial circle often mistakenly attributed to the iris but

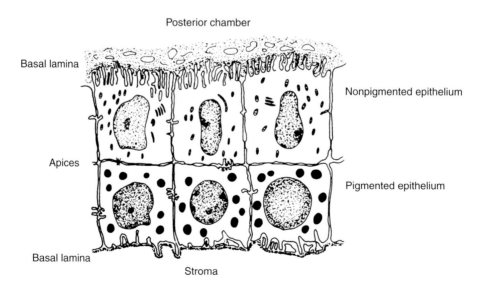

Figure 2-18 Ciliary epithelium. *(Illustration by Thomas A. Weingeist, PhD, MD.)*

actually located posterior to the anterior chamber angle recess, in the ciliary body. The major veins drain posteriorly through the vortex system, although some drainage also occurs through the intrascleral venous plexus and the episcleral veins into the limbal region.

Ciliary Muscle

Three layers of fibers have been described in the ciliary muscle (Fig 2-19):

1. longitudinal
2. radial
3. circular

Most of the ciliary muscle is made up of an outer layer of longitudinal fibers that attach to the scleral spur. The radial muscle fibers arise in the midportion of the ciliary body, and the circular fibers are located in the innermost portion. Clinically, the 3 groups of muscle fibers function as a unit. Presbyopia is associated with age-related changes in the lens (discussed in the section Lens, later in the chapter) rather than to changes in the ciliary muscle. Even so, the muscle does change with age, with increasing amounts of connective tissue between the muscle bundles and a loss of elastic recoil after contraction.

The ciliary muscles behave like other smooth, nonstriated muscle fibers. Ultrastructural studies reveal that they contain multiple myofibrils with characteristic electron-dense

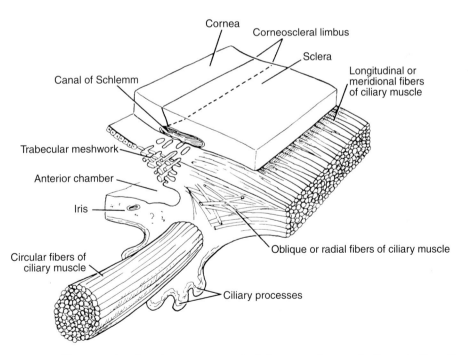

Figure 2-19 Diagram showing the arrangement of the smooth muscle fibers in the ciliary body. Note the relationship of the ciliary body to the iris, the anterior chamber, the Schlemm canal, and the corneoscleral limbus. *(Reproduced with permission from Snell RS, Lemp MA. Clinical Anatomy of the Eye. Cambridge, MA: Blackwell Scientific Publications; 1989.)*

attachment bodies, mitochondria, glycogen particles, and a prominent nucleus. The smooth muscle cells are surrounded by a basal lamina separated from the cell membrane by a 300 Å space. Bundles of fibers are surrounded by a thin fibroblastic sheath rather than by collagen. The muscle is rich in type VI collagen, which forms a sheath around the anterior elastic tendons. These tendons insert into the scleral spur and around the tips of the oblique and circular muscle fibers as they insert into the trabecular meshwork.

> Streeten BW. The ciliary body. In: Duane TD, Jaeger EA, eds. *Biomedical Foundations of Ophthalmology.* Philadelphia: Lippincott; 1995.

Both myelinated and nonmyelinated nerve fibers are observed throughout the ciliary muscle. Innervation is mainly derived from parasympathetic fibers of CN III via the short ciliary nerves. Approximately 97% of these ciliary fibers are directed to the ciliary muscle, and about 3% to the iris sphincter. Sympathetic fibers have also been observed and may play a role in relaxing the muscle. Cholinergic drugs contract the ciliary muscle. Because some of the muscle fibers form tendinous attachments to the scleral spur, their contraction increases aqueous flow by opening up the spaces of the trabecular meshwork.

Choroid

The choroid, the posterior portion of the uveal tract, nourishes the outer portion of the retina (Fig 2-20). It averages 0.25 mm in thickness and consists of 3 layers of vessels:

1. the choriocapillaris, the innermost layer
2. a middle layer of small vessels
3. an outer layer of large vessels

Perfusion of the choroid comes from both the long and the short posterior ciliary arteries and from the perforating anterior ciliary arteries. Venous blood drains through the vortex system. Blood flow through the choroid is high compared to that of other tissues. As a result, the oxygen content of choroidal venous blood is only 2%–3% less than that of arterial blood.

Bruch's Membrane

Bruch's membrane is a PAS-positive lamina resulting from the fusion of the basal laminae of the retinal pigment epithelium (RPE) and the choriocapillaris of the choroid (Fig 2-21). It extends from the margin of the optic disc to the ora serrata, and ultrastructurally it has 5 elements:

1. basal lamina of the RPE
2. inner collagenous zone
3. thicker, porous band of elastic fibers
4. outer collagenous zone
5. basal lamina of the choriocapillaris

Bruch's membrane, therefore, consists of a series of connective tissue sheets that are highly permeable to small molecules such as fluorescein. Defects in Bruch's membrane develop

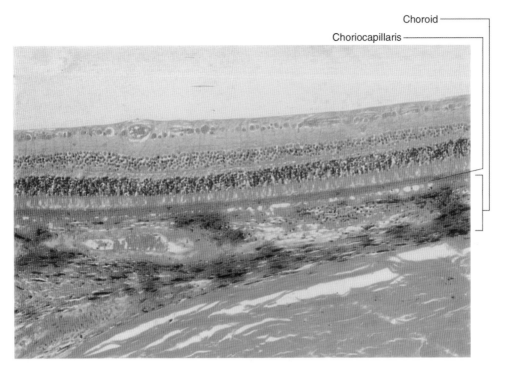

Figure 2-20 Choroid. The choriocapillaris lies just below the retinal pigment epithelium. Beneath are a middle and outer vascular layer and multiple dendritic melanocytes (H&E ×32). *(Courtesy of Thomas A. Weingeist, PhD, MD.)*

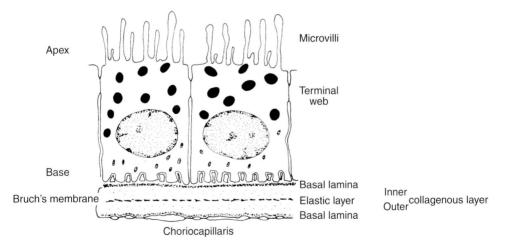

Figure 2-21 Retinal pigment epithelium and Bruch's membrane. *(Illustration by Thomas A. Weingeist, PhD, MD.)*

spontaneously in myopia or pseudoxanthoma elasticum, or they result from trauma or inflammation. Subretinal neovascular membranes can arise as a result of these defects, and they can lead to disciform macular changes as part of exudative age-related macular degeneration and ocular histoplasmosis syndrome.

Choriocapillaris

The choriocapillaris is a continuous layer of large capillaries (40–60 μm in diameter) lying in a single plane beneath the RPE (Fig 2-22). The vessel walls are extremely thin and contain multiple fenestrations, especially on the surface facing the retina (Fig 2-23). Pericytes are located along the outer wall.

The middle and outer choroidal vessels are not fenestrated. The large vessels, typical of small arteries elsewhere, possess an internal elastic lamina and smooth muscle cells in the media. As a result, small molecules such as fluorescein, which diffuse across the endothelium of the choriocapillaris, do not leak through medium and large choroidal vessels. Abundant melanocytes as well as occasional macrophages, lymphocytes, mast cells, and plasma cells appear throughout the choroidal stroma. The intercellular space contains collagen fibers and nerve fibers. The degree of pigmentation observed ophthalmoscopically in the ocular fundus primarily depends on the number of pigmented melanocytes in the choroid. Melanosomes are absent from the RPE and choroid of albinos. In lightly pigmented eyes, pigmentation in the choroid is sparse compared with that of darkly pigmented eyes. The degree of pigmentation in the choroid must be considered when one is performing photocoagulation, because it influences the absorption of laser energy.

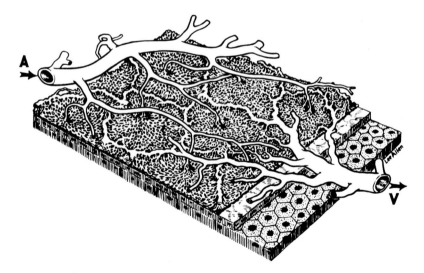

Figure 2-22 Lobular pattern of choriocapillaris. Note that the retinal pigment epithelium is internal to the choriocapillaris. *A* = choroidal arteriole, *V* = choroidal venule. *(Reproduced with permission from Hayreh SS. The choriocapillaris. Albrecht Von Graefes Arch Klin Exp Ophthalmol. 1974;192(3):165–179.)*

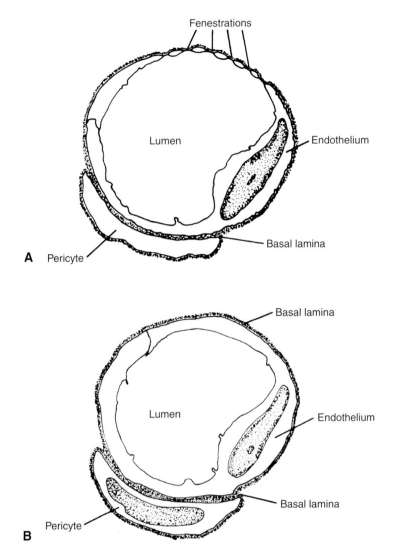

Figure 2-23   A, Fenestrated choroidal capillary. **B,** Nonfenestrated retinal capillary. *(Illustration by Thomas A. Weingeist, PhD, MD.)*

Lens

The lens is a biconvex structure located directly behind the posterior chamber and pupil (Fig 2-24). The lens contributes 20 D of the 60 D of focusing power of the average adult eye. The equatorial diameter is 6.5 mm at birth and increases in the first 2 to 3 decades of life, remaining in the region of 9–10 mm in diameter in late life. The anteroposterior width of the lens is about 3 mm at birth and increases after the second decade of life to about 6 mm at age 80 years. This growth is accompanied by a shortening of the anterior

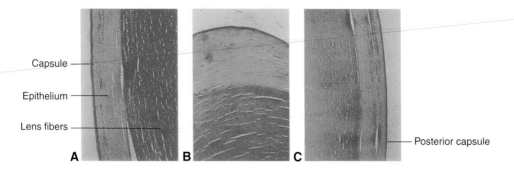

Capsule

Epithelium

Lens fibers

A   **B**   **C**

Posterior capsule

Figure 2-24 **A,** Lens: anterior capsule, epithelium, and lens fibers. **B,** Equator of the lens. Note the nuclei within the lens bow and the zonular fibers. **C,** Posterior lens capsule. Note the absence of lens epithelium (H&E ×32). *(Courtesy of Thomas A. Weingeist, PhD, MD.)*

radius of curvature of the lens, which would increase its optical power if it were not for a compensatory change in the refractive gradient across the lens substance.

In youth, accommodation for near vision is achieved by ciliary muscle contraction, which moves the ciliary muscle mass forward and inward. This contraction relaxes zonular tension and allows the lens to assume a globular shape, causing a shortening of its anterior curvature. The increased lens thickness during accommodation is entirely due to a change in nuclear shape. With age, accommodative power is steadily lost. Adolescents have 12–16 D of accommodation, decreasing to 2 D at age 50. Causes of this power loss include the increased size of the lens, altered mechanical relationships, and an increased stiffness of the lens nucleus secondary to changes in the crystalline proteins of the fiber cytoplasm. Other factors, such as alterations in the geometry of zonular attachments with age and changes in lens capsule elasticity, may also play a role.

The lens has certain unusual features. It lacks innervation and is avascular. After regression of the hyaloid vasculature during embryogenesis, the lens depends totally on the aqueous and vitreous for its nourishment. From embryonic life on, it is entirely enclosed by a basal lamina, the lens capsule. BCSC Section 11, *Lens and Cataract,* discusses the lens in depth.

Capsule

The lens is surrounded by a basal lamina, the lens capsule, which is a product of the lens epithelium (Fig 2-25). It is rich in type IV collagen and other matrix proteins. Synthesis of the anterior lens capsule (which overlies the epithelium) proceeds throughout life, so that its thickness increases, whereas that of the posterior capsule remains relatively constant. Values of 15.5 μm for the thickness of the anterior capsule and 2.8 μm for the posterior capsule have been cited for the adult lens.

Morphologically, the lens capsule consists of fine filaments arranged in lamellae, parallel to the surface. The anterior lens capsule contains a fibrogranular material, identified as laminin, which is absent from the posterior capsule at the ultrastructural level. The thinness of the posterior capsule creates a potential for rupture during cataract surgery.

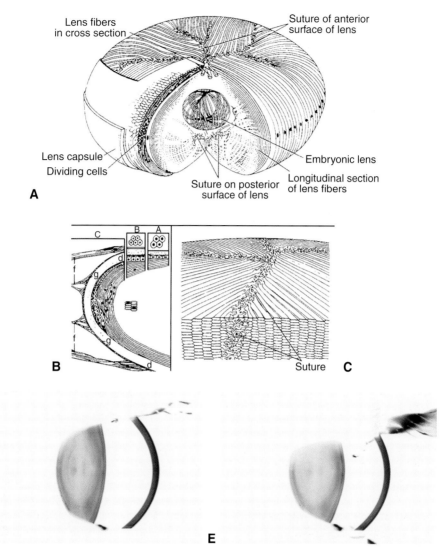

Figure 2-25 Organization of the lens. At areas where lens cells converge and meet, sutures are formed. **A,** Cutaway view of the adult lens showing embryonic lens inside. The embryonal nucleus has a Y-shaped suture at both the anterior and posterior poles; in the adult lens cortex, the organization of the sutures is more complex. At the equator, the lens epithelium can divide, and the cells become highly elongated and ribbonlike, sending processes anteriorly and posteriorly. As new lens cells are formed, older cells come to lie in the deeper parts of the cortex. **B,** The diagram shows, in cross section and corresponding surface view, the difference in lens fibers at the anterior *(A)*, intermediate *(B)*, and equatorial *(C)* zones. The lens capsule, or basement membrane of the lens epithelium *(d)*, is shown in relation to the zonular fibers *(f)* and their attachment to the lens *(g)*. **C,** The diagram shows a closer view of lens sutures. **D** and **E,** Optical sections of a young adult human lens (25-year-old female) demonstrated by Scheimpflug photography. The cornea is to the right. **D,** Lens in the nonaccommodative state. **E,** Lens during accommodation—note that the anterior radius of curvature is shortened in the latter case. *(Parts A–C reproduced with permission from Kessel RG, Kardon RH.* Tissues and Organs: A Text-Atlas of Scanning Electron Microscopy. *San Francisco: WH Freeman; 1979. Parts D and E courtesy of Jane Koretz.)*

Epithelium

The lens epithelium lies beneath the anterior and equatorial capsule, but it is absent under the posterior capsule. The basal aspects of the cells abut the lens capsule without specialized attachment sites. The apices of the cells face the interior of the lens, and the lateral borders interdigitate, with practically no intercellular space. Each cell contains a prominent nucleus but relatively few cytoplasmic organelles.

Regional differences in the lens epithelium are important. The central zone represents a stable population of cells whose numbers slowly decline with age. An intermediate zone of smaller cells shows occasional mitoses. Peripherally, there are meridional rows of cuboidal pre-equatorial cells that form the germinative zone of the lens. Here, cells undergo mitotic division, elongate anteriorly and posteriorly, and form the differentiated fiber cells of the lens. In the human lens, cell division continues throughout life and is responsible for the continued growth of the lens. Germinative cells left behind after phacoemulsification can give rise to posterior capsular opacification as a result of aberrant proliferation and cell migration.

Fibers

The lens has an outer cortex and an inner nucleus. The nucleus is the part of the fiber mass that is formed at birth, and the cortex forms as new fibers are added postnatally. In optical section with the slit lamp, lamellar zones of discontinuity are visible, differentiating the adult cortex into deep and superficial regions. The fiber cells are hexagonal in cross section, are spindle-shaped, and possess numerous interlocking fingerlike projections (Fig 2-26). Apart from the most superficial cortical fibers, the cytoplasm is homogeneous and contains few organelles. The high refractive index of the lens results from the high concentration of lens crystallins (α, β, and γ) in the fiber cytoplasm. The lens sutures are formed by the interdigitation of the anterior and posterior tips of the spindle-shaped fibers. In the fetal lens, this forms the anterior Y-shaped suture and the posterior inverted Y-shaped suture. As the lens ages, further branches are added to the sutures, each new set of branch points corresponding to the appearance of a fresh optical zone of discontinuity.

Zonules (Suspensory Ligaments)

The lens is held in place by a system of zonular fibers that originate from the basal laminae of the nonpigmented epithelium of the pars plana and pars plicata of the ciliary body. These fibers chiefly attach to the lens capsule anterior and posterior to the equator. Each zonular fiber is made up of multiple filaments of fibrillin that merge with the equatorial lens capsule. In Marfan syndrome, mutations in the fibrillin gene lead to weakening of the zonule and subluxation of the lens.

Streeten BW. Anatomy of the zonular apparatus. In: Duane TD, Jaeger EA, eds. *Biomedical Foundations of Ophthalmology*. Philadelphia: Harper & Row; 1992.

When the eye is focused for distance, the zonule is under tension and the lens form is relatively flattened. During accommodation, contraction of the ciliary muscle moves the proximal attachment of the zonule forward and inward so that the lens becomes more globular and the eye adjusts for near vision (see Fig 2-26).

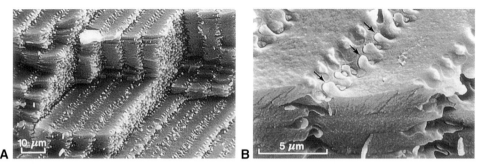

Figure 2-26 **A** and **B,** Scanning electron micrographs of the relationship of lens fiber packing and interdigitation *(arrows in B)*. *(Reproduced with permission from Kessel RG, Kardon RH. Tissues and Organs: A Text-Atlas of Scanning Electron Microscopy. San Francisco: WH Freeman; 1979.)*

Retina

The *fundus oculi* is the part of the eye that is visible on ophthalmoscopy, including the retina and its vessels and the *optic nerve head* (or *optic disc*). The *macula,* 5–6 mm in diameter, lies between the temporal vascular arcades. At the macula's center lies the *fovea,* rich in cones and responsible for color vision and the highest visual acuity. In the far periphery, the *ora serrata* (the junction between the retina and the pars plana) can be seen by gonioscopy or indirect ophthalmoscopy. The reddish color of the fundus is due to the transmission of light reflected from the posterior sclera through the capillary bed of the choroid.

The *retina* is a thin, transparent structure that develops from the inner and outer layers of the optic cup. In cross section, from outer to inner retina, its layers are

- RPE and its basal lamina
- rod and cone inner and outer segments
- external limiting membrane
- outer nuclear layer (nuclei of the photoreceptors)
- outer plexiform layer
- inner nuclear layer
- inner plexiform layer
- ganglion cell layer
- nerve fiber layer (axons of the ganglion cells)
- internal limiting membrane

The retina is also discussed in BCSC Section 12, *Retina and Vitreous.*

Retinal Pigment Epithelium

The structure of the outer pigmented epithelial layer is relatively simple compared with that of the overlying inner, or neurosensory, retina. The RPE consists of a monolayer of hexagonal cells that extends anteriorly from the optic disc to the ora serrata, where it merges with the pigmented epithelium of the ciliary body. Its structure is deceptively simple considering its many functions:

- vitamin A metabolism
- maintenance of the outer blood–retina barrier

- phagocytosis of the photoreceptor outer segments
- absorption of light (reduction of scatter)
- heat exchange
- formation of the basal lamina
- production of the mucopolysaccharide matrix surrounding the outer segments
- active transport of materials in and out of the RPE

Like other epithelial and endothelial cells, the RPE cells are polarized. The basal aspect is intricately folded and provides a large surface of attachment to the thin basal lamina that forms the inner layer of Bruch's membrane (see Fig 2-21). The apices have multiple villous processes that engage with the photoreceptor outer segments, embedded in a mucopolysaccharide matrix (interphotoreceptor matrix) containing chondroitin-6-sulfate, sialic acid, and hyaluronic acid. Separation of the RPE from the neurosensory retina is called *retinal detachment.*

Contiguous RPE cells are firmly attached by a series of lateral, intercellular junctional complexes. The *zonulae occludentes* and *zonulae adherentes* not only provide structural stability but also play an important role in maintaining the outer blood–retina barrier. Zonulae occludentes consist of fused plasma membranes forming a circular band or belt between adjacent cells. A small intercellular space is present between zonulae adherentes.

The retina and RPE show important regional differences (Fig 2-27). The retina is thickest in the papillomacular bundle near the optic nerve (0.23 mm) and thinnest in the foveola (0.10 mm) and ora serrata (0.11 mm). RPE cells vary from 10 to 60 μm in diameter. Compared with RPE cells in the periphery, RPE cells in the fovea are taller and thinner, they contain more melanosomes, and their melanosomes are larger. These characteristics account in part for the decreased transmission of choroidal fluorescence observed during fundus fluorescein angiography. Cells in the periphery are shorter, broader, and less pigmented. The eye of a fetus or infant contains between 4 and 6 million RPE cells. Although the surface area of the eye increases appreciably with age, the increase in the number of RPE cells is relatively small. No mitotic figures are apparent within the RPE of the normal adult eye.

The cytoplasm of the RPE cells contains multiple round and ovoid pigment granules *(melanosomes).* These organelles develop in situ during formation of the optic cup and first appear as nonmelanized premelanosomes. Their development contrasts sharply with that of the pigment granules in uveal melanocytes, which are derived from the neural crest and later migrate into the uvea.

Lipofuscin granules probably arise from the discs of photoreceptor outer segments and represent residual bodies arising from phagosomal activity. This so-called wear-and-tear pigment is less electron-dense than the melanosomes, and its concentration increases gradually with age. Histologically, it stains with Sudan stain and exhibits a golden yellow autofluorescence.

Phagosomes are membrane-enclosed packets of disc outer segments that have been engulfed by the RPE. Several stages of disintegration are evident at any given time. In some species, shedding and degradation of the membranes of rod and cone outer segments follow a diurnal rhythm synchronized with daily fluctuations of environmental light.

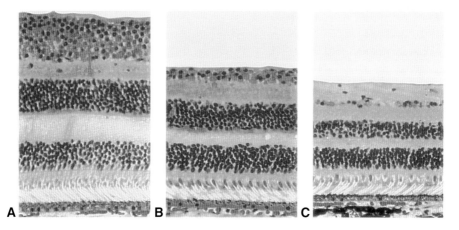

Figure 2-27 Regional differences in the retina. **A,** Papillomacular bundle. **B,** Macula. **C,** Peripheral retina. (H&E, all same magnification). *(Courtesy of Thomas A. Weingeist, PhD, MD.)*

The cytoplasm of the RPE also contains numerous mitochondria (involved in aerobic metabolism), rough-surfaced endoplasmic reticulum, a Golgi apparatus, and a large round nucleus.

Throughout life, incompletely digested residual bodies, lipofuscin pigment, phagosomes, and other material are excreted beneath the basal lamina of the RPE. These contribute to the formation of *drusen,* which are accumulations of this extracellular material. They can vary in size and are commonly classified by their funduscopic appearance as either hard or soft drusen. They are typically located between the basement membrane of the RPE cells and the inner collagenous zone of Bruch's membrane.

Neurosensory Retina

The neurosensory retina is composed of neuronal, glial, and vascular elements (Fig 2-28).

Neuronal elements

The photoreceptor layer of the neurosensory retina consists of highly specialized neuroepithelial cells called *rods* and *cones.* Each photoreceptor cell consists of an outer and an inner segment. The outer segments, surrounded by a mucopolysaccharide matrix, make contact with the apical processes of the RPE. Tight junctions or other intercellular connections do not exist between the photoreceptor cell outer segments and the RPE. The factors responsible for keeping these layers in apposition are poorly understood but probably involve active transport.

The rod photoreceptor consists of an outer segment that contains multiple laminated discs resembling a stack of coins and a central connecting cilium. The microtubules of the cilium have a "9 plus 0" cross-sectional configuration rather than the "9 plus 2" configuration found in motile cilia. The rod inner segment is subdivided into 2 additional elements: an outer ellipsoid containing a large number of mitochondria and an inner myoid containing a large amount of glycogen; the myoid is continuous with the main cell body, where the nucleus is located (Fig 2-29). The inner portion of the cell contains the *synaptic*

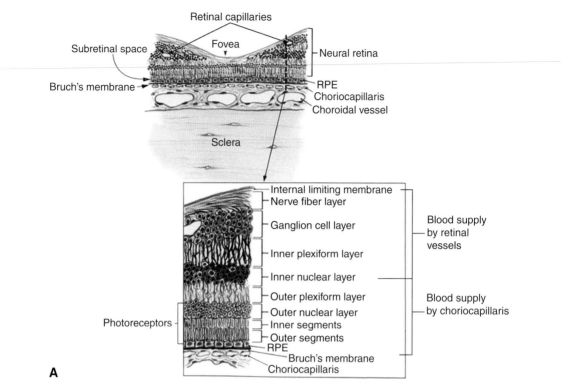

Figure 2-28   A, Schematic cross section of retina demonstrating layers of retina and approximate location of blood supply to these layers.

(continues)

body, or *spherule,* of the rod, which is formed by a single invagination that accommodates 2 horizontal cell processes and 1 or more central bipolar dendrites (Fig 2-30). The outer segments of the cones have a different morphology depending on their location in the retina.

The extrafoveal cone photoreceptors of the retina have conical ellipsoids and myoids, and their nuclei tend to be closer to the external limiting membrane than are the nuclei of the rods. Although the structure of the outer segments of the rods and cones is similar, at least 1 important difference exists. Rod discs are not attached to the cell membrane; they are discrete structures. Cone discs are attached to the cell membrane and are thought to be renewed by membranous replacement. The cone *synaptic body,* or *pedicle,* is more complex than the rod spherule. Cone pedicles synapse with other rods and cones as well as with horizontal and bipolar cell processes. Foveal cones have cylindrical inner segments like rods but otherwise are cytologically identical to extrafoveal cones. Horizontal cells make synaptic connections with many rod spherules and cone pedicles; they also extend cell processes horizontally throughout the outer plexiform layer. Bipolar cells are oriented vertically. Their dendrites synapse with either rod or cone synaptic bodies, and their axons make synaptic contact with ganglion cells and amacrine cells in the inner plexiform layer.

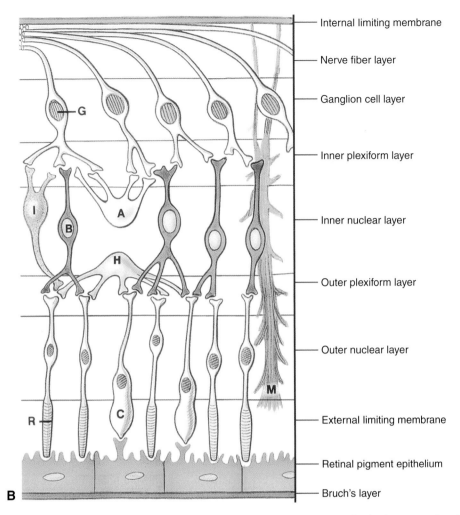

Internal limiting membrane

Nerve fiber layer

Ganglion cell layer

Inner plexiform layer

Inner nuclear layer

Outer plexiform layer

Outer nuclear layer

External limiting membrane

Retinal pigment epithelium

Bruch's layer

Figure 2-28   B, Schematic diagram of cell types and histologic layers in the human retina. The basic relationship between rod *(R)* and cone *(C)* photoreceptors as well as bipolar *(B)*, horizontal *(H)*, amacrine *(A)*, inner plexiform cell *(I)*, and ganglion *(G)* neurons is depicted. Note that the Müller cell *(M)* extends across almost the whole thickness of the retina; the apical processes of Müller cells form the external limiting membrane; the foot processes of Müller cells partially form the internal limiting membrane. *(Part A modified with permission from D'Amico DJ. Diseases of the retina. N Engl J Med. 1994;331:95–106. Illustration B by Christine Gralapp.)*

The axons of the ganglion cells bend to become parallel to the inner surface of the retina, where they form the nerve fiber layer and later the axons of the optic nerve. Each optic nerve has more than 1 million optic nerve fibers. The nerve fibers from the temporal retina follow an arcuate course around the macula to enter the superior and inferior poles of the optic disc. The papillomacular fibers travel straight to the optic nerve from the fovea. The nasal axons also pursue a radial course. The visibility of the nerve fibers is enhanced when they are viewed ophthalmoscopically using green (red-free) illumination.

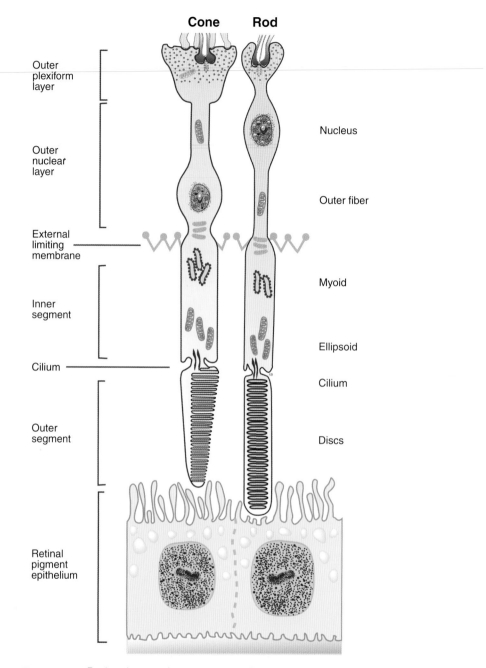

Cone   Rod

Outer plexiform layer

Outer nuclear layer

External limiting membrane

Inner segment

Cilium

Outer segment

Retinal pigment epithelium

Nucleus

Outer fiber

Myoid

Ellipsoid

Cilium

Discs

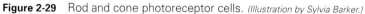

Figure 2-29   Rod and cone photoreceptor cells. *(Illustration by Sylvia Barker.)*

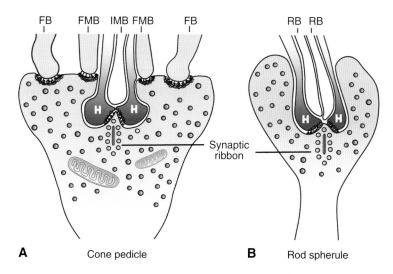

Figure 2-30 Synaptic bodies of photoreceptors. *H* = horizontal cell processes. **A,** Cone pedicle with synapses to several types of bipolar cells. *FB* = flat bipolar, *FMB* = flat midget bipolar, *IMB* = invaginating midget bipolar. **B,** Rod spherule with synapses to bipolar cells. *RB* = rod bipolar. *(Illustration by Sylvia Barker.)*

The neuronal elements and their connections in the retina are highly complex. Many types of bipolar, amacrine, and ganglion cells exist. The neuronal elements of more than 120 million rods and 6 million cones are interconnected, and signal processing within the neurosensory retina is significant.

Glial elements

Müller cells are glial cells that extend vertically from the external limiting membrane inward to the internal limiting membrane. Their nuclei are located in the inner nuclear layer. Müller cells, along with the other glial elements (the fibrous and protoplasmic astrocytes and microglia), provide structural support and nutrition to the retina.

Recent studies have provided evidence of the importance of Müller cells in retinal development and metabolism. Immunohistochemistry has shown that these cells contain cellular retinaldehyde–binding proteins, glutamine, taurine, and glutamine synthetase. Müller cells have also been shown to be involved in degradation of the neurotransmitters glutamate and gamma-aminobutyric acid (GABA). The presence of messenger RNA coding for carbonic anhydrase II implies that these cells also are important in buffering carbon dioxide liberated into the extracellular space by neurosensory elements of the retina. The production of insulin and growth factors by these cells may also be important in retinal metabolism.

The retina. In: Bron AJ, Tripathi RC, Tripathi BJ, eds. *Wolff's Anatomy of the Eye and Orbit.* 8th ed. London: Chapman & Hall; 1997.

Vascular elements

The inner portion of the retina is perfused by branches of the central retinal artery. In 30% of eyes and 50% of people, a cilioretinal artery, branching from the ciliary circulation, also supplies part of the inner retina. This cilioretinal artery, when present, contributes to some portion of the macular circulation in approximately 15% of people, but it may supply any portion of the retina.

The retinal blood vessels are analogous to the cerebral blood vessels and maintain the inner blood–retina barrier. This physiologic barrier is due to the single layer of nonfenestrated endothelial cells, whose tight junctions are impervious to tracer substances such as fluorescein and horseradish peroxidase. A basal lamina covers the outer surface of the endothelium. The basement membrane contains an interrupted layer of pericytes, or mural cells, surrounded by their own basement membrane material.

Müller cells and other glial elements are generally attached to the basal lamina of retinal blood vessels. Retinal blood vessels lack an internal elastic lamina and the continuous layer of smooth muscle cells found in other vessels in the body. Smooth muscle cells are occasionally present in vessels near the optic nerve head. They become a more discontinuous layer as the retinal arterioles pass farther out to the peripheral retina. The retinal blood vessels do not ordinarily extend deeper than the middle limiting membrane. Where venules and arterioles cross, they share a common basement membrane. Venous occlusive disorders are common at an arteriovenous crossing.

Stratification of the neurosensory retina

The neurosensory retina can be subdivided into several layers (see Fig 2-28).

The outermost layer, which is located next to the RPE, is the *external limiting membrane (ELM)*. It is not a true membrane and is formed by the attachment sites of adjacent photoreceptors and Müller cells. It is highly fenestrated.

The *outer plexiform layer (OPL)* is made up of the interconnections between the photoreceptor synaptic bodies and the horizontal and bipolar cells. In the macular region, the OPL is thicker and contains more fibers, because the axons of the rods and cones become longer and more oblique as they deviate from the fovea. In this region, the OPL is known as the *Henle fiber layer* (Fig 2-31). At the edge of the foveola, it lies almost parallel with the internal limiting membrane.

The *inner nuclear layer (INL)* contains nuclei of bipolar, Müller, horizontal, and amacrine cells.

The next region is formed by a zone of desmosome-like attachments in the region of the synaptic bodies of the photoreceptor cells. The retinal blood vessels ordinarily do not extend beyond this point.

The *inner plexiform layer (IPL)* consists of axons of the bipolar and amacrine cells and dendrites of the ganglion cells and their synapses.

The *ganglion cell layer (GCL)* is made up of the cell bodies of the ganglion cells that lie near the inner surface of the retina.

The *nerve fiber layer (NFL)* is formed by axons of the ganglion cells. Normally, these axons do not become myelinated until after they pass through the lamina cribrosa of the optic nerve.

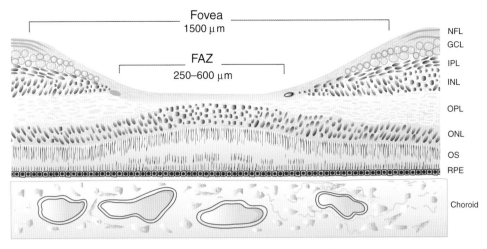

Figure 2-31 Schematic section through the fovea. *FAZ* = foveal avascular zone, *GCL* = ganglion cell layer, *INL* = inner nuclear layer, *IPL* = inner plexiform layer, *NFL* = nerve fiber layer, *ONL* = outer nuclear layer, *OPL* = outer plexiform layer/Henle fiber layer, *OS* = outer segments of the photoreceptors, *RPE* = retinal pigment epithelium. *(Illustration by Sylvia Barker.)*

Like the ELM, the *internal limiting membrane (ILM)* is also not a true membrane. It is formed by the footplates of the Müller cells and attachments to the basal lamina. The basal lamina of the retina is smooth on the vitreal side but appears undulating on the retinal side, where it follows the contour of the Müller cells. The thickness of the basal lamina varies.

Drexler W, Morgner U, Ghanta RK, Kärtner FX, Schuman JS, Fujimoto JG. Ultrahigh-resolution ophthalmic optical coherence tomography. *Nature Med.* 2001;7(4):502–507.

Overall, cells and their processes in the retina are oriented perpendicular to the plane of the RPE in the middle and outer layers but parallel to the retinal surface in the inner layers. For this reason, deposits of blood or exudates tend to form round blots in the outer layers (where small capillaries are found) and linear or flame-shaped patterns in the nerve fiber layer. At the fovea, the outer layers also tend to be parallel to the surface (Henle fiber layer). As a result, radial or star-shaped patterns may arise when these extracellular spaces are filled with serum and exudate.

Macula

The terms *macula, macula lutea, posterior pole, area centralis, fovea,* and *foveola* have created confusion among anatomists and clinicians. Clinical retina specialists tend to regard the macula as the area within the temporal vascular arcades. Histologically, it is the region with more than 1 layer of ganglion cell nuclei (see Fig 2-28; Figs 2-32, 2-33). See also BCSC Section 12, *Retina and Vitreous.*

Orth DH, Fine BS, Fagman W, Quirk TC. Clarification of foveomacular nomenclature and grid for quantitation of macular disorders. *Trans Sect Ophthalmol Am Acad Ophthalmol Otolaryngol.* 1977;83(3 Pt 1):OP506–514.

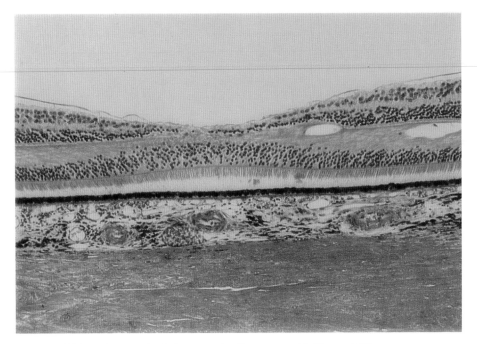

Figure 2-32 Light micrograph of the macula. Compare with Figure 2-31. *(Courtesy of Thomas A. Weingeist, PhD, MD.)*

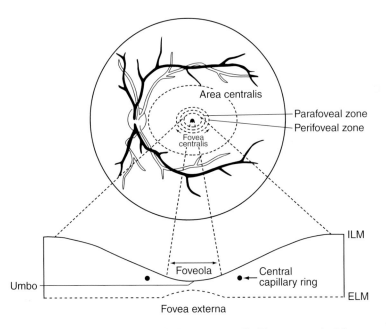

Figure 2-33 Anatomical macula; also called *area centralis*. The anatomical fovea and foveola are contained within the center of the macula. *ELM* = external limiting membrane, *ILM* = internal limiting membrane.

The name *macula lutea* ("yellow spot") derives from the yellow color of the central retina in dissected cadaver eyes; this color is due to the presence of carotenoid pigments, chiefly located in the Henle fiber layer. Two major pigments have been identified—zeaxanthin and lutein—whose proportions vary with distance from the fovea: the lutein to zeaxanthin ratio is 1:2.4 in the central area (0.25 mm from the fovea) and greater than 2:1 in the periphery (2.2–8.7 mm from the fovea). This variation in pigment ratio corresponds to the rod-to-cone ratio. Lutein is more concentrated in rod-dense areas of the retina; zeaxanthin is more concentrated in cone-dense areas. Lipofuscin, the yellow age pigment, has been observed in the cytoplasm of the perifoveal ganglion cells by electron microscopy.

The *fovea* is a concave central retinal depression approximately 1.5 mm in diameter; it is comparable in size to the optic nerve head (see Fig 2-31). Its margins are clinically inexact, but in younger subjects the fovea is evident ophthalmoscopically as an elliptical light reflex that arises from the slope of the thickened ILM of the retina. From this point inward, the basal lamina rapidly decreases in thickness as it dives down the slopes of the fovea toward the depths of the foveola, where it is barely visible, even by electron microscopy.

Around the fovea is the *parafovea*, 0.5 mm wide, where the GCL, the INL, and the OPL are thickest; surrounding this zone is the most peripheral region of the macula, the *perifovea*, 1.5 mm wide.

The masking of choroidal fluorescence observed in the macula during fundus fluorescein angiography is caused partly by xanthophyll pigment and partly by the higher melanin pigment content of the foveal RPE.

The *foveola* is a central depression within the fovea, located approximately 4.0 mm temporal and 0.8 mm inferior to the center of the optic disc. It is approximately 0.35 mm across and 0.10 mm in thickness at its center. The borders of the foveola merge imperceptibly with the fovea. The nuclei of the photoreceptor cells in the region of the foveola bow forward toward the ILM to form the fovea externa. Usually, only photoreceptors, Müller cells, and other glial cells are present in this area. Occasionally, light microscopy reveals ganglion cell nuclei just below the ILM.

The photoreceptor layer of the foveola is made up entirely of cones, whose close packing accounts for the high visual acuity for which this small area is responsible. The foveal cones are shaped like rods but possess all the cytologic characteristics of extramacular cones. The outer segments are oriented parallel to the visual axis and perpendicular to the plane of the RPE. In contrast, the peripheral photoreceptor cell outer segments are tilted toward the entrance pupil.

The *foveal avascular zone (FAZ)*, or capillary-free zone (see Fig 2-31; Fig 2-34), is an important clinical landmark in the treatment of subretinal neovascular membranes by laser photocoagulation. Its location is approximately the same as that of the foveola, and its appearance in fundus fluorescein angiograms varies greatly. The diameter of the FAZ varies from 250 to 600 μm or more; often, a truly avascular, or capillary-free, zone cannot be identified.

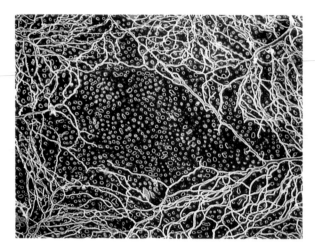

Figure 2-34 Scanning electron micrograph of a retinal vascular cast at the fovea, showing the foveal avascular zone and underlying choriocapillaris.

Ora Serrata

The ora serrata is the boundary between the retina and the pars plana. Its distance from the Schwalbe line is between 5.75 mm nasally and 6.50 mm temporally. In myopia, this distance is greater; in hyperopia, it is shorter. Bruch's membrane extends anteriorly, beyond the ora serrata, but is modified because there is no choriocapillaris in the ciliary body.

At the ora serrata, the diameter of the eye is 20 mm and the circumference is 63 mm; at the equator, the diameter is 24 mm and the circumference is 75 mm. Topographically, the ora serrata is relatively smooth temporally and serrated nasally. Retinal blood vessels end in loops before reaching the ora serrata.

The ora serrata is in a watershed zone between the anterior and posterior vascular system, which may in part explain why peripheral retinal degeneration is relatively common. The peripheral retina in the region of the ora serrata is markedly attenuated. The photoreceptors are malformed, and the overlying retina frequently appears cystic in paraffin sections (Blessig-Iwanoff cysts) (Fig 2-35).

Vitreous

The vitreous cavity occupies four fifths of the volume of the globe. The transparent vitreous humor is important to the metabolism of the intraocular tissues because it provides a route for metabolites used by the lens, ciliary body, and retina. Its volume is close to 4.0 mL. Although it has a gel-like structure, the vitreous is 99% water. Its viscosity is approximately twice that of water, mainly due to the presence of the mucopolysaccharide hyaluronic acid (Fig 2-36).

At the ultrastructural level, fine collagen fibrils (chiefly type II) and cells have been identified in the vitreous. The origin and function of these cells are unknown. They have been termed *hyalocytes* and probably represent modified histiocytes, glial cells, or

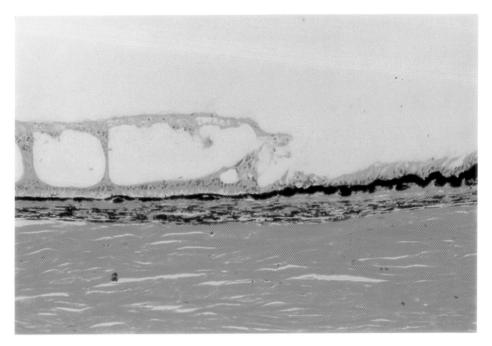

Figure 2-35 Ora serrata. Note the malformed appearance of the peripheral retina and the cystic changes at the junction between the pars plana and the retina (H&E ×32). *(Courtesy of Thomas A. Weingeist, PhD, MD.)*

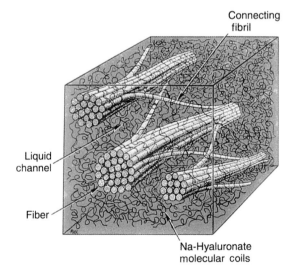

Connecting
fibril

Liquid
channel

Fiber

Na-Hyaluronate
molecular coils

Figure 2-36 Three-dimensional depiction of the molecular organization of the vitreous, showing the dissociation between hyaluronic acid molecules and collagen fibrils. The fibrils are packed into bundles, and the hyaluronic acid forms molecular "coils" that fill the intervening spaces to provide channels of liquid vitreous. *(Reproduced with permission from Sebag J, Balazs EA. Morphology and ultrastructure of human vitreous fibers.* Invest Ophthalmol Vis Sci. *1989;30(8):1867–1871.)*

fibroblasts. The fibrils at the vitreous base merge with the basal lamina of the nonpigmented epithelium of the pars plana and the ILM of the retina.

The vitreous adheres to the retina peripherally at the vitreous base, which extends from 2.0 mm anterior to the ora serrata to approximately 4.0 mm posterior to the ora serrata. Additional attachments exist at the disc margin, at the perimacular region, along the retinal vessels, and at the periphery of the posterior lens capsule. The vitreous becomes more fluid with age and frequently separates from the inner retina (posterior vitreous detachment) (Fig 2-37). The associated peripheral retinal traction is a potential cause of rhegmatogenous retinal detachment (Figs 2-38 through 2-40).

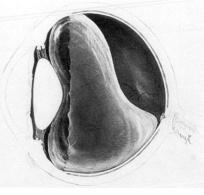

Figure 2-37 Typical posterior vitreous detachment. The cortical vitreous initially separates from the retina in the posterior pole and the superior quadrants. The detachment may then progress farther anteriorly until reaching the posterior margin of the vitreous base in the inferior quadrants. *(Reproduced with permission from Michels RG, Wilkinson CP, Rice TA, eds.* Retinal Detachment. *St Louis: Mosby; 1990.)*

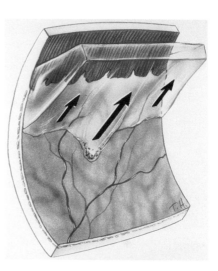

Figure 2-38 Localized posterior extension of the vitreous base with firm underlying area of vitreoretinal attachment may result in greater traction in that area *(large arrow)* than along the adjacent vitreous base *(smaller arrows)*. *(Reproduced with permission from Michels RG, Wilkinson CP, Rice TA, eds.* Retinal Detachment. *St Louis: Mosby; 1990.)*

Figure 2-39 A, Traction from the posterior vitreous surface on a site of firm vitreoretinal attachment is the usual mechanism causing a retinal break. **B,** Persistent traction on the flap of the retinal tear and fluid currents in the vitreous cavity contribute to retinal detachment. *(Reproduced with permission from Michels RG, Wilkinson CP, Rice TA, eds.* Retinal Detachment. *St Louis: Mosby; 1990.)*

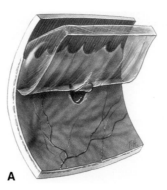

A

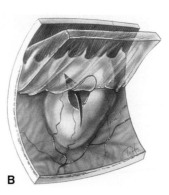

B

Lund-Andersen H, Sander B. The vitreous. In: Kaufman PL, Alm A, eds. *Adler's Physiology of the Eye.* 10th ed. St Louis: Mosby; 2003:293–316.

During embryonic development, regression of the hyaloid vasculature results in the formation of an S-shaped channel (the Cloquet canal), which passes sinuously from a point slightly nasal to the posterior pole of the lens (Mittendorf dot; Fig 2-41) to the margin of the optic nerve head. Remnants of this fetal vasculature may be observed clinically on the nerve head in the adult (vascular loops and Bergmeister papilla).

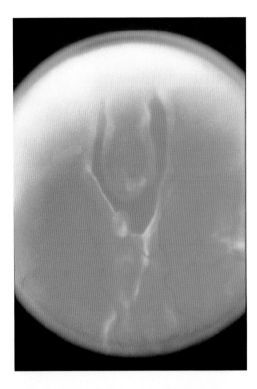

Figure 2-40 Fundus photo of a flap retinal tear with associated retinal detachment. *(Courtesy of James Folk, MD.)*

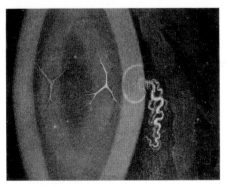

Figure 2-41 Mittendorf dot. In some individuals, a remnant of the hyaloid vasculature is visible on the posterior pole of the lens, as a normal variant. *(Reproduced with permission from Thiel R.* Atlas of Diseases of the Eye. *Amsterdam: Elsevier; 1963.)*

CHAPTER 3

Cranial Nerves: Central and Peripheral Connections

Cranial nerves (CN) I–VI are depicted in Figure 3-1 in relation to the bony canals and arteries at the base of the skull. The reader may find it useful to refer back to this figure as each of the cranial nerves is discussed. CN VII is discussed later in the chapter. For further study, BCSC Section 5, *Neuro-Ophthalmology*, describes the cranial nerves and their function and dysfunction in detail.

Cranial Nerve I (Olfactory)

Cranial nerve I originates from small olfactory receptors in the mucous membrane of the nose. Unmyelinated CN I fibers pass from these receptors in the nasal cavity through the cribriform plate of the ethmoidal bone and enter the ventral surface of the olfactory bulb, where they form the nerve.

The olfactory tract runs posteriorly from the bulb, beneath the frontal lobe of the brain in a groove (or sulcus) and lateral to the gyrus rectus (Fig 3-2). The gyrus rectus forms the anterolateral border of the suprasellar cistern. Meningiomas arising from the arachnoid cells in this area can produce important ophthalmic signs and symptoms associated with loss of olfaction.

Cranial Nerve II (Optic Nerve)

The optic nerve consists of more than 1 million axons that originate in the ganglion cell layer of the retina and extend toward the occipital cortex. The optic nerve may be divided into the following topographic areas:

- intraocular region of the optic nerve: optic disc, or nerve head; prelaminar area; and laminar area
- intraorbital region (located within the muscle cone)
- intracanalicular region (located within the optic canal)
- intracranial region (ending in the optic chiasm)

See Table 3-1 for a summary of regional differences. The organization of the optic nerve is similar to that of the white matter of the brain. Developmentally, the optic nerve is part of the brain, and its fibers are surrounded by glial (and not Schwann cell) sheaths. The optic

Figure 3-1 View from the right parietal bone looking downward into the skull base, showing the relationship between the bony canals **(A)**, nerves **(B)**, and arteries **(C)** at the base of the skull. The orbits are located to the right, out of the picture (the roof of the orbits is just visible). The floor of the right middle cranial fossa is in the lower part. **A,** AC = anterior clinoid, ACF = anterior cranial fossa, CC = carotid canal, FO = foramen ovale, FR = foramen rotundum, MCF = middle cranial fossa, OF = optic foramen, PC = posterior clinoid, SOF = superior orbital fissure, ST = sella turcica. **B,** I = olfactory nerve; II = optic nerve; III = oculomotor nerve; IV = trochlear nerve; V = trigeminal nerve, with ophthalmic V_1, maxillary V_2, and mandibular V_3 divisions; VI = abducens nerve; TG = trigeminal ganglion. **C,** $ACoA$ and *arrowhead* = anterior communicating artery, BA = basilar artery, ICA = internal carotid artery, MCA = middle cerebral artery, OA = ophthalmic artery, PCA = posterior cerebral artery, $PCoA$ = posterior communicating artery. *(Reproduced with permission from Zide BM, Jelks GW, eds. Surgical Anatomy of the Orbit. New York: Raven; 1985.)*

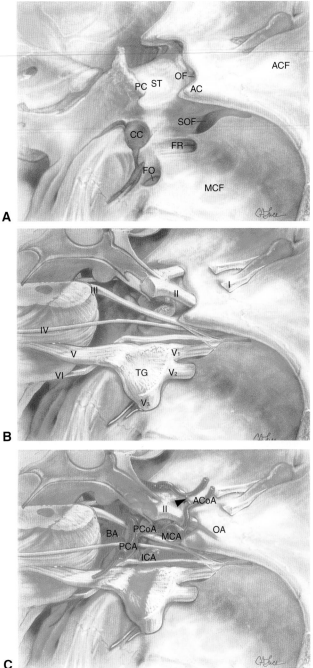

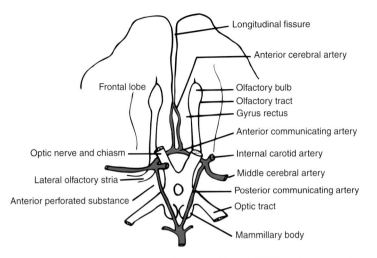

Figure 3-2 Inferior surface of the brain, depicting CN I and CN II and surrounding structures. *(Illustration by Thomas A. Weingeist, PhD, MD.)*

Table 3-1 Regional Differences in the Optic Nerve

Segment	Length (mm)	Diameter (mm)	Blood Supply
Intraocular	1.0		Retinal arterioles
optic disc prelaminar laminar		1.5 × 1.75	Branches of posterior ciliary arteries
Intraorbital	25	3–4	Intraneural branches of central retinal artery; pial branches from CRA and choroid
Intracanalicular	4–10		Ophthalmic artery
Intracranial	10	4–7	Branches of internal carotid and ophthalmic arteries

nerve varies in length from 35 to 55 mm and averages 40 mm. Part of the intraocular portion of the optic nerve is visible ophthalmoscopically as the optic nerve head, or optic disc. The intraorbital portion is 25–30 mm long, which is greater than the distance between the back of the globe and the optic canal (18 mm). For this reason, when the eye is in the primary position, the optic nerve runs a sinuous course.

Intraocular Region

The optic nerve head is the principal site of many congenital and acquired ocular diseases; therefore, detailed knowledge of its anatomy is important for the practicing ophthalmologist. Its anterior surface is visible ophthalmoscopically as the *optic disc,* an oval structure measuring 1.5 mm horizontally and 1.75 mm vertically, with a cup-shaped depression, the *physiologic cup,* located slightly temporal to its geometric center. The main branches of the central retinal artery (CRA) and central retinal vein (CRV) pass through the center of the cup. The optic nerve head can be described in 4 parts:

1. superficial nerve fiber layer
2. prelaminar area
3. laminar area
4. retrolaminar area

Superficial nerve fiber layer

As the nonmyelinated ganglion cell axons enter the nerve head, they retain their retinotopic organization, with fibers from the upper retina above and those from the lower retina below. Fibers from the temporal retina are lateral; those from the nasal side are medial. Macular fibers, constituting about one third of the nerve, are laterally placed. In the nerve head, foveal fibers are located peripherally and peripapillary fibers, centrally.

Prelaminar area

The ganglion cell axons that enter the nerve head are supported by a "wicker basket" of astrocytic glial cells and segregated into bundles, or *fascicles,* that pass through the lamina cribrosa. These astrocytes invest the optic nerve and form continuous circular tubes that enclose groups of nerve fibers throughout their intraocular and intraorbital course, separating them from connective tissue elements at all sites. No Müller cells are present in the nerve head, but the astrocytes form an internal limiting membrane (ILM) that covers the surface of the nerve head and is continuous with that of the retina. Astrocytes make up 10% of the nerve head volume.

When the optic nerve is damaged, axons and supporting glial elements can be lost, resulting in pathologic enlargement of the optic cup. This cupping may be the first objective sign of damage from glaucoma. The retinal layers terminate as they approach the edge of the optic disc. The Müller cells that make up the ILM are replaced by astrocytes. The pigment epithelium may be exposed at the temporal margin of the disc to form a narrow pigmented crescent. When the pigment epithelium and choroid fail to reach the temporal margin, crescents of partial or absent pigmentation can be seen. The relationship of the choroid to the prelaminar portion of the optic nerve partly accounts for the staining of the disc normally observed in late phases of fluorescein fundus angiography. The disc vessels do not leak, but the choroidal capillaries are freely permeable to fluorescein, which can therefore diffuse into the lamina.

Laminar area

The *lamina cribrosa* comprises approximately 10 connective tissue plates, which are integrated with the sclera and whose pores transmit the axon bundles. The openings are wider above than below, which may imply less protection from the mechanical effects of pressure in glaucoma. The lamina contains type I and type III collagens, abundant elastin, and laminin and fibronectin. Astrocytes surround the axon bundles, and small blood vessels are present. The lamina cribrosa serves the following functions: scaffold for the optic nerve axons, point of fixation for the CRA and CRV, and reinforcement of the posterior segment of the globe.

Retrolaminar area

Behind the lamina cribrosa, the optic nerve increases to 3 mm in diameter as a result of myelination of the nerve fibers and the presence of oligodendroglia and the surrounding meningeal sheaths (pia, arachnoid, and dura) (Fig 3-3). The retrolaminar nerve continues proximally (as the intraorbital part of the optic nerve) to the apex of the orbit. The axoplasm of the neurons contains neurofilaments, microtubules, mitochondria, and smooth endoplasmic reticulum.

Intraorbital Region

Annulus of Zinn

The intraorbital part of the optic nerve lies within the muscle cone. Before passing into the optic canal, the nerve is surrounded by the annulus of Zinn, which is formed by the origins of the rectus muscles. The superior rectus and the medial rectus partially originate from the sheath of the optic nerve. This connection may partly explain why patients with retrobulbar neuritis complain of pain on eye movement. At the optic canal, the dural sheath of the nerve fuses to the periosteum, completely immobilizing the nerve.

Meningeal sheaths

The *pia mater* is the innermost layer of the optic nerve sheath. It is a vascular connective tissue coat, covered with meningothelial cells, which sends numerous septa into the optic nerve, dividing its axons into bundles. The septa continue throughout the intraorbital and intracanalicular regions of the nerve and end just before the chiasm. They contain collagen, elastic tissue, fibroblasts, nerves, and small arterioles and venules (Fig 3-4). They provide mechanical support for the nerve bundles and nutrition to the axons and glial cells. A mantle of astrocytic glial cells prevents the pia and septa from direct contact with nerve axons.

The *arachnoid mater,* which is composed of collagenous tissue, small amounts of elastic tissue, and meningothelial cells, lines the dura mater and is connected to the pia across the subarachnoid space by vascular trabeculae. The subarachnoid space ends anteriorly at the level of the lamina cribrosa. Posteriorly, it is usually continuous with the subarachnoid space of the brain. Because the central retinal vessels cross this space, a rise in intracranial pressure can compress the retinal vein and raise the venous pressure within the retina above the intraocular pressure. This situation causes the loss of spontaneous venous pulsation at the nerve head. Such an absence of pulsation may clinically indicate raised intracranial pressure.

The thick *dura mater* encases the brain and makes up the outer layer of the meningeal sheath of the optic nerve. It is 0.3–0.5 mm thick and consists of dense bundles of collagen and elastic tissue that fuse anteriorly with the outer layers of the sclera.

The meninges of the optic nerve are supplied by sensory nerve fibers, which account in part for the pain experienced by patients with retrobulbar neuritis and other inflammatory optic nerve diseases.

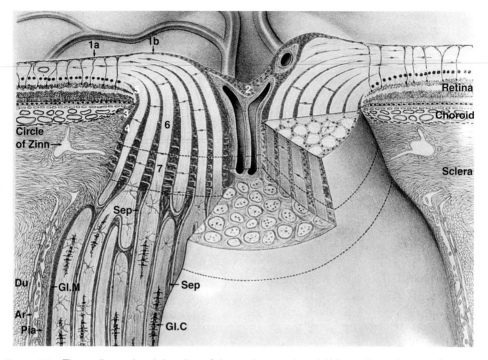

Figure 3-3   Three-dimensional drawing of the optic nerve head. Where the retina terminates at the optic disc edge, the Müller cells *(1a)* are continuous with the astrocytes, forming the internal limiting membrane *(1b)*. *(2)* The optic nerve cup. At the posterior termination of the choroid on the temporal side, the border tissue of Elschnig *(3)* lies between the astrocytes surrounding the optic nerve canal *(4)* and the stroma of the choroid. On the nasal side, the choroidal stroma is directly adjacent to the astrocytes surrounding the nerve. This collection of astrocytes surrounding the canal is known as the "border tissue," which is continuous with a similar glial lining *(5)* at the termination of the retina. The nerve fibers of the retina are segregated into approximately 1000 fascicles by astrocytes *(6)*. On reaching the lamina cribrosa, or cribriform plate *(upper dotted line)*, the nerve fascicles *(7)* and their surrounding astrocytes are separated from each other by connective tissue. The cribriform plate is an extension of scleral collagen and elastic fibers through the nerve. The external choroid also sends some connective tissue to the anterior part of the lamina. At the external part of the lamina cribrosa *(lower dotted line)*, the nerve fibers become myelinated, and columns of oligodendrocytes and a few astrocytes are present within the nerve fascicles. The bundles continue to be separated by connective tissue septa all the way to the chiasm *(Sep)*. The septa are derived from the pia mater. This connective tissue is also derived from the pia mater and is known as the "septal tissue." A mantle of astrocytes *(Gl.M)*, continuous anteriorly with the border tissue, surrounds the nerve along its orbital course. The dura *(Du)*, arachnoid *(Ar)*, and pia mater *(Pia)* are shown. The nerve fibers are myelinated. Within the bundles, the cell bodies of astrocytes and oligodendrocytes form a column of nuclei *(Gl.C)*. The central retinal vessels are surrounded by a perivascular connective tissue throughout its course in the nerve. This connective tissue blends with the connective tissue of the lamina cribrosa and is called the "central supporting connective tissue strand" here. *(Reproduced with permission from Anderson DR, Hoyt WF. Ultrastructure of intraorbital portion of human and monkey optic nerve. Arch Ophthalmol. 1969;82(4):507.)*

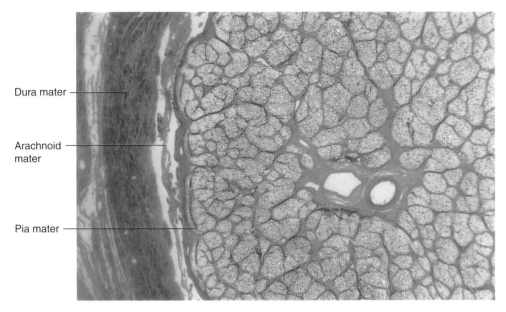

Dura mater

Arachnoid
mater

Pia mater

Figure 3-4 Meningeal sheaths. The dura mater, the outer layer, is composed of collagenous connective tissue. The arachnoid mater, the middle layer, is made up of fine collagenous fibers arranged in a loose meshwork lined by endothelial cells. The innermost layer, the pia mater, is made up of fine collagenous and elastic fibers and is highly vascularized. Elements from both the arachnoid and the pia are continuous with the optic nerve septa (Masson trichrome ×64). *(Courtesy of Thomas A. Weingeist, PhD, MD.)*

Intracanalicular Region

Within the optic canal, the blood supply of the optic nerve is derived from pial vessels originating from the ophthalmic artery. The optic nerve and surrounding arachnoid are tethered to the periosteum of the bony canal within the intracanalicular region. Blunt trauma, particularly over the eyebrow, can transmit the force of injury to the intracanalicular region, causing shearing and interruption of the blood supply to the nerve in this area, which is called *indirect traumatic optic neuropathy*. In addition, optic nerve edema in this area can produce a compartment syndrome, further compromising the function of the optic nerve within the confined space of the optic canal.

Intracranial Region

After passing through the optic canals, the 2 optic nerves lie above the ophthalmic arteries, above and medial to the internal carotid arteries (ICAs). The anterior cerebral arteries cross over the optic nerves and are connected by the anterior communicating artery, which completes the anterior portion of the circle of Willis. The optic nerves then pass posteriorly over the cavernous sinus to join in the optic chiasm. The chiasm then divides into right and left optic tracts, which end in their respective lateral geniculate bodies. From these bodies arise the geniculocalcarine pathways (or optic radiations), which pass to each primary visual cortex. Lesions at different locations along the visual pathway produce characteristic visual field defects that help to localize the site of damage (Fig 3-5).

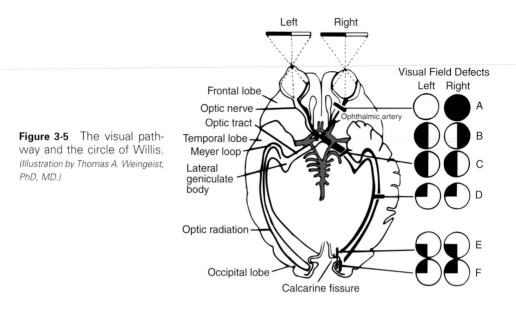

Figure 3-5 The visual pathway and the circle of Willis. *(Illustration by Thomas A. Weingeist, PhD, MD.)*

Blood Supply of the Optic Nerve

The ophthalmic artery lies below the optic nerve. The CRA and, usually, 2 long posterior ciliary arteries branch off from the ophthalmic artery once it has entered the muscle cone at the annulus of Zinn.

The blood supply of the optic nerve varies from one segment of the nerve to another. Although the blood supply can vary widely, a basic pattern has emerged from a multitude of studies.

The arterial supply of the optic nerve head is as follows: the retrolaminar nerve is supplied chiefly by pial vessels and short posterior ciliary vessels, with some help from the CRA and recurrent choroidal arteries. The lamina is supplied by short posterior ciliary arteries or by branches of the arterial circle of Haller and Zinn (circle of Zinn-Haller). This circle arises from the paraoptic branches of the short posterior ciliary arteries and is usually embedded in the sclera around the nerve head. It is often incomplete and may be divided into a superior and an inferior half. There is no supply from the CRA in this region.

The prelaminar nerve is supplied by the short posterior ciliary arteries (cilioretinal arteries, if present) and recurrent choroidal arteries, although their relative contribution is debated. The nerve fiber layer is supplied by the CRA (Figs 3-6, 3-7). The posterior ciliary arteries are terminal arteries, and the area where the respective capillary beds from each artery meet has been termed the *watershed zone*. When perfusion pressure drops, the tissue lying within this area is the most vulnerable to ischemia. Consequences can be significant when the entire optic nerve head or a part of it lies within the watershed zone.

The intraorbital region of the optic nerve is supplied proximally by the pial vascular network and by neighboring branches of the ophthalmic artery. Distally, it is also supplied by intraneural branches of the CRA. Most anteriorly, short posterior ciliary arteries and occasional peripapillary choroidal arteries contribute.

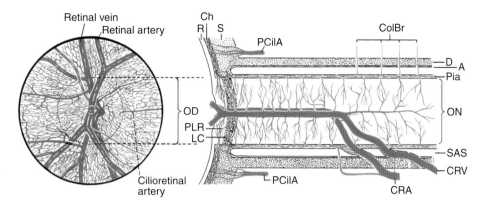

Figure 3-6 Diagram of blood supply of the optic nerve head and intraorbital optic nerve. A = arachnoid, Ch = choroid, $ColBr$ = collateral branches, CRA = central retinal artery, CRV = central retinal vein, D = dura, LC = lamina cribrosa, OD = optic disc, ON = optic nerve, $PCilA$ = posterior ciliary arteries, PLR = prelaminar region, R = retina, S = sclera, SAS = subarachnoid space. *(Reproduced with permission from Hayreh SS. Anatomy and physiology of the optic nerve head. Trans Am Acad Ophthalmol Otolaryngol. 1974;78(2):OP240–254.)*

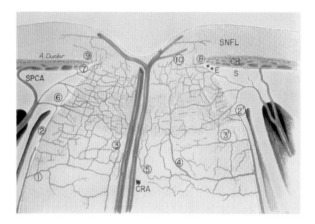

Figure 3-7 Vascular supply of the optic nerve head. **Retrolaminar:** *1,* pial supply; *2,* recurrent short posterior ciliary arterioles; *3,* pial-derived longitudinal arterioles; *4,* large pial vessels; *5,* branches of CRA; *6,* scleral short posterior arteries. **Prelaminar:** *7,* branch of short posterior ciliary artery enters nerve; *8,* occasional choroidal supply; *9,* choriocapillary anastomosis and epipapillary and peripapillary branches of the CRA; *10,* both epipapillary and peripapillary branches of the CRA anastomose with prelaminar vessels in this area. *CRA* = central retinal artery, *SNFL* = superficial nerve fiber layer, *SPCA* = short posterior ciliary arteries. *(Reprinted from Lieberman MF, Maumenee AE, Green WR. Histologic studies of the vasculature of the anterior optic nerve. Am J Ophthalmol. 1976;82(3):405–423, © 1976, with permission from Elsevier Science.)*

The intracanalicular region of the optic nerve is supplied almost exclusively by the ophthalmic artery.

The intracranial region of the optic nerve is supplied primarily by branches of both the ICA and the ophthalmic artery.

Central retinal artery and vein

The lumen of the CRA is surrounded by nonfenestrated endothelial cells with typical zonulae occludentes like those in retinal vessels. The CRA, however, differs from retinal arterioles in that it contains a fenestrated internal elastic lamina and an outer layer of smooth muscle cells surrounded by a thin basement membrane. The retinal arterioles have no internal elastic lamina, and they lose their smooth muscle cells shortly after entering the retina. The CRV consists of endothelial cells, a thin basal lamina, and a thick collagenous adventitia.

Chiasm

The optic chiasm makes up part of the anterior inferior floor of the third ventricle. It is surrounded by pia and arachnoid and is richly vascularized. The chiasm is approximately 12 mm wide, 8 mm long in the anteroposterior direction, and 4 mm thick. The extramacular fibers from the inferonasal retina cross anteriorly in the chiasm at the Wilbrand knee before passing into the optic tract. Extramacular supranasal fibers cross directly to the opposite tract. Extramacular temporal fibers remain uncrossed in the chiasm and optic tract. The macular projections are located centrally in the optic nerve and constitute 80%–90% of the total volume of the optic nerve and the chiasmal fibers. The temporal macular fibers pursue a direct course through the chiasm as a bundle of uncrossed fibers. Nasal macular fibers cross in the posterior part of the chiasm. Approximately 53% of the optic nerve fibers are crossed, and 47% are uncrossed.

Optic Tract

Each optic tract contains ipsilateral temporal and contralateral nasal fibers from the optic nerves. Fibers (both crossed and uncrossed) from the upper retinal projections travel medially in the optic tract; lower projections move laterally. The macular fibers adopt a dorsolateral orientation as they course toward the lateral geniculate body.

Lateral Geniculate Body

The lateral geniculate body, or nucleus, is the synaptic zone for the higher visual projections. It is an oval, caplike structure that receives approximately 70% of the optic tract fibers within its 6 alternating layers of gray and white matter. Layers 1, 4, and 6 of the lateral geniculate body contain axons from the contralateral optic nerve. Layers 2, 3, and 5 arise from the ipsilateral optic nerve. The 6 layers, numbered consecutively from below upward, give rise to the optic radiations.

Optic Radiations

The optic radiations connect the lateral geniculate body with the cortex of the occipital lobe. The fibers of the optic radiations leave the lateral geniculate body and wind around the temporal horn of the lateral ventricle, approaching the anterior tip of the temporal lobe (the so-called loop of Meyer). They then sweep backward toward the visual area of the occipital lobe. Damage to the optic radiation in the anterior temporal lobe gives rise to a wedge-shaped, upper homonymous "pie in the sky" visual field defect.

Visual Cortex

The visual cortex, the thinnest area of the human cerebral cortex, has 6 cellular layers and occupies the superior and inferior lips of the calcarine fissure on the posterior and medial surfaces of the occipital lobes. Macular function is extremely well represented in the visual cortex and occupies the most posterior position at the tip of the occipital lobe. The most anterior portion of the calcarine fissure is occupied by contralateral nasal retinal fibers only. The posterior cerebral artery, a branch of the basilar artery, supplies the visual cortex almost exclusively. The blood supply to the occipital lobe does show anatomical variation, however, with the middle cerebral artery making a contribution in some individuals.

Trobe JD. *The Neurology of Vision.* New York: Oxford University Press; 2001:1–42.

Cranial Nerve III (Oculomotor)

Although CN III contains only 24,000 fibers, it supplies all the extraocular muscles except the superior oblique and the lateral rectus. It also carries cholinergic innervation to the pupillary sphincter and the ciliary muscle.

Cranial nerve III arises from a complex group of cells in the rostral midbrain, or mesencephalon, at the level of the superior colliculus. This nuclear complex lies ventral to the periaqueductal gray matter, is immediately rostral to the CN IV nuclear complex, and is bounded inferolaterally by the medial longitudinal fasciculus.

The CN III nucleus consists of several distinct, large motor cell subnuclei, each of which subserves the extraocular muscle it innervates (Fig 3-8). Except for a single central

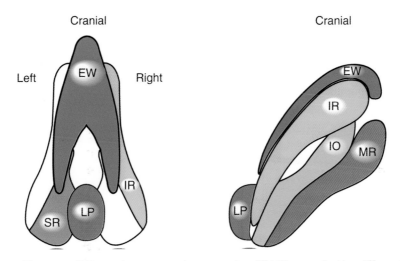

Figure 3-8   Diagram of the oculomotor nuclear complex (CN III), supplied by different subnuclei. Note that a central caudal nucleus supplies both levator muscles and that the nucleus for each superior rectus supplies the contralateral muscle. *EW* = Edinger-Westphal nucleus, *IO* = nucleus to the inferior oblique muscle, *IR* = nucleus to the inferior rectus muscle, *LP* = nucleus to the levator palpebrae muscle, *MR* = nucleus to the medial rectus muscle, *SR* = nucleus to the superior rectus muscle. *(Illustration by Sylvia Barker.)*

caudal nucleus that serves both levators, the cell groups are paired. Fibers from the superior rectus cross in the caudal aspect of the nucleus and therefore supply the contralateral superior rectus muscles.

The Edinger-Westphal nucleus is cephalad and dorsomedial in location. It provides the parasympathetic preganglionic efferent innervation to the ciliary muscle and pupillary sphincter. The most ventral subnuclei supply the medial rectus muscles. A subnucleus for ocular convergence has been described but is not found consistently in primates.

The fascicular portion of CN III travels ventrally from the nuclear complex, through the red nucleus, between the medial aspects of the cerebral peduncles, and through the corticospinal fibers. It exits in the interpeduncular space. In the subarachnoid space, CN III passes below the posterior cerebral artery and above the superior cerebellar artery, the 2 major branches of the basilar artery (Fig 3-9). The nerve travels forward in the interpeduncular cistern lateral to the posterior communicating artery and penetrates the arachnoid between the free and attached borders of the tentorium cerebelli. Aneurysms that affect CN III commonly occur at the junction of the posterior communicating artery and the ICA. The nerve pierces the dura on the lateral side of the posterior clinoid process, initially traversing the roof of the cavernous sinus. It runs along the lateral wall of the cavernous sinus and above CN IV and enters the orbit through the superior orbital fissure.

Cranial nerve III usually divides into superior and inferior divisions after passing through the annulus of Zinn in the orbit. Alternatively, it may divide within the anterior cavernous sinus. The nerve maintains a topographic organization even in the midbrain, so that lesions almost anywhere along its course may cause a divisional nerve palsy.

The superior division of CN III innervates the superior rectus and levator palpebrae muscles. The larger inferior division splits into 3 branches to supply the medial and inferior rectus muscles and the inferior oblique.

The parasympathetic fibers wind around the periphery of the nerve, enter the inferior division, and course through the branch that supplies the inferior oblique muscle. They join the ciliary ganglion, where they synapse with the postganglionic fibers, which emerge as many short ciliary nerves. These pierce the sclera and travel through the choroid to innervate the pupillary sphincter and the ciliary muscle. The superficial location of these

Figure 3-9 Cross section through the midbrain at the level of the CN III nucleus. Note the relationship between CN III and the posterior cerebral, superior cerebellar, and posterior communicating arteries. *CA* = cerebral aqueduct, *CC* = crus cerebri (includes corticospinal tract), *IPF* = interpeduncular fossa, *MLF* = medial longitudinal fasciculus, *ON* = oculomotor nucleus, *PAG* = periaqueductal gray, *RN* = red nucleus, *SN* = substantia nigra.

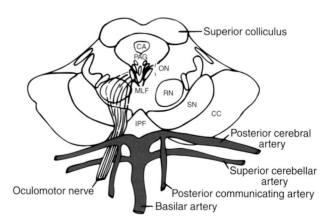

fibers makes them more vulnerable to compression, such as from an aneurysm, than to ischemia. Pupillary dilation is a sensitive (and commonly early) sign of compression.

Pathways for the Pupil Reflexes

Light reflex

The light reflex consists of a simultaneous and equal constriction of the pupils in response to illumination of one or the other eye. The afferent pupillary pathway coincides with that of the visual pathway and includes a decussation of nasal fibers in the chiasm. At the posterior part of the optic tract, the pupillary fibers leave the visual fibers and pass to the lateral side of the midbrain to reach the pretectal nuclei at the level of the superior colliculus. Here, efferent fibers arise and pass to the Edinger-Westphal nuclei, decussating partially (both ventral to the aqueduct and dorsally, in the posterior commissure). Preganglionic parasympathetic fibers leave each Edinger-Westphal nucleus and run in the oculomotor nerve as it leaves the brainstem. The fibers spiral downward to lie medially in the nerve at the level of the petroclinoid ligament and inferiorly in the inferior division of the third nerve as it enters the orbit. These fibers synapse in the ciliary ganglion and give rise to postganglionic myelinated short ciliary nerves, about 3%–5% of which are pupillomotor. The rest are designated for the ciliary muscle and are concerned with the near reflex.

Near reflex

The near reflex is a synkinesis that occurs when attention is changed from distance to near. This reflex includes accommodation, pupil constriction, and convergence. The reflex is initiated in the occipital association cortex, from which impulses descend along corticofugal pathways to relay in pretectal and possibly tegmental areas. From these relays, fibers pass to the Edinger-Westphal nuclei, the motor nuclei of the medial rectus muscles, and the nuclei of CN VI. Fibers for the near reflex approach the pretectal nucleus from the ventral aspect, so that with compressive dorsal lesions of the optic tectum there is sparing of the near pupil reflex relative to the light reflex (light–near dissociation). Efferent fibers for accommodation follow the same general pathway as those for the light reflex, but their final distribution (via the short ciliary nerves) is to the ciliary muscle.

Cranial Nerve IV (Trochlear)

Cranial nerve IV contains the fewest nerve fibers (approximately 3400) of any cranial nerve, but it has the longest intracranial course (75 mm). The nerve nucleus is located in the caudal mesencephalon at the level of the inferior colliculus near the periaqueductal gray matter, ventral to the aqueduct of Sylvius. It is continuous with the caudal end of the CN III nucleus and differs histologically from the CN III nucleus only in the smaller size of its cells. Like the CN III nucleus, it is bounded ventrolaterally by the medial longitudinal fasciculus.

The fascicles of CN IV curve dorsocaudally around the periaqueductal gray matter and decussate completely in the superior medullary velum. The nerves exit the brainstem just beneath the inferior colliculus. Thus, CN IV is the only cranial nerve that is completely decussated and the only motor nerve to exit dorsally from the nervous system. As it curves around the brainstem in the ambient cistern, CN IV runs from beneath the free edge of the tentorium, passes between the posterior cerebral and superior cerebellar arteries, and then pierces the dura mater to enter the cavernous sinus.

Cranial nerve IV travels beneath CN III and above the ophthalmic division of CN V in the lateral wall of the cavernous sinus. Cranial nerve IV enters the orbit through the superior orbital fissure outside the annulus of Zinn and runs superiorly to innervate the superior oblique muscle. Because of its location outside the muscle cone, CN IV is usually not affected by injection of retrobulbar anesthetics.

Cranial Nerve V (Trigeminal)

Cranial nerve V, the largest cranial nerve, possesses both sensory and motor divisions. The sensory portion subserves the greater part of the scalp, forehead, face, eyelids, eye, lacrimal gland, extraocular muscles, ear, dura mater, and tongue. The motor portion innervates the muscles of mastication through branches of the mandibular division.

The CN V nuclear complex extends from the midbrain to the upper cervical segments, often as caudal as C4. It consists of the following 4 nuclei, from above downward:

1. mesencephalic nucleus
2. main sensory nucleus
3. spinal nucleus and tract
4. motor nucleus located in the pons

Important interconnections exist between the different subdivisions of the CN V sensory nuclei and the reticular formation (Fig 3-10).

Mesencephalic Nucleus

The mesencephalic nucleus mediates proprioception and deep sensation from the masticatory, facial, and extraocular muscles. The nucleus extends inferiorly into the posterior pons as far as the main sensory nucleus.

Main Sensory Nucleus

The main sensory nucleus lies in the pons, lateral to the motor nucleus. It is continuous with the mesencephalic nucleus (above) and with the spinal nucleus (below). It receives its input from ascending branches of the sensory root, and it serves light touch from the skin and mucous membranes. The sensory root of CN V, upon entering the pons, divides into an ascending tract and a descending tract. The former terminates in the main sensory nucleus, and the latter ends in the spinal nucleus.

Spinal Nucleus and Tract

The spinal nucleus and tract extend through the medulla to C4. The nucleus receives pain and temperature afferents from the descending spinal tract, which also carries cutaneous

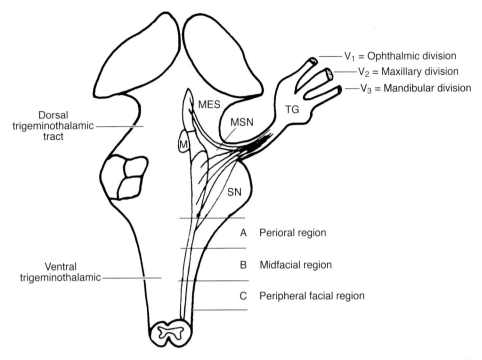

Figure 3-10 Cranial nerve V complex (dorsal view of brainstem). *M* = motor nucleus, *MES* = mesencephalic nucleus, *MSN* = main sensory nucleus, *SN* = spinal nucleus and tract, *TG* = trigeminal ganglion. *A, B,* and *C* are portions of the caudal spinal nucleus that correspond to concentric areas of the face: *A,* perioral; *B,* midface, including eyes; *C,* peripheral face and scalp.

components of CN VII, CN IX, and CN X that serve sensations from the ear and external auditory meatus. The sensory fibers from the ophthalmic division of CN V (V₁) terminate in the most ventral portion of the spinal nucleus and tract. Fibers from the maxillary division (V₂) end in the midportion of the spinal nucleus (in a ventral-dorsal plane). The fibers from the mandibular division (V₃) end in the dorsal parts of the nucleus.

The cutaneous territory of each of the CN V divisions is represented in the spinal nucleus and tract in a rostral-caudal direction. Fibers from the perioral region are thought to terminate most rostrally in the nucleus; fibers from the peripheral face and scalp end in the caudal portion. The zone between them, the midfacial region, is projected onto the central portion of the nucleus. This "onionskin" pattern of cutaneous sensation has been derived from clinical studies in patients with damage to the spinal nucleus and tract (Fig 3-11). Damage to the trigeminal sensory nucleus at the level of the brainstem causes bilateral sensory loss in concentric areas of the face, with the sensory area surrounding the mouth in the center. If a patient verifies this distribution of sensory loss, then the lesion is in the brainstem. Conversely, sensory loss that follows the peripheral distribution of the trigeminal sensory divisions (ophthalmic, maxillary, and mandibular) indicates the lesion lies in CN V after it exits the brainstem.

Brodal A. *Neurological Anatomy in Relation to Clinical Medicine.* 3rd ed. New York: Oxford; 1981: 524–529.

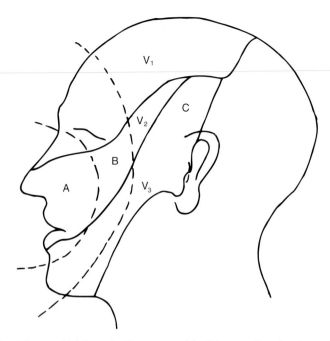

Figure 3-11 Cranial nerve V (trigeminal): pattern of facial sensation. Lesions of the trigeminal sensory nucleus in the brainstem result in an onionskin distribution of altered sensation (sections *A, B,* and *C*) delineated by the *dashed lines*; lesions of the ophthalmic *(V₁),* maxillary *(V₂),* and mandibular *(V₃)* nerves result in the pattern of sensory loss delineated by the *solid lines.* *(Illustration by Thomas A. Weingeist, PhD, MD.)*

Axons from the main sensory, spinal, and portions of the mesencephalic nuclei relay sensory information to higher sensory areas of the brain. The axons cross the midline in the pons and ascend to the thalamus along the ventral and dorsal trigeminothalamic tracts. They terminate in the nerve cells of the ventral posteromedial nucleus of the thalamus. These cells in turn send axons through the internal capsule to the postcentral gyrus of the cerebral cortex.

Motor Nucleus

The motor nucleus is located medial to the main sensory nucleus in the pons. It receives fibers from both cerebral hemispheres, the reticular formation, the red nucleus, the tectum, the medial longitudinal fasciculus, and the mesencephalic nucleus. A monosynaptic reflex arc is formed by cells from the mesencephalic nucleus and the motor nucleus. The motor nucleus sends off axons that form the motor root, which eventually supplies the muscles of mastication (pterygoid, masseter, temporalis), the tensor tympani, the tensor veli palatini, the mylohyoid, and the anterior belly of the digastric.

The intracranial fifth nerve emerges from the upper lateral portion of the ventral pons, passes over the petrous apex, forms the *trigeminal ganglion,* and then divides into 3 branches. The trigeminal ganglion, also called the *gasserian* or *semilunar ganglion,* contains the cells of origin of all the CN V sensory axons. The crescent-shaped ganglion occupies a recess in the dura mater posterolateral to the cavernous sinus. This recess, called the Meckel cave, is near the apex of the petrous part of the temporal bone in the middle cranial fossa. Medially, the trigeminal ganglion is close to the ICA and the posterior cavernous sinus.

Divisions of Cranial Nerve V

The 3 divisions of CN V are the ophthalmic (V_1), the maxillary (V_2), and the mandibular (V_3).

CN V₁

The ophthalmic division enters the cavernous sinus lateral to the ICA and courses beneath CN III and CN IV. Within the sinus, it gives off a tentorial-dural branch, which supplies sensation to the cerebral vessels, dura mater of the anterior fossa, cavernous sinus, sphenoid wing, petrous apex, Meckel cave, tentorium cerebelli, falx cerebri, and dural venous sinuses. CN V_1 passes into the orbit through the superior orbital fissure and divides into 3 branches: frontal, lacrimal, and nasociliary.

The frontal nerve divides into the supraorbital and the supratrochlear nerves, which provide sensation for the medial portion of the upper eyelid and the conjunctiva, forehead, scalp, frontal sinuses, and side of the nose.

The lacrimal nerve innervates the lacrimal gland and the neighboring conjunctiva and skin. It was once suggested that postganglionic parasympathetic lacrimal secretory fibers, arising in the pterygopalatine ganglion, were carried to the lacrimal gland via a zygomaticotemporal connection with the lacrimal nerve. However, it is now thought more likely that the gland receives its parasympathetic supply directly, from the retro-orbital plexus (discussed later in the chapter).

The nasociliary nerve supplies sensation through nasal branches to the middle and inferior turbinates, septum, lateral nasal wall, and tip of the nose. The infratrochlear branch serves the lacrimal drainage system, the conjunctiva, and the skin of the medial canthal region. Long ciliary nerves carry sensory fibers from the ciliary body, the iris, and the cornea and provide the sympathetic innervation to the dilator muscle of the iris. Sensation from the globe is carried by short ciliary nerves. The CN V fibers pass through the ciliary ganglion to join the nasociliary nerve. The ciliary nerves also contain postganglionic parasympathetic fibers from the ganglion to the pupillary sphincter and the ciliary muscle.

CN V₂

The maxillary division leaves the trigeminal ganglion to exit the skull through the foramen rotundum, which lies below the superior orbital fissure. CN V_2 courses through the pterygopalatine fossa into the inferior orbital fissure, then runs through the infraorbital canal as the infraorbital nerve. After exiting the infraorbital foramen, CN V_2 divides into an inferior palpebral branch supplying the lower eyelid, a nasal branch for the side of the nose, and a superior labial branch for the upper lip. The teeth, maxillary sinus, roof of the mouth, and soft palate are also innervated by branches of the maxillary division.

CN V₃

The mandibular division contains both sensory and motor fibers. It exits the skull through the foramen ovale and provides motor input for the masticatory muscles. Sensation is supplied to the mucosa and skin of the mandible, lower lip, tongue, external ear, and tympanum.

> Standring S, ed. *Gray's Anatomy: The Anatomical Basis of Clinical Practice.* 39th ed. Edinburgh, New York: Elsevier Churchill Livingstone; 2005.

Cranial Nerve VI (Abducens)

The nucleus of CN VI is situated in the floor of the fourth ventricle, beneath the facial colliculus, in the caudal pons. Fibers of CN VII pass over or loop around the CN VI nucleus and exit in the cerebellopontine angle. The medial longitudinal fasciculus lies medial to the CN VI nucleus. The fascicular portion of the nerve runs ventrally through the paramedian pontine reticular formation and the pyramidal tract and leaves the brainstem in the pontomedullary junction (Fig 3-12).

Cranial nerve VI takes a vertical course along the ventral face of the pons and is crossed by the anterior inferior cerebellar artery. It continues through the subarachnoid space along the surface of the clivus, surrounded by the Batson venous plexus, to perforate the dura mater below the crest of the petrous portion of the temporal bone, approximately 2 cm below the posterior clinoid process. It then passes intradurally through or around the inferior petrosal sinus and beneath the petroclinoid (Gruber) ligament through the Dorello canal, where it enters the cavernous sinus. In the cavernous sinus, CN VI runs

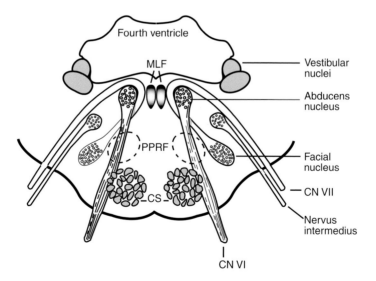

Figure 3-12 Cross section of the pons at the level of the CN VI (abducens) nucleus. *CS =* corticospinal tract, *MLF =* medial longitudinal fasciculus, *PPRF =* pontine paramedian reticular formation. *(Illustration by Sylvia Barker.)*

below and lateral to the carotid artery and may transiently carry sympathetic fibers from the carotid plexus. It passes through the superior orbital fissure within the annulus of Zinn and innervates the lateral rectus muscle on its ocular surface.

Cranial Nerve VII (Facial)

Cranial nerve VII is a complex mixed sensory and motor nerve. The motor root contains special visceral efferent fibers that innervate the muscles of facial expression. The so-called sensory root of CN VII is the nervus intermedius, which contains special visceral afferent, general somatic afferent, and general visceral efferent fibers. The special *visceral afferent fibers,* which convey the sense of taste from the anterior two thirds of the tongue, terminate centrally in the nucleus of the tractus solitarius. The general *somatic afferent fibers* convey sensation from the external auditory meatus and the retroauricular skin; centrally, they enter the spinal nucleus of CN V. The general visceral efferent fibers provide preganglionic parasympathetic innervation by way of the sphenopalatine and submandibular ganglia to the lacrimal, submaxillary, and sublingual glands.

The motor nucleus of CN VII is a cigar-shaped column, 4 mm long, located in the caudal third of the pons. It is ventrolateral to the CN VI nucleus, ventromedial to the spinal nucleus of CN V, and dorsal to the superior olive. Four distinct subgroups within the nucleus innervate specific facial muscles; the ventral portion of the intermediate group probably supplies axons to the orbicularis oculi. The part of the nucleus supplying the upper half of the face receives corticobulbar input from both cerebral hemispheres. The lower half of the face is influenced by corticobulbar fibers from the opposite cerebral hemisphere.

Fibers from the motor nucleus course dorsomedially to approach the floor of the fourth ventricle and then ascend immediately dorsal to the CN VI nucleus. At the rostral end of the CN VI nucleus, the main facial motor fibers arch over its dorsal surface (forming the internal genu of CN VII) and then pass ventrolaterally between the spinal nucleus of CN V and the CN VII nucleus to exit the brainstem at the pontomedullary junction. The bulge formed by the CN VII genu in the floor of the fourth ventricle is the facial colliculus (Fig 3-13).

The sensory nucleus of CN VII is the rostral portion of the tractus solitarius, sometimes known as the *gustatory nucleus.* It lies lateral to the motor and parasympathetic nuclei in the caudal pons. Sensations of taste from the anterior two thirds of the tongue are carried by special visceral afferent fibers to this nucleus. The impulses travel along the lingual nerve and chorda tympani; the cell bodies for these impulses are located in the geniculate ganglion. They eventually reach the brain through the nervus intermedius.

Cranial nerve VII, the nervus intermedius, and CN VIII (acoustic) pass together through the lateral pontine cistern in the cerebellopontine angle and enter the internal auditory meatus in a common meningeal sheath. Cranial nerve VII and the intermedius nerve then enter the fallopian canal, the longest bony canal traversed by any cranial nerve (30 mm).

Cranial nerve VII can be divided into 3 segments in its course through this canal. After passing anterolaterally for a short distance known as the *labyrinthine segment,* the nerves bend sharply at the geniculate ganglion and are then directed dorsolaterally past the tympanic cavity. This 90° bend, known as the *tympanic segment,* is the external genu of

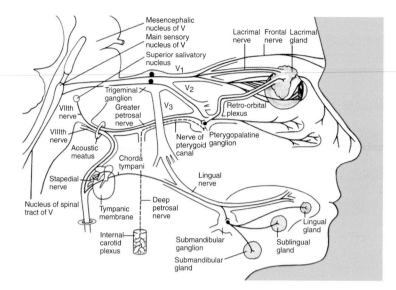

Figure 3-13 Lacrimal reflex arc (after Kurihashi). The afferent pathway is provided by the first and second divisions of CN V. The efferent path proceeds from the lacrimal nucleus (close to the superior salivary nucleus) via CN VII (nervus intermedius), through the geniculate ganglion, the greater superficial petrosal nerve, and the nerve of the pterygoid canal (where it is joined by sympathetic fibers from the deep petrosal nerve). The nerve passes to the pterygopalatine ganglion, where it synapses with postganglionic fibers. These fibers reach the lacrimal gland directly, via the retro-orbital plexus of nerves. The fibers carry cholinergic and vasoactive intestinal polypeptide (VIP)-ergic fibers to the gland. *(From Bron AJ, Tripathi RC, Tripathi BJ.* Wolff's Anatomy of the Eye and Orbit. *8th ed. London: Chapman & Hall; 1997.)*

CN VII. Two parasympathetic branches from the superior salivatory and lacrimal nuclei leave the nerve at the tympanic segment: the greater superficial petrosal nerve and a small filament that joins the inferior petrosal nerve. The third segment, the *mastoid segment,* of the nerve is directed straight down toward the base of the skull. The stapedius nerve leaves, and the chorda tympani joins CN VII in the mastoid segment. The CN VII trunk then exits the skull at the stylomastoid foramen and separates into a large temporofacial and a small cervicofacial division between the superficial and deep lobes of the parotid gland. This area of branching is known as the *pes anserinus.*

The temporofacial division gives rise to the temporal, zygomatic, and buccal branches. The cervicofacial division is the origin of the marginal mandibular and colli branches. However, anastomoses and branching patterns are numerous. Commonly, the temporal branch supplies the upper half of the orbicularis oculi, and the zygomatic branch supplies the lower half. The frontalis, corrugator supercilii, and pyramidalis muscles are usually innervated by the temporal branch.

The parasympathetic outflow originates in the superior salivatory nucleus and the lacrimal nucleus, both of which lie posterolateral to the motor nucleus and which probably receive afferent fibers from the hypothalamus. The superior salivatory nucleus also receives input from the olfactory system. The hypothalamic fibers reaching the lacrimal nucleus may mediate emotional tearing, and there is supranuclear input from the cortex and the limbic system. Reflex lacrimation is controlled by afferents from the sensory nuclei of CN V. These preganglionic parasympathetic fibers pass peripherally as part of the nervus intermedius and divide into 2 groups near the external genu of CN VII. The lacrimal group of fibers passes to the pterygopalatine ganglion in the greater superficial petrosal nerve. The salivatory group of fibers projects through the chorda tympani nerve to the submandibular ganglion to innervate the submandibular and sublingual salivary glands.

The greater superficial petrosal nerve extends forward on the anterior surface of the petrous temporal bone to join the deep petrosal nerve (sympathetic) and form the nerve of the pterygoid canal. This nerve enters the pterygopalatine fossa; joins the pterygopalatine ganglion; and gives rise to unmyelinated postganglionic fibers that innervate the globe, lacrimal gland, glands of the palate, and nose. Those parasympathetic fibers destined for the orbit enter it via the inferior orbital fissure. Here, they are joined by sympathetic fibers from the carotid plexus and form a retro-orbital plexus of nerves, whose rami oculares supply orbital vessels or enter the globe to supply the choroid and anterior segment structures. Some of these fibers enter the globe directly; others enter via connections with the short ciliary nerves. The rami oculares also supply the lacrimal gland.

Cavernous Sinus

The cavernous sinus is an interconnected series of venous channels located just posterior to the orbital apex and lateral to the sphenoidal air sinus and pituitary fossa (Fig 3-14). The following structures are located within the venous cavity:

- the ICA surrounded by the sympathetic carotid plexus
- CN III, CN IV, and CN VI
- the ophthalmic and maxillary divisions of CN V

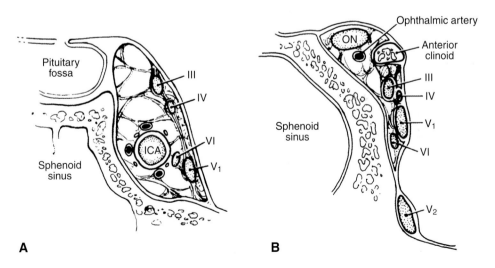

Figure 3-14 Cavernous sinus, coronal sections **(A)** at the level of the pituitary fossa and **(B)** at the level of the anterior clinoid process. *ICA* = internal carotid artery, *ON* = optic nerve. *(Reproduced by permission from Doxanas MT, Anderson RL. Clinical Orbital Anatomy. Baltimore: Williams & Wilkins; 1984.)*

Other Venous Sinuses

The cavernous sinus is only 1 part of an interconnecting series of venous channels that carry blood away from the brain and drain into the internal jugular veins. Other venous sinuses include the superior sagittal, transverse, straight, sigmoid, and petrosal. The various components of the venous system are depicted in Figure 3-15. Thrombosis in any

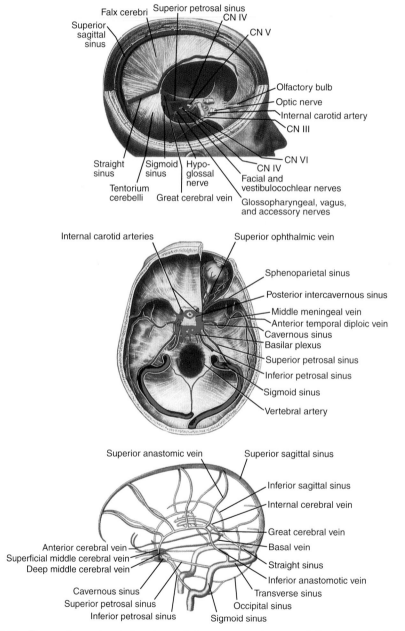

Figure 3-15 Three-dimensional drawings of the venous sinuses of the brain, their interconnections, and the relationship to the dura. *(Reproduced with permission from Williams PL, Warwick R. Gray's Anatomy. 38th ed. Edinburgh: Churchill Livingstone; 1995.)*

portion of the venous sinuses can lead to increased venous pressure and may cause intracranial hypertension and papilledema.

Circle of Willis

The major arteries supplying the brain are the right and left ICAs (which distribute blood primarily to the rostral portion of the brain) and the right and left vertebral arteries (which join to form the basilar artery). The basilar artery primarily distributes blood to the brainstem and posterior portion of the brain. These arteries interconnect at the base of the brain at the circle of Willis (Fig 3-16). These interconnections help to distribute blood to all regions of the brain, even when a portion of the system becomes occluded.

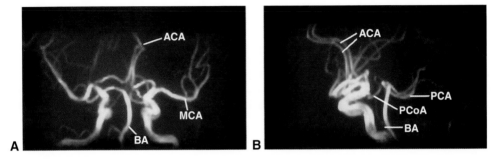

Figure 3-16 **A,** Magnetic resonance angiogram showing the circle of Willis in an anteroposterior view. **B,** Same patient shown in an oblique view. *ACA* = anterior cerebral artery, *BA* = basilar artery, *MCA* = middle cerebral artery, *PCA* = posterior cerebral artery, *PCoA* = posterior communicating artery. *(Courtesy of T. Talli, MD, and W. Yuh, MD.)*

PART II

Embryology

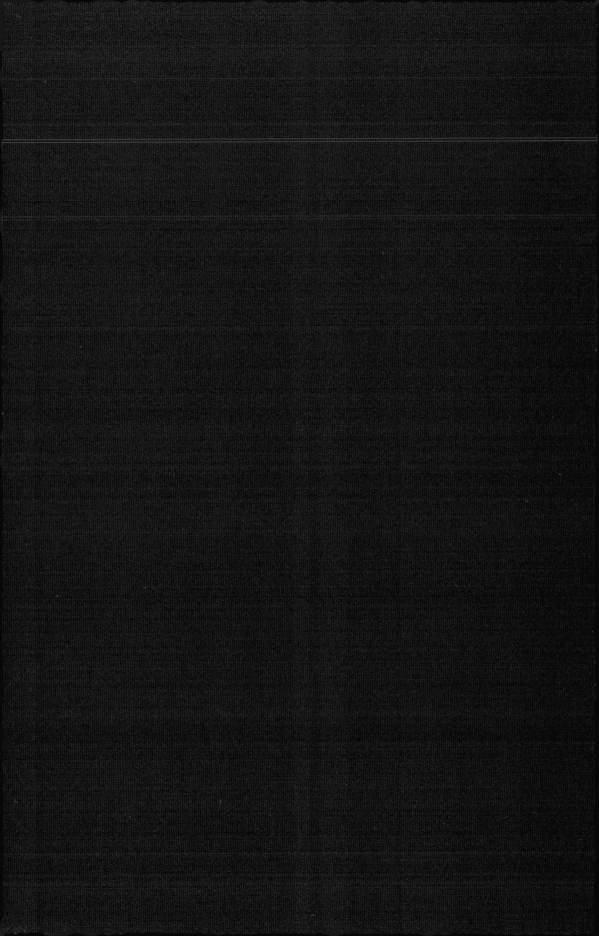

CHAPTER 4

Ocular Development

Introduction

Experimental studies conducted in recent decades have revolutionized our understanding of ocular development. Consequently, the original treatises on the growth and differentiation of the eye have been modified. The classic *germ layer theory* depicted the epithelium of the cornea, the retina, and the neural components of the uveal tract as derived from ectoderm and the remainder of the ocular structures as derived from mesoderm.

Although this general schema is still used, it is currently recognized that the embryonic and fetal development of the human eye involves a series of sequential events, including inductive interactions and morphogenetic movement of cells from distant regions of the embryo. The primary tissues involved in these processes are the head epidermis, neuroectoderm, and mesenchyme. Three elements have been identified as making important contributions to the genesis of the eye:

1. growth factors
2. homeobox genes
3. neural crest cells

Each is described separately in the following sections, but interaction among these elements is also crucial. Part III of this volume, Genetics, also discusses some of the concepts reviewed in this chapter.

Growth Factors

The process of *induction* is mediated by tissue communication through macromolecules that act as chemical signals. Growth factors are now known to be active in the earliest stages of embryonic development. They are a class of trophic substances that participate in the control of normal development by modulating the migration, proliferation, and differentiation of cells. These molecules act at nanomolar concentrations by binding with high affinity to specific receptor sites localized in the plasma membrane of the target cell.

The embryonic genome is not transcribed until the stage of midblastula transition, which takes place several hours after fertilization. The messenger RNAs (mRNA) for the growth factors involved in the earliest aspects of the growth and differentiation of the fertilized egg are endogenous and are supplied from maternal sources until the embryonic tissues become able to synthesize them de novo.

These growth factors include

- fibroblast growth factor (FGF)
- transforming growth factor βs (TGF-β_1 and TGF-β_2)
- insulin-like growth factor I (IGF-I)

Experimental studies have revealed that when cells of the animal cap are exposed to FGF, they are induced to differentiate into posterior mesoderm that is destined to form tissues of the caudal region. However, TGF-βs induce animal cap cells to differentiate into mesoderm that forms structures in the head region, including the eye.

Growth factors also regulate the levels of expression of homeobox genes, which function as a mechanism for controlling the establishment of the overall arrangement of the eye as an organ. Visual acuity requires a precise spatial arrangement of tissues of the eye; thus, it is critical that homeobox genes be expressed at the appropriate level and time.

Some growth factors are crucial in directing the migration and developmental patterns of cranial neural crest cells by influencing the synthesis and degradation of the extracellular matrix. Various components of the extracellular matrix act as morphogenetic factors that facilitate a complex series of integrated tissue interactions, movements, and shape changes, especially during the earliest stages of morphogenesis of the optic vesicle and lens.

Differentiation of the various ocular tissues appears to be at least partly controlled by a variety of growth factors. For example, the FGFs induce the neuroectodermal cells that line the inner wall of the optic cup to develop as neural retina; FGF is also responsible for certain aspects of differentiation of the lens epithelial cells into lens fibers. However, the differentiation of lens epithelial cells immediately anterior to the equator—as well as their mitotic activity—is promoted by the IGFs. The synergistic action of multiple trophic factors appears to be a significant regulatory tool for initiating cellular activities and for limiting abnormal development.

Tripathi BJ, Tripathi RC, Livingston AM, Borisuth NS. The role of growth factors in the embryogenesis and differentiation of the eye. *Am J Anat.* 1991;192(4):442–471.

Homeobox Genes

Homeobox genes contain a distinctive segment of DNA, approximately 180 base pairs in length, that shows similarity in the sequence of the nucleotides. This region is termed the homeobox (from the Greek *homoios* ["like, resembling"] and *box* [the extent of the conserved sequence]). The homeobox encodes an almost identical sequence of approximately 60 amino acids, the *homeodomain,* in the protein products of these genes. Because they control the activity of many subordinate genes, homeobox genes are considered "master" genes. Conserved evolutionarily, these genes are present throughout the plant and animal kingdoms. The function of homeobox genes is mediated by the homeodomain, which recognizes and binds to specific DNA sequences in the subordinate genes, thereby activating or repressing their expression. Thus, these genes act as selector genes, or "master switches," encoding transcription factors. Transcription factors regulate mRNA production by other genes. On the basis of the pattern of homeobox gene expression, which is restricted both spatially and temporally during the earliest stages of development, the vertebrate embryo can be subdivided anteriorly to posteriorly into fields of cells that have different developmental capacities. This organizational plan precedes the formation of any specific organ or structures. The fact that homeobox genes are located on the chromosomes in the same order in which they are expressed along the anteroposterior axis of the embryo indicates that they are activated sequentially. The same homeobox genes are expressed again later in embryogenesis, apparently to specify the identity of a particular cell. Experimental evidence suggests that homeobox genes are activated not only by growth factors—especially FGFs and TGF-βs—but also by retinoic acid, a direct derivative of vitamin A. Too much or too little vitamin A is teratogenic.

—Hox genes activated by FGF, TGF-β, and retinoic acid

Investigations in several vertebrate species have revealed the involvement of specific homeobox genes in the development of the eye. For example, expression of the *PAX6* gene marks the location of the lens-competent region in the head ectoderm before the optic vesicle can be recognized. During the early stages of eye development, 2 *HOX* genes are expressed with a distinct spatial and temporal relationship. The *HOX8.1* gene is expressed in the surface ectoderm, in a region destined to form the corneal epithelium, and in the optic vesicle, where the retina will differentiate before invagination occurs. *HOX7.1*, which is expressed after the formation of the optic cup, marks the region of the future ciliary body. Subsequently, the *PAX6* gene has a role in the expression of tissue-specific genes in the eye. For example, it induces differentiation of progenitor cells into neurons in the retina, as well as the expression of zeta (ζ)-crystallins in lens epithelial cells.

—PAX6 prior to optic vesicles then later in differentiation

Hsiung F, Moses K. Retinal development in Drosophila: specifying the first neuron. *Hum Mol Gen.* 2002;11(10):1207–1214.

Nguyen M, Arnheiter H. Signaling and transcriptional regulation in early mammalian eye development: a link between FGF and MITF. *Development.* 2000;127(16):3581–3591.

Neural Crest Cells

Neural crest cells arise from neuroectoderm located at the crest of the neural folds at approximately the same time that the folds fuse to form the neural tube. They are a transient population of cells; after they migrate to different regions of the embryo, differentiation occurs. Most mesenchymal cells of the facial primordia are derived from the neural crest. Crest cells do not arise from the region of the forebrain. However, neural crest cells from the diencephalic, mesencephalic, and rhombencephalic regions migrate anteriorly along the dorsum of the embryo. Crest cells that originate from the posterior midbrain form the maxillary primordia, and those from the hindbrain form the mandibular primordia. The crest cells from the diencephalon contribute to the tissue of the frontonasal mass; later, they are joined by cells from the anterior midbrain that migrate to and settle around the optic vesicles. The anterior flexure of the embryo aids the migration of neural crest cells ventrad and cephalad.

The extracellular matrix has a significant role in directing the migration of neural crest cells. Molecules such as fibronectin promote migration, whereas others, such as proteoglycans, are inhibitory. The positive and negative cues that the crest cells encounter during migration appear to guide the cells along the correct pathways to the appropriate destination. Because the synthesis and secretion of extracellular matrix molecules such as

—ECM molecules either promote or inhibit migration of neural crest cells

collagen, fibronectin, and proteoglycans can be influenced by growth factors, especially TGF-βs, cytokines also have a role in regulating the migration of crest cells.

Early in development, neural crest cells are pluripotent, and their final differentiation is considerably influenced by local factors. Crest cells from the hindbrain normally form the connective tissue of the visceral arch and contribute to the formation of the cranial sensory ganglia. However, if these hindbrain neural crest cells are grafted in place of the posterior diencephalic and mesencephalic crest population, they differentiate appropriately into ocular, orbital, and facial tissues.

Neural crest cells make a major contribution to the connective tissue components of the eye and orbit. Notable exceptions include the striated fibers of the extraocular muscles and the endothelial cells that line all blood vessels of the eye and orbit. Both of these exceptions arise from mesoderm (Table 4-1).

Table 4-1 **Derivatives of Embryonic Tissues**

=== ECTODERM ===

Neuroectoderm
  Neurosensory retina
  Retinal pigment epithelium
  Pigmented ciliary epithelium
  Nonpigmented ciliary epithelium
  Pigmented iris epithelium
  Sphincter and dilator muscles of iris
  Optic nerve, axons, and glia
  Vitreous
Cranial Neural Crest Cells
  Corneal stroma and endothelium
  Sclera (see also mesoderm)
  Trabecular meshwork
  Sheaths and tendons of extraocular muscles
  Connective tissues of iris
  Ciliary muscles
  Choroidal stroma
  Melanocytes (uveal and epithelial)
  Meningeal sheaths of the optic nerve
  Schwann cells of ciliary nerves
  Ciliary ganglion
  All midline and inferior orbital bones, as well as parts of orbital roof and lateral rim
  Cartilage
  Connective tissue of orbit
  Muscular layer and connective tissue sheaths of all ocular and orbital vessels
Surface Ectoderm
  Epithelium, glands, cilia of skin of eyelids and caruncle
  Conjunctival epithelium
  Lens
  Lacrimal gland
  Lacrimal drainage system
  Vitreous

=== MESODERM ===

  Fibers of extraocular muscles
  Endothelial lining of all orbital and ocular blood vessels
  Temporal portion of sclera
  Vitreous

Ito Y, Yeo JY, Chytil A, et al. Conditional inactivation of Tgfbr2 in cranial neural crest causes cleft palate and calvaria defects. *Development.* 2003;130(21):5269–5280.

Neurocristopathy

Congenital and developmental anomalies that involve cells derived from the neural crest have been grouped together under the term *neurocristopathies*. Most of these abnormalities result from defects in either the migration of neural crest cells or their terminal differentiation. Several conditions are common in combination with ocular defects, especially those of the anterior segment:

- craniofacial and dental malformations
- middle-ear deafness
- malformations of the skull, shoulder girdle, and upper spine

Primary cleft palate can be produced by extirpation of the neural folds prior to crest cell migration. The median face malformation (severe orbital hypertelorism) is thought to result from an impaired midline coalescence of the frontonasal process.

Honkanen RA, Nishimura DY, Swiderski RE, et al. A family with Axenfeld-Rieger syndrome and Peters anomaly caused by a point mutation (Phe112Ser) in the FOXC1 gene. *Am J of Ophthalmol.* 2003;135(3):368–375.

Tripathi BJ, Tripathi RC, Wisdom JE. Embryology of the anterior segment of the human eye. In: Ritch R, Shields MB, Krupin T, eds. *The Glaucomas.* 2nd ed. St Louis: Mosby; 1996:1.

Embryogenesis

In the 2 weeks after fertilization, the impregnated ovum undergoes a series of repeated cell divisions and, through repositioning and reorientation of the cells, becomes sequentially morula, blastula, and gastrula (Fig 4-1). Only the inner cell mass, a small number of cells derived from the fertilized ovum, differentiates subsequently into the embryo. The outer cell mass, or trophoblast, forms the placenta and support tissues. The formation of the epiblast and hypoblast from the inner cell mass precedes gastrulation, a process that results in the establishment of the 3 primary germ layers: *ectoderm, mesoderm,* and *endoderm* (Fig 4-2).

Cells of the epiblast in the medial region of the embryonic disc begin to proliferate at the caudal end, which causes the development of a thickening known as the *primitive streak.* The cells of the primitive streak migrate both laterally and cephalad beneath the epiblast, where they give rise to the mesenchymal cells of the intraembryonic mesoderm. The cells that remain in the epiblast are now recognized as the embryonic ectoderm. Some cells of the primitive streak invade the hypoblast and laterally displace most of these cells to give rise to the embryonic endoderm. The primitive streak elongates by the addition of cells at the caudal end and thus establishes the axial orientation of the embryo. The cranial end of the primitive streak enlarges as the primitive node. Mesenchymal cells that migrate cranially from this site form the medial notochordal process, which develops into the primitive mesenchymal axial skeleton (or *notochord*) of the embryo. The development of the notochord induces the overlying ectoderm to differentiate into neuroectoderm that becomes identified as the *neural plate.* The brain and the eye develop from the most anterior region of the neural plate.

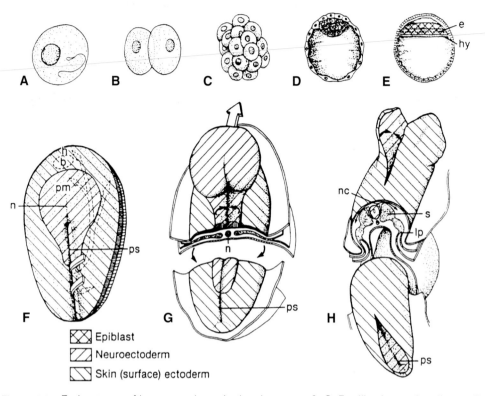

Figure 4-1 Early stages of human embryonic development. **A–C,** Fertilization and earliest cell divisions to morula stage. **D,** Sectioned blastocyst. A fluid-filled cavity has formed, and cells that will form the embryo (the darker area indicates the inner cell mass) are distinct from cells that will develop into support tissues (eg, the placenta). **E,** Embryo-forming cells have now separated into 2 layers: the epiblast *(e)* and hypoblast *(hy)*. **F,** Dorsal view of an embryo that is slightly more advanced than the sectioned embryo illustrated in **E.** Gastrulation movements *(arrows)* bring cells from the upper layer through the primitive streak *(ps)* into the potential space between the 2 layers to form the middle germ layer (mesoderm). Mesodermal cells fail to penetrate between the ectoderm and endoderm at the oral plate (*b* = buccopharyngeal membrane), which later forms the embryonic partition between the oral and pharyngeal cavities. At this stage, the heart primordium *(h)* lies anterior to the oral plate. The notochord *(n)* is formed from the anterior (cephalic) end of the primitive streak. The prochordal mesoderm *(pm)* is subjacent to the neural plate on the region between *n* and *b.* **G,** Early stages of neural tube folding and closure, and folding of the lateral body walls *(solid arrows)*. The anterior neural plate has begun to "overgrow" *(open arrow)* the heart primordium and future oral region, including the buccopharyngeal membrane. **H,** Embryo folding is nearing completion. Migration of cranial neural crest cells *(nc)* in the hindbrain region has been initiated. In contrast to the trunk crest cells, most of those forming in the head region migrate laterally—under the surface ectoderm but superficial to the somites *(s)* and the lateral plate *(lp)* of the mesoderm. *(Reproduced with permission from Serafin D, Georgiade NG. Pediatric Plastic Surgery. St Louis: Mosby; 1984.)*

Growth of the lateral part of the neural plate results in folds that develop upward and outward, parallel to the neural groove from the head to the caudal region. At this stage, neuroectoderm lines the inner folds, and surface ectoderm covers the outer surface of the folds. The neuroectodermal cells at the apex of the folds proliferate and produce a population of neural crest cells, which contribute extensively to the tissues of the eye (Fig 4-3).

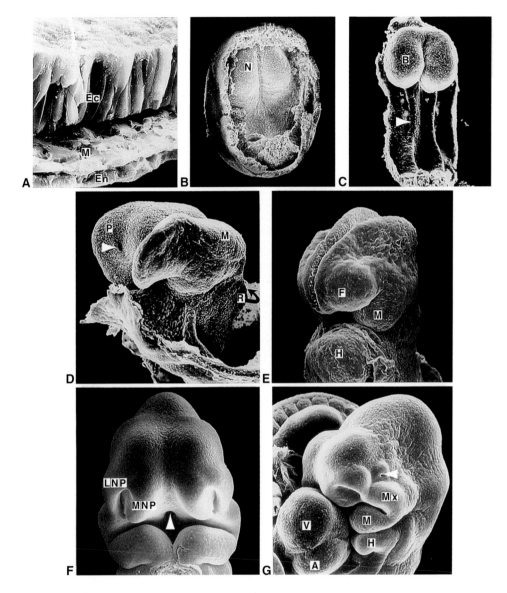

Figure 4-2 Normal craniofacial development. **A,** A parasagittal section through the cranial aspect of a gastrulation-stage mouse embryo. The cells of the 3 germ layers—ectoderm *(Ec)*, mesoderm *(M)*, and endoderm *(En)*—have distinct morphologies. **B,** The developing neural plate *(N)* is apparent in a dorsal view of this presomite mouse embryo. **C,** Neural folds *(arrowhead)* can be seen in the developing spinal cord region. The lateral aspects of the brain *(B)* region have not yet begun to elevate in this mouse embryo in the head-fold stage. **D,** Three regions of the brain can be distinguished at this 6-somite stage: prosencephalon *(P)*, mesencephalon *(M)*, and rhombencephalon *(R, curved arrow)*. Optic sulci *(arrowhead)* are seen as evaginations from the prosencephalon. **E,** The neural tube has not yet fused in this 12-somite embryo. The stomodeum, or primitive oral cavity, is bordered by the frontonasal prominence *(F)*, the first visceral arch (mandibular arch, *M*), and the developing heart *(H)*. **F,** Medial and lateral nasal prominences *(MNP, LNP)* surround olfactory pits in this 36-somite mouse embryo. The Rathke pouch *(arrowhead)* can be distinguished in the roof of the stomodeum. **G,** In this lateral view of a 36-somite mouse embryo, the first and second (hyoid, *H*) visceral arches are apparent. The region of the first arch consists of maxillary *(Mx)* and mandibular *(M)* components. Note the presence of the eye with its invaginating lens *(arrowhead)*. Atrial *(A)* and ventricular *(V)* heart chambers can be distinguished. *(Reproduced with permission from Sulik KK, Johnston MC. Embryonic origin of holoprosencephaly: interrelationship of the developing brain and face. Scan Electron Microsc. 1982;(Pt 1):311.)*

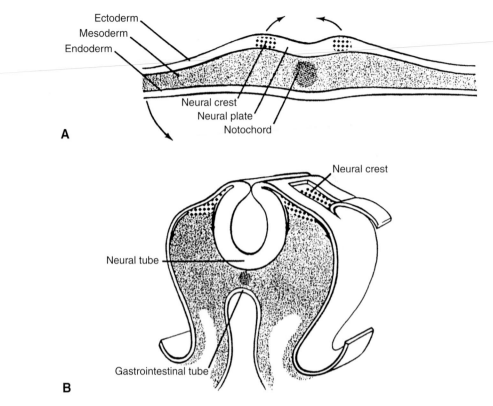

Figure 4-3 Cross sections through embryos before **(A)** and after **(B)** the onset of migration of crest cells *(diamond pattern)*. The ectoderm has been peeled back in **B** to show the underlying neural crest cells. *(Reproduced with permission from Johnston MC, Sulik KK. Development of face and oral cavity. In: Bhaskar SN, ed. Orban's Oral Histology and Embryology. 11th ed. St Louis: Mosby; 1991.)*

The cephalic neural folds grow and expand markedly. At the end of the third week after conception, the neural folds begin to close to form the neural tube. This process starts in the midregion of the embryo and proceeds anteriorly and posteriorly at the same time. As the neural tube closes, 3 events important to the development of the eye and orbit occur simultaneously (Fig 4-4):

1. Optic pits develop from the optic sulci, small depressions present in the cephalic neuroectoderm.
2. Neural crest cells begin to migrate.
3. As the anterior neural tube closes, it flexes ventrally.

Organogenesis of the Eye

The chronology of ocular development is given in Table 4-2. The optic sulci are first recognizable as slight, curved indentations in the widest part of each neural fold just internal to the peak of the ridge. The long axis of the depression is roughly parallel to that of the

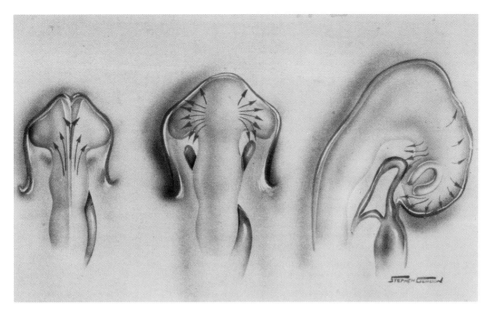

Figure 4-4 Migration of cranial neural crest cells from dorsal diencephalic and mesencephalic regions. **Left,** Cells begin migration anteriorly as tube closes. **Center,** Crest cells move in waves around the optic vesicle and lose continuity with the surface cells. **Right,** The neural tube flexes ventrally, carrying the optic cup and crest cells ventrally. *(Redrawn from M. Johnston, 1966.)*

neural groove. The optic pits, formed of a single layer of neuroectoderm, develop from the continued evagination of the sulci. As the neural tube closes, the pits deepen and become optic vesicles, which appear as symmetric, hollow, hemispheric outgrowths on the lateral sides of what is now the forebrain vesicle. The optic vesicles remain attached to, and continuous with, the neural tube by optic stalks composed of neuroectodermal cells (Fig 4-5). The expansion and ballooning that take place in the hollow optic vesicle do not occur in the stalk, which remains as a tubular link from the cavity of the vesicle to that of the diencephalon.

As the optic vesicle approaches the outer wall of the embryo, a focal thickening of the cells, the *lens placode,* develops in the surface ectoderm, which has been primed by lens-bias signals during earlier embryogenesis. In the fourth week, invagination of the lens placode leads to formation of the *lens vesicle,* which initially remains attached to the surface ectoderm by the lens stalk. Simultaneously, differential growth and movement of the cells of the optic vesicle result in the invagination of its temporal and lower walls and the formation of the optic cup.

The outer layer of the optic cup evolves as a monolayer of cells, the *retinal pigment epithelium (RPE).* The inner, invaginated layer will differentiate into the neurosensory retina. Initially, the cup is incomplete in its inferior portion (Fig 4-6). The indentation, or fissure, between the folds or margins of the cup is called the *embryonic fissure* (previously the *choroidal,* or *fetal, fissure*). Invagination pushes the neuroectodermal cells originally near the surface deep into the cup near the outer layer. Invagination produces a fold in

Table 4-2 Chronology of Embryonic and Fetal Development of the Eye

22 days	Optic primordium appears in neural folds (1.5–3.0 mm).
25 days	Optic vesicle evaginates. Neural crest cells migrate to surround vesicle.
28 days	Vesicle induces lens placode.
Second month	Invagination of optic and lens vesicles. Hyaloid artery fills embryonic fissure. Closure of embryonic fissure begins. Pigment granules appear in retinal pigment epithelium. Primordia of lateral rectus and superior oblique muscles grow anteriorly. Eyelid folds appear. Retinal differentiation begins with nuclear and marginal zones. Migration of retinal cells begins. Neural crest cells of corneal endothelium migrate centrally. Corneal stroma follows. Cavity of lens vesicle is obliterated. Secondary vitreous surrounds hyaloid system. Choroidal vasculature develops. Axons from ganglion cells migrate to optic nerve. Glial laminal cribrosa forms. Bruch's membrane appears.
Third month	Precursors of rods and cones differentiate. Anterior rim of optic vesicle grows forward, and ciliary body starts to develop. Sclera condenses. Vortex veins pierce sclera. Eyelid folds meet and fuse.
Fourth month	Retinal vessels grow into nerve fiber layer near optic disc. Folds of ciliary processes appear. Iris sphincter develops. Descemet's membrane forms. Schlemm's canal appears. Hyaloid system starts to regress. Glands and cilia develop.
Fifth month	Photoreceptors develop inner segments. Choroidal vessels form layers. Iris stroma is vascularized. Eyelids begin to separate.
Sixth month	Ganglion cells thicken in macula. Recurrent arterial branches join the choroidal vessels. Dilator muscle of iris forms.
Seventh month	Outer segments of photoreceptors differentiate. Central fovea starts to thin. Fibrous lamina cribrosa forms. Choroidal melanocytes produce pigment. Circular muscle forms in ciliary body.
Eighth month	Chamber angle completes formation. Hyaloid system disappears.
Ninth month	Retinal vessels reach the periphery. Myelination of fibers of optic nerve is complete to lamina cribrosa. Pupillary membrane disappears.

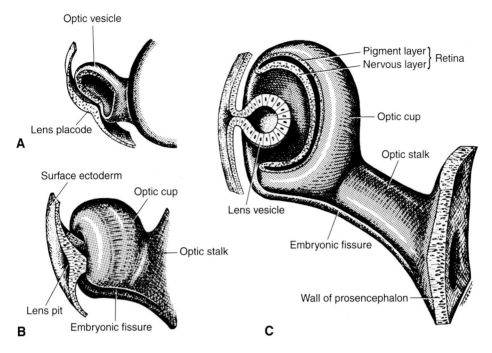

Optic vesicle

Lens placode

A

Surface ectoderm

Optic cup

Optic stalk

Lens pit

B

Embryonic fissure

Pigment layer ⎫
Nervous layer ⎬ Retina

Optic cup

Optic stalk

Lens vesicle

Embryonic fissure

Wall of prosencephalon

C

Figure 4-5 Diagram of the development of the human optic cup. The optic vesicle and cup have been partly cut away in **A** and **C**, and the lens vesicle is sectioned for clarity. **A,** 4.5-mm embryo (27 days). **B,** 5.5-mm embryo. **C,** 7.5-mm embryo (28 days). *(Reproduced from Tripathi RC, Tripathi BJ. Comparative physiology and anatomy of the aqueous outflow pathway. In: Davson H, ed. The Eye. 3rd ed. Orlando: Academic Press; 1984.)*

the neuroectoderm anteriorly, adjacent to the lens, called the *rim* of the optic cup. At first, the 2 layers of the developing cup have a small space between them, the *optic ventricle*; however, as invagination proceeds and the inner and outer layers become juxtaposed, the cavity of the optic ventricle progressively narrows. Basement membrane lines both the outer and the inner layers of the cup. The apices of the cells in both layers meet end to end as the ventricle narrows. The ventricle cavity remains throughout life as a potential space, the subretinal space.

The embryonic fissure extends from the rim of the cup near the lens to the distal optic stalk. This fissure allows vessels of the hyaloid system to be incorporated within the eye (Fig 4-7). To complete the entire wall of the globe, the 2 lips of the embryonic fissure meet and fuse. Closure begins in the midregion of the cup near the equator of the globe and proceeds anteriorly to the rim and posteriorly down the stalk, enclosing the hyaloid artery. This process occasionally gives rise to a bridge coloboma with a posterior and peripheral component separated by a band of normal tissue. The inner and outer layers of the cup meet end to end. Because the primitive cells are still labile, they seal the fissure without evidence of a seam or scar. Incomplete or inadequate closure produces a coloboma of the iris, ciliary body, choroid, or optic disc, depending on the extent of the failed closure and secondary attempts to close the defect (Fig 4-8).

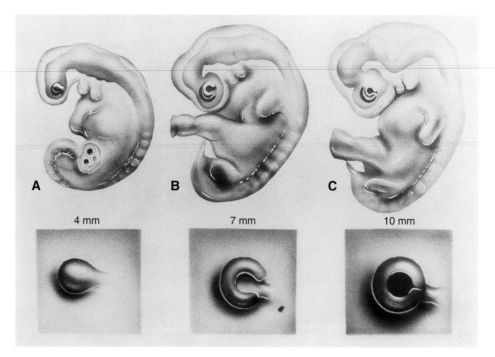

Figure 4-6 Ocular and somatic development. **A,** Flexion of the neural tube and ballooning of the optic vesicle. **B,** Upper-limb buds appear as the optic cup and embryonic fissure emerge. **C,** Completion of the optic cup with closure of the fissure. Convolutions appear in the brain, and leg buds appear. The size of the fetus is given. *Lower sequence:* optic vesicle; optic cup with open embryonic fissure; cup with fissure closing.

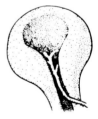

Figure 4-7 Optic cup and stalk with open embryonic fissure below. The hyaloid artery from the dorsal ophthalmic artery enters the cavity through the posterior aspect of the embryonic fissure. The rim of the optic cup is above. The lens is not shown.

Neurosensory Retina

The neurosensory, or neural, retina arises from the inner layer of neuroectodermal cells of the optic cup (Fig 4-9). Differentiation of this cell layer begins early, and within 1 month of fertilization, mitotic activity has produced 3–4 compact rows of cells that rapidly increase in number. The nuclei segregate at the outer two thirds of the primordial retina toward the outer layer of the optic cup. This region is recognized as the *primitive zone.* The ciliated apices of the cells are directed outward into the rapidly shrinking cavity of the optic ventricle. The inner third of the developing retina is initially devoid of nuclei and is termed the *inner marginal zone;* it eventually differentiates into the nerve fiber layer. The primitive and marginal zones are recognizable only until the seventh week of gestation. Little

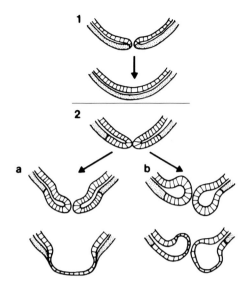

Figure 4-8 Closure of lips of the embryonic fissure. *1,* Normal closure: Inner layers (neurosensory retina) and outer layers (*dotted area,* RPE) meet and merge. Basement membrane forms on both surfaces. *2,* Coloboma formation: Ectropion of the inner retina at the lips of the fissure results in imperfect fusion; pigment epithelium is displaced laterally by cells of the neurosensory retina. *a,* A simple coloboma results in a defective retina and RPE. The uvea and sclera (not shown) are thin and dysgenic. *b,* In a cystic coloboma, the primary vesicular cavity enlarges adjacent to the point of defective closure.

Figure 4-9 Development of the retina and optic nerve. **A,** *Right,* The fetal neurosensory retina develops from neuroectoderm as ganglion cells migrate from the outer primitive zone of closely packed nuclei to the inner marginal zone of fibrils. A few axons from ganglion cells grow toward the optic nerve. RPE begins melanization in the posterior pole. *Left,* A cross section shows the fetal optic nerve with a center of vacuolating primitive cells through which axons from the ganglion cells will grow toward the brain. Neural crest cells as mesenchyme loosely ring the nerve. The hyaloid artery enters the vitreous (fifth week). **B,** *Right,* The migration of nuclei results in 3 nuclear and plexiform layers. *Left,* A cross section of the optic nerve shows axons of ganglion cells *(black dots)* migrating through vacuolating cells, first in the periphery of the nerve. Neural crest cells condense to meningeal sheaths of optic nerve (seventh week).

is known about the stimuli that initiate and direct the complex migration and subsequent differentiation of the primitive neuroepithelial cells into the retina.

Differentiation of the retina begins in the center of the optic cup and gradually extends peripherally toward its rim. Neural and glial cells develop simultaneously. By the fifth week of gestation, the putative ganglion and Müller cells have migrated from the outer neuroepithelial layers toward the vitreous cavity. As a result, the nuclei of the neuroblastic cells become segregated as 2 distinct layers, the inner and outer neuroblastic layers. These 2 layers are separated by a region of tangled cell processes known as the *transient nerve fiber layer of Chievitz,* which becomes the definitive inner plexiform layer between weeks 9 and 12 of gestation (except in the macula, where it persists until birth). At 9–12 weeks, the 4 major horizontal layers of the retina become distinguishable.

The ganglion cells are the first cells of the retina to become clearly differentiated. Their axonal processes and dendritic trees begin to develop at about the sixth week of gestation. Axons from ganglion cells nearest the posterior pole are the first to enter the optic stalk and induce formation of the optic nerve. The number of ganglion cells increases rapidly between weeks 15 and 17 of gestation, then decreases between weeks 18 and 30 because of apoptosis. The ganglion cell somas grow larger with advancing gestational age.

The processes of the Müller cells extend from the inner basal lamina of the optic vesicle toward the optic ventricle. As soon as the photoreceptors enlarge and become morphologically distinct as cones, the development of junctional complexes on adjacent lateral surfaces of these cells and of the Müller cell processes gives rise to the external limiting membrane.

Photoreceptors arise from the outermost layer of neuroblastic cells. Mitotic activity, abundant in the outer neuroblastic layers in weeks 4–12, ceases in the central retina by week 15 of gestation, and differentiation of the cones begins in the region of the putative fovea. The cilia on the apices of the cells that had invaginated the adjacent RPE disappear, and precursors of outer segments gradually develop. Initially, cylindrical cytoplasmic processes extend toward the apical region of the RPE cells.

Differentiation of cone outer segments begins at 5 months, when multiple infoldings develop in the plasma membrane of the processes. The folds separate from the plasma membrane, and their orientation as flattened, lamellar discs parallels the development of the horizontal cells. The cell bodies of the rods are dispersed among the cones and are first recognizable by their dark nuclei with condensed peripheral chromatin. The rod outer segments develop during the seventh month of gestation.

Amacrine cells are identified by their large, round, pale-staining nuclei. They are first seen scattered at the inner border of the outer neuroblastic layer by week 14 of gestation. Bipolar cells do not differentiate until week 23. The bipolar dendrites extend to the outer plexiform layer by week 25, at which time the horizontal cells probably differentiate.

Fovea

Differentiation of the neurons, photoreceptors, and glial cells in the fovea occurs early because this region is the focal point for the centraperipheral development of the retina.

The different cell types, as well as many synapses and intercellular junctions, are already established by 15 weeks of gestation. Thinning of the ganglion cell and inner nuclear layers begins at 24–26 weeks of gestation and gives rise to the earliest recognizable depression in the area of the macula.

The foveal pit becomes more prominent by the seventh month as a result of the marked thinning of the inner nuclear layer. An acellular fibrous zone is now present on both the nasal and temporal sides of the fovea. By this time, major changes have occurred in the cones: the width of the inner segments has decreased, whereas their length has increased, as has the length of the fibers of the Henle fiber layer. Only 2 layers of ganglion cells remain at 8 months, and the inner nuclear layer at the foveola is reduced to 3 rows or fewer because of lateral displacement. At birth, axons of bipolar cells that pass to the inner plexiform layers constitute the prominent transient layer of Chievitz. Relocation of all layers to the periphery of the foveal slope, which leaves the nuclei of the cones uncovered in the foveola, occurs by 4 months after birth. However, remodeling of the elements of the fovea continues until nearly 4 years of age, at which time the transient layer of Chievitz is lost completely.

> Tripathi BJ, Tripathi RC. Development of the human eye. In: Bron AJ, Tripathi RC, Tripathi BJ, eds. *Wolff's Anatomy of the Eye and Orbit.* 8th ed. London: Chapman & Hall; 1997.

Retinal Pigment Epithelium

Mitotic activity continues in the pseudostratified, columnar epithelial cells that constitute the outer wall of the optic cup up to the sixth week of gestation. The apical borders of adjacent cells are already joined by zonulae occludentes and zonulae adherentes junctional complexes. At week 6, melanogenesis begins; concurrently, the cilia that had been present on the inner cell surface (ie, adjacent to the developing neurosensory retina) disappear. The RPE cells are the first in the body to produce melanin. Whether in the retina or in the choroid, the stages of melanin production are the same: premelanosomes gradually become melanosomes.

Differentiation of the RPE begins at the posterior pole and proceeds anteriorly, so that by 8 weeks of gestation the RPE is organized as a single layer of hexagonal columnar cells located posteriorly. The cells become tall and cuboidal during the third and fourth months, and the terminal web becomes well established at the lateral apical borders. The RPE is thought to be fully functional at this stage. The increase in surface area of the RPE (which takes place after birth to accommodate the subsequent growth of the globe) is achieved by enlargement and expansion of individual cells.

The basement membrane of the RPE becomes the inner portion of Bruch's membrane; the outer layer of Bruch's membrane, also basement membrane, is laid down by the choriocapillaris layer. The embryonic pigment epithelial cells have a profound inductive influence on the development of the choroid, sclera, and neurosensory retina. In areas where pigment epithelium does not form, as sometimes happens along the line of closure of the embryonic fissure, the underlying choroid, sclera, and retina are hypoplastic (see Fig 4-8). The nature of the inductive stimulus is not known.

Optic Nerve

The optic nerve develops from the optic stalk, the original connection between the optic vesicle and the forebrain. Initially, the stalk is composed of an inner zone of closely packed neuroectodermal cells surrounded by a less compact layer of undifferentiated neural crest cells. Late in the sixth week of gestation, some cells of the inner region vacuolate and degenerate, and nerve fibers from the ganglion cells migrate through the spaces thus created. Other cells of the inner zone differentiate as glial cells. By the seventh week, the optic disc contains the hyaloid artery, which is surrounded by axons and covered by a mantle of glial cells, many of which disappear by the seventh month. The glial cells also give rise to the glial elements of the lamina cribrosa during the eighth week of gestation. Differentiation of the neural crest cells into the pia, arachnoid, and dura mater of the optic nerve begins in the seventh week, but the sheaths become well defined only after the fourth month.

The number of axons increases rapidly: by 10–12 weeks of gestation, some 1.9 million axons are present in the optic nerve, rising to 3.7 million by 16 weeks. Later, attrition of axons causes the number of fibers to drop to approximately 1.1 million, which establishes the adult condition by 33 weeks. The loss of axons parallels the degeneration of ganglion cells in the fetal retina and may be related to the segregation of terminals as discrete laminae in the dorsal lateral geniculate body.

As the axons grow toward the lateral geniculate body, partial crossover occurs at the optic chiasm. Cells located at the chiasm midline (probably radial glial cells) express certain repulsive or inhibitory molecules that provide a guidance cue by acting specifically on ipsilateral projecting axons.

Myelination starts in the chiasm at the seventh month of gestation, proceeds toward the eye, and ceases at the lamina cribrosa by about 1 month after birth. Occasionally, medullated fibers develop in the retina. They appear on ophthalmoscopic examination as a flat, serrated white patch on the inner surface of the retina. The medullation is usually interrupted at the lamina, but occasionally it is continuous across the lamina from nerve to retina.

Some fetuses demonstrate a response to light as early as the eighth week of gestation, which indicates that at least some central nervous system pathways are established. By 5 months, 50% of the growth of the optic nerve and disc has occurred; by birth, 75%; and before 1 year of age, 95%.

Lens

One of the earliest events in embryogenesis is determination of lens development. The interaction that takes place between the surface ectoderm and the underlying chordamesoderm during midgastrulation imparts a lens-forming bias on an extensive region of head ectoderm. Next, the anlage of the eye conveys an inductive signal to the ectoderm, which determines the region of the presumptive lens. The mesoderm beneath the putative lens ectoderm transmits another signal late in gastrulation (but when the neural plate is still open) that potentiates the fate of the tissue that will become the lens. Finally, by invoking the final phase of determination and enhancing differentiation during neurulation, the optic vesicle designates the specific region of the head ectoderm that will become the lens. The surface ectoderm can respond to the influence of the optic vesicle only during a precise period of development.

The lens is first apparent at about 27 days' gestation as a disc-shaped thickening of surface epithelial cells over the optic vesicle. This lens placode and its thin basal lamina are separated from the basal lamina of the optic vesicle by a narrow space containing fine filaments that have a role in the gradual invagination of the lens placode to form the lens vesicle. Initially, the vesicle, consisting of a single layer of cells with apices directed inward, is covered by a basal lamina that seals anteriorly to complete the formation of the lens capsule (Fig 4-10). Ultimately, the lens vesicle separates from the surface epithelium at about 33 days' gestation. The area of lens separation from the surface ectoderm heals without

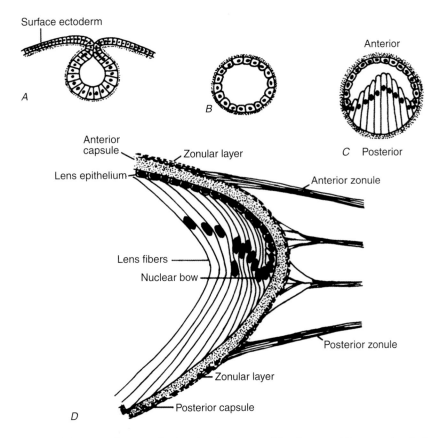

Figure 4-10 Diagram of stages in the development of the lens and its capsule. *A,* Formation of the lens vesicle from invagination of surface ectoderm together with its basal lamina in an embryo corresponding to 32 days' gestation. *B,* Separation of the vesicle from the surface ectoderm and its surrounding basal lamina. *C,* Obliteration of the lens vesicle cavity by elongation of posterior cells at about 35 days' gestation. *D,* Equatorial region of the fully formed lens. Attachment of zonular fibers to the anterior, posterior, and equatorial regions of the lens periphery becomes apparent at approximately 5½ weeks' gestation. Note the change in polarity of cells from anterior to posterior regions of the lens. *(Modified from Tripathi RC, Tripathi BJ. Anatomy of the human eye. In: Davson H, ed. The Eye. 3rd ed. Orlando: Academic Press; 1984.)*

residuum. The epithelial cells deposit additional basal lamina material, which forms the lens capsule. Initially, the posterior capsule is more prominent than the anterior capsule. The lens capsule isolates the lens constituents immunologically within the globe.

During closure of the lens vesicle, DNA synthesis decreases in the cells that form the posterior half of the lens; simultaneously, specific lens proteins *(crystallins)* are synthesized. By 45 days' gestation, the posterior cells, or primary lens fibers, have lengthened to fill the cavity of the vesicle from posterior to anterior. The posterior cells of the vesicle account for most of the growth of the lens during the first 2 months of embryogenesis. The primary fibers form the compact core of the lens, known as the *embryonic nucleus.*

The pre-equatorial epithelial cells retain their mitotic activity throughout life, producing secondary lens fibers. These fibers are displaced inward between the capsule and the embryonic nucleus and meet on the vertical planes, the lens *sutures.* The first suture marking the fetal nucleus is shaped like a Y anteriorly and an inverted Y posteriorly. The basic anatomy of the lens is established after the first layer of secondary fibers has been laid down at the seventh week of gestation.

At first, the lens is spherical, but it becomes ellipsoid with the addition of secondary fibers. As secondary fibers are added, the sutures become more complex and dendriform. In the third month, the innermost fibers mature; cytoplasmic fibrillar material increases and cellular organelles decrease. The nuclei of the deeper cells, at first homogeneous and dense, are lost; the chromatin and ribosomes disintegrate. The equatorial diameter of the unfixed human lens measures 2 mm at 12 weeks and 6 mm at 35 weeks. Both the growth and the maturation of lenticular fibers continue throughout life. BCSC Section 11, *Lens and Cataract,* discusses the development of the lens in detail.

The zonular apparatus begins to develop after the tertiary vitreous has formed. The ciliary epithelial cells then synthesize collagen fibrils of the zonular fibers. By the fifth month of gestation, as they increase in number, strength, and coarseness, the fibers reach the lens and merge with the anterior and posterior capsule.

Vitreous

Between the fourth and fifth weeks of gestation, the space between the lens vesicle and the inner layer of the optic cup becomes filled with fibrils, mesenchymal cells, and vascular channels of the hyaloid system. Together, these elements constitute the *primary vitreous* (Fig 4-11). Initially, the fibrillar content is of ectodermal origin, being derived from the fibrils already in place between the invaginating lens placode and the inner layer of the optic cup. The mesenchymal cells are mostly mesodermal in origin, having invaded the cavity of the optic cup with the hyaloid vessel through the patent optic fissure. However, some mesenchymal cells are derived from neural crest cells that migrated over the rim of the cup. The vascular primary vitreous attains its maximum development by 2 months' gestation.

The development of the *secondary vitreous* begins soon after the primary vitreous is established. The secondary vitreous is avascular and consists of type II collagen fibrils and hyalocytes, which are presumed to be derived from mesenchymal cells of the primary vitreous that differentiated into monocytes. The content of hyaluronic acid in the vitreous

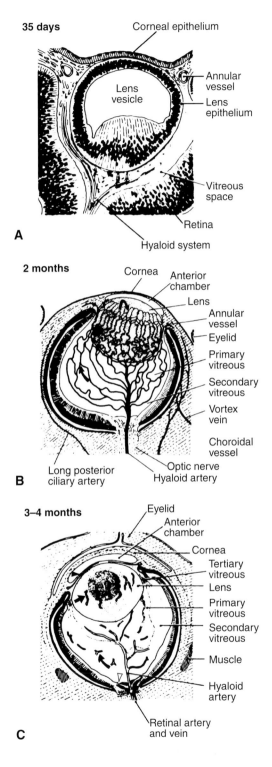

35 days

Corneal epithelium

Lens vesicle

Annular vessel

Lens epithelium

Vitreous space

Retina

A

Hyaloid system

2 months

Cornea

Anterior chamber

Lens

Annular vessel

Eyelid

Primary vitreous

Secondary vitreous

Vortex vein

Choroidal vessel

Optic nerve

Long posterior ciliary artery

Hyaloid artery

B

3–4 months

Eyelid

Anterior chamber

Cornea

Tertiary vitreous

Lens

Primary vitreous

Secondary vitreous

Muscle

Hyaloid artery

Retinal artery and vein

C

Figure 4-11 Main features in vitreous development and the regression of the hyaloid system shown in drawings of sagittal sections. **A,** At 35 days, hyaloid vessels and their branches, the vasa hyaloidea propria, occupy the space between the lens and the neural ectoderm. A capillary net joins the capsula perilenticularis fibrosa, which is composed of ectodermal fibrils associated with vasoformative mesenchyme from the periphery. The ground substance of the primary vitreous is finely fibrillar. **B,** By the second month, the vascular primary vitreous reaches its greatest extent. Arborization of the vasa hyaloidea propria *(curved arrow)* fills the retrolental area and is embedded in collagen fibrils. An avascular secondary vitreous of more finely fibrillar composition forms a narrow zone between the peripheral (outer) branches of the vasa hyaloidea propria and the retina. The *bent arrow* (at top) points to the vessel of the pupillary membrane. The drawing is a composite of embryos at 15–30 mm. **C,** During the fourth month, hyaloid vessels and the vasa hyaloidea propria, together with the tunica vasculosa lentis, atrophy progressively, with the smaller peripheral channels regressing first. The *curved arrow* points to remnants of involuted vessels of the superficial portion of the vasa hyaloidea propria in the secondary vitreous. The *black arrowhead (upper left)* indicates the pupillary membrane (not sketched). The *straight arrow* points to the remnants of the atrophied capsulopupillary vessels. Zonular fibers (tertiary vitreous) begin to stretch from the growing ciliary region toward the lens capsule. Vessels through the center of the optic nerve connect with the hyaloid artery and vein and send small loops into the retina *(open arrowhead).* The drawing is a composite of fetuses at 75–110 mm. *(Reproduced with permission from Cook CS, Ozanics V, Jakobiec FA. Prenatal development of the eye and its adnexa. In: Tasman W, Jaeger EA, eds.* Duane's Foundations of Clinical Ophthalmology. *Philadelphia: Lippincott; 1991.)*

is very low during the prenatal period but increases after birth. Initially, the secondary vitreous occupies only a narrow space between the retina and the posterior limit of the primary vitreous. The continued development of the secondary vitreous, until the end of the third month, is related to the regression of the hyaloid system and the simultaneous retraction of the primary vitreous. Remnants of the atrophied hyaloid system and primary vitreous remain throughout life as the Cloquet canal.

Between the third and fourth months of gestation, collagen fibrils of the secondary vitreous condense and become attached to the internal limiting membrane at the rim of the optic cup. The condensation of fibrils extends to the lens equator and constitutes the tertiary vitreous. The zonular apparatus of the lens ultimately develops anterior to these collagen fibrils.

Choroid

The development of the choroid begins at the anterior region of the optic cup and proceeds posteriorly toward the optic stalk. Choroidal development is associated with the condensation of neural crest cells around the cup that differentiate into cells of the choroidal stroma. Endothelium-lined blood spaces appear in this mesenchymal tissue and first coalesce as the embryonic annular vessel at the rim of the optic cup. During the fourth and fifth weeks of gestation, the choriocapillaris begins to differentiate. The choriocapillary network is formed by mesodermal cells that come in contact with the RPE, which is differentiating simultaneously.

The embryonic eye is completely invested with a primitive layer of capillaries at the beginning of the sixth week of gestation. Adjacent endothelial cells are joined by punctate junctional complexes and zonulae occludentes. Characteristic diaphragmed fenestrations develop in the endothelium between the seventh and ninth weeks. At the same time, the basal lamina becomes defined as a continuous layer of extracellular material surrounding the capillaries. Toward the RPE, this basal lamina constitutes the fifth layer of Bruch's membrane.

The network of vascular channels is supplied by vessels from the internal carotid artery and, later, by the primitive ophthalmic arteries. The channels drain into 2 main blood spaces, the superior orbital and inferior orbital venous plexuses, and from there into what will become the cavernous sinuses. By the end of the second month of gestation, short ciliary arteries enter the capillary coat. Arteries can be distinguished by narrow lumina and walls 2 or more cells thick; veins are larger and lined only by endothelium.

Definite layering of the choroidal vasculature begins in the third month, when the outer layer of large vessels develops. Mainly venous, this layer receives small efferent branches of the choriocapillaris and connects with the vortex veins, which eventually perforate the neighboring sclera. During the fourth month of gestation, the anterior ciliary and long posterior ciliary arteries form the major arterial circle of the iris. Recurrent branches extend from this vessel into the ciliary body by the end of the fifth month. (However, the final anastomosis with the arterial circulation of the choroid is not established until the eighth month.) During the fifth month of gestation, the third layer of medium-sized arterioles develops between the choriocapillaris and the outer layer of large vessels. This layer is initially confined to the level of the equator and reaches the developing ciliary body only at the sixth month.

The choroidal stroma is demarcated by the sclera at the end of the third month of gestation. Initially, the stroma consists of a loosely organized framework of collagen fibrils and abundant fibroblasts. Elastic tissue is laid down during the fourth month. Melanosomes appear between weeks 24 and 27 of gestation, most notably in the melanocytes of the outer choroid and suprachoroid. Melanocytes differentiate from neural crest cells. Melanogenesis proceeds anteriorly from the optic disc to the ora serrata. A few immature melanosomes can be found in the choroidal melanocytes at birth.

Cornea and Sclera

The separation of the lens vesicle from the surface ectoderm initiates the development of the cornea (Fig 4-12). By the end of the fifth week of gestation, the ectoderm consists of 2 layers of epithelial cells that rest on a thin basal lamina (Fig 4-13). Detachment of the lens vesicle induces the basal layer of epithelial cells to secrete collagen fibrils and glycosaminoglycans, which occupy the space between the lens and the corneal epithelium and constitute the primary stroma. Mesenchymal cells migrate from the margins of the rim of the optic cup along the posterior surface of the primary stroma. The first of 3 successive waves of ingrowth, these neural crest–derived cells form the corneal endothelium.

At 5–6 weeks of gestation, the cornea consists of the following:

- a superficial squamous and a basal cuboidal layer of epithelial cells
- a primary stroma
- a double layer of endothelial cells posteriorly

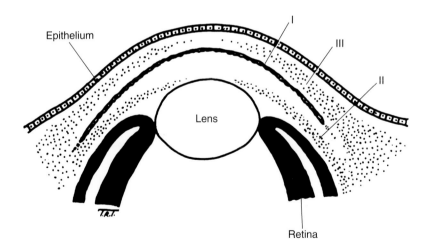

Figure 4-12 Three successive waves of ingrowth of neural crest cells associated with differentiation of the anterior chambers. *I*, First wave forms the corneal endothelium. *II*, Second wave forms the iris and part of the pupillary membrane. *III*, Third wave forms keratocytes. *(Reproduced with permission from Tripathi BJ, Tripathi RC, Wisdom J. Embryology of the anterior segment. In: Ritch R, Shields MB, Krupin T, eds. The Glaucomas. 2nd ed. St Louis: Mosby; 1996.)*

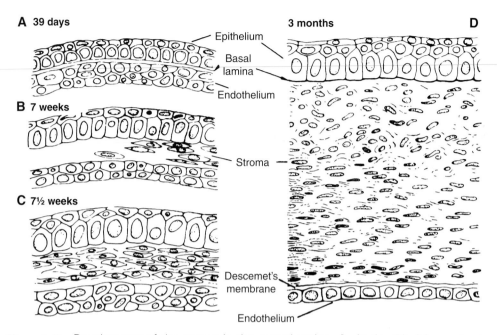

Figure 4-13 Development of the cornea in the central region. **A,** At day 39, 2-layered epithelium rests on the basal lamina and is separated from the endothelium (2–3 layers) by a narrow acellular space. **B,** At week 7, mesenchymal cells from the periphery migrate into the space between the epithelium and endothelium. **C,** Mesenchymal cells (future keratocytes) are arranged in 4–5 incomplete layers by 7½ weeks; a few collagen fibrils are present among the cells. **D,** By 3 months, the epithelium has 2–3 layers of cells, and the stroma has about 25–30 layers of keratocytes that are arranged more regularly in the posterior half. Thin, uneven Descemet's membrane lies between the most posterior keratocytes and the now-single layer of endothelium. *(Reproduced with permission from Cook CS, Ozanics V, Jakobiec FA. Prenatal development of the eye and its adnexa. In: Tasman W, Jaeger EA, ed. Duane's Foundations of Clinical Ophthalmology. Philadelphia: Lippincott; 1991.)*

Further development of the stroma is preceded by the ingrowth of another wave of mesenchymal cells from the rim of the optic cup, which proceeds in 2 directions. The cells of the posterior extension grow between the lens epithelium and the corneal endothelium and are destined to form the primary pupillary membrane. Concurrently, hydration of the hyaluronic acid component of the primary stroma causes swelling that seems to make space available for the next migratory wave of cells. At approximately 7 weeks' gestation, the anterior extension of mesenchymal cells migrates into the corneal stroma. These cells differentiate into keratocytes that secrete type I collagen fibrils and form the matrix of the mature (or secondary) corneal stroma.

When the stroma attains its maximum width, it is approximately double the normal postembryonic width. Dehydration (especially of hyaluronic acid) and compression of the connective tissue cause the later reduction in thickness. Morphogenesis of keratocytes begins in the posterior stroma and proceeds anteriorly. The cells synthesize proteoglycans and collagen fibrils, which are organized as lamellae. Each lamella continues to grow by the formation of additional fibrils (interstitial growth); simultaneously, successive layers of lamellae are added (appositional growth). As the lamellae increase in length and width, the diameter and thickness of the cornea enlarge.

The endothelium in the central region of the cornea becomes a single layer of flattened cells by the third month of gestation. The cells rest on an interrupted basal lamina, which is the future Descemet's membrane. At this stage in development, Descemet's membrane consists of 2 zones: the *lamina densa,* toward the stroma, and the *lamina lucida,* adjacent to the endothelium. Subsequent growth of Descemet's membrane forms a unique organization that is recognized as the *fetal banded zone,* which attains a maximum thickness of about 3 μm at birth. In postnatal life, the posterior nonbanded zone of Descemet's membrane is composed of a homogeneous, fibrillogranular material. This region continues to thicken with age.

By the middle of the fourth month of gestation, the apices of adjacent endothelial cells are joined by zonulae occludentes. This development corresponds with the onset of aqueous humor production by the ciliary processes. Late in the fourth month, the acellular Bowman's zone of the anterior stroma is formed. It is thought that the most superficial keratocytes synthesize and lay down the collagen fibrils and ground substance as they migrate somewhat posteriorly in the stroma.

The diameter of the unfixed cornea measures 2 mm at 12 weeks' gestation, 4.5 mm at 17 weeks, and 9.3 mm at 35 weeks'.

The sclera is formed by mesenchymal cells that condense around the optic cup. Most of these cells are derived from the neural crest. However, those in the caudal region of the sclera are probably derived from paraxial mesoderm that lies juxtaposed to the caudomedial surface of the optic cup throughout the period of crest cell migration. The sclera develops anteriorly before the seventh week of gestation and gradually extends posteriorly. The alignment of cells into parallel layers and the deposition of collagen fibrils are evidence of differentiation. Deposits of elastin and glycosaminoglycans are added to the extracellular matrix at a later stage. By the third month of gestation, some undifferentiated mesenchymal cells have migrated between the nerve fibers in the optic nerve. These cells become oriented transversely and synthesize extracellular matrix materials to form the lamina cribrosa.

Anterior Chamber, Angle, Iris, and Ciliary Body

The anterior chamber is first recognizable as the slitlike space that results after the ingrowth of the first wave of mesenchymal cells and the posterior extension of the second wave. By approximately 7 weeks' gestation, the angle of the anterior chamber is occupied by a nest of loosely organized mesenchymal cells of neural crest origin. These cells will develop into the trabecular meshwork. At the posterior aspect of the angle, mesodermal cells are developing into the vascular channels of the pupillary membrane. Loosely organized mesenchymal cells and the pigment epithelium of the forward-growing optic cup are also present in this region.

Anteriorly, cells that resemble the corneal endothelium form a layer that extends to the angle recess; these cells meet the anterior surface of the developing iris, thus demarcating the angle of the anterior chamber by week 15 of gestation. Beginning at the third month of gestation and continuing for a considerable time after birth (up to the age of 4 years), the angle recess progressively deepens (Fig 4-14). It also appears to be repositioned posteriorly because of the differential growth rate of adjacent tissues.

Initially, no demarcation exists between the mesenchymal cells that will form the trabecular meshwork and those that will differentiate into the ciliary muscle. The extracellular matrix of the trabecular beams is synthesized and deposited by the differentiating trabecular cells beginning at week 15 and continuing up to the eighth month of gestation. Even as early as 12–14 weeks' gestation, the cellular layer that lines the trabecular meshwork on its anterior chamber aspect is perforated by gaps of 2–8 μm in diameter. As development proceeds, these gaps become larger, and eventually the open spaces of the meshwork directly communicate with the anterior chamber.

The Schlemm canal develops from a small plexus of venous canaliculi by the end of the third month of gestation. Derived from mesodermal mesenchyme, these channels function initially as blood vessels. Other mesenchymal cells surround the canal during the fourth month of gestation. These cells and their secreted extracellular matrix materials will form juxtacanalicular tissue. Characteristic vacuolar configurations begin to appear in the endothelial cells that line the Schlemm canal at approximately the beginning of the fifth month. Their development corresponds to the onset of aqueous humor circulation. The canal begins to function as an aqueous sinus rather than as a blood vessel.

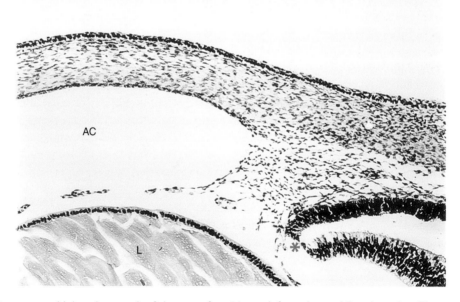

Figure 4-14 Light micrograph of the eye of an 11-week fetus in meridional section. The angular region is poorly defined at this stage and is occupied by loosely arranged, spindle-shaped cells. The Schlemm canal is unrecognizable, and ciliary muscles and ciliary processes are not yet formed; the latter are derived from neural ectodermal fold *(asterisk)*. Corneal endothelium appears continuous with the cellular covering of the primitive iris. *AC* = anterior chamber, *L* = lens. (Original magnification ×230.) *(Reproduced with permission from Tripathi RC, Tripathi BC. Functional anatomy of the anterior chamber angle. In: Tasman W, Jaeger EA, eds.* Duane's Foundations of Clinical Ophthalmology. *Philadelphia: Lippincott; 1991.)*

Differentiation of the ciliary epithelium occurs in the 2 layers of neuroectoderm just behind the advancing optic cup. Late in the third month, longitudinal indentations appear in the outer pigmented layer. Between the third and fourth months, the inner, nonpigmented, layer starts to follow the contour and adhere to the pigmented layer. These radial folds, approximately 75 in number, are the beginning of the ciliary processes.

At week 10 of gestation, precursor ciliary muscle cells are identified as an accumulation of mesenchymal cells between the primitive ciliary epithelium and the anterior sclera condensation at the margin of the optic cup. Differentiation, which begins in the outermost (sclerad) cells during week 12, is evident from the myofilaments that surround plaques of dense bodies along the plasmalemma. The meridional part of the muscle becomes organized during the fifth month, followed by the circular and radial parts. The circular muscle continues to develop for at least 1 year after birth.

The development of the iris is associated with the formation of the anterior portion of the tunica vasculosa lentis. At approximately the sixth week of gestation, vascular channels of this embryonic structure are present as blind outgrowths from the annular vessel that encircles the rim of the optic cup. The developing vessels extend into the mesenchymal cells that cover the anterior lens surface and will ultimately be incorporated into the iris stroma. The most anterior region of the tunica vasculosa lentis is replaced subsequently by the pupillary membrane. At the end of the third month of gestation, after the future ciliary processes have formed, both walls of the optic cup (at its margin) grow forward beneath the pupillary membrane and mesenchymal cells. The mesenchymal tissue of the iris differentiates earlier than does the neuroectoderm. Cells in the developing stroma become fibroblast-like and secrete collagen fibrils and other components of the extracellular matrix.

The earliest differentiation of the sphincter muscle from the anterior layer of epithelium (the forward extension of the RPE) occurs at 3 months' gestation. However, myofibrils are not synthesized until the fifth month, and the muscle does not come to lie free in the stroma until the eighth month of gestation. The dilator muscle is not apparent until the sixth month, and differentiation of the myoepithelial cells continues after birth.

Pigmentation of the posterior epithelial layer of the iris, which is a continuation of the nonpigmented layer of the ciliary body and hence of the neurosensory retina, begins at the pupillary margin at midterm and proceeds toward the periphery. It ceases at the iris root by the end of the seventh month.

The pupillary portion of the tunica vasculosa lentis is resorbed during the sixth month of gestation. The remains of an incomplete arteriovenous anastomosis at the ciliary end of the sphincter muscle demarcate the collarette. The pupillary membrane atrophies near term.

The iris is still immature at birth. Much of the extracellular matrix is yet to be laid down in the stroma. The collarette is closer to the pupil in the newborn eye than it is in the adult eye.

Vascular System

The development of the vascular system of the eye and orbit is complex. Many vessels are transitory, arising and regressing in response to the changing needs of the embryonic eye.

Vascular channels from the internal carotid artery develop in the mesenchyme around the optic vesicle late in the fourth week. Primitive dorsal and ventral ophthalmic arteries bud inward from the carotid and join a loose reticulum of capillaries around the optic vesicle. The system is drained into the future cavernous sinuses by way of plexuses. The early vessels are primarily ocular. A transient vessel, the stapedial artery, arises from the carotid to supply the expanding orbit. Later, the distal part of the stapedial artery is annexed to the ophthalmic artery.

The hyaloid artery is a branch of the primitive dorsal ophthalmic artery that arises at the juncture of the optic stalk and the optic cup at the time of closure of the embryonic fissure. The annular vessel that develops at the rim of the optic cup is supplied by the dorsal and ventral arteries. When incorporated in the optic cup, the hyaloid system extends toward and around the lens to join the annular vessel. Together with the tunica vasculosa lentis, the hyaloid system nourishes the interior of the developing eye.

The primitive dorsal ophthalmic artery becomes the definitive ophthalmic artery of the orbit at the sixth week of gestation. It supplies the temporal long posterior ciliary artery, the short posterior ciliary arteries, and the central retinal artery. The primitive ventral ophthalmic artery almost disappears; only a portion remains as the long posterior nasal ciliary artery.

The major arterial circle of the iris develops in the mesenchyme that surrounds the optic cup. It is located slightly lateral and anterior to the annular vessel and is formed by a coalescence of branches from the long ciliary arteries. Vascular twigs with little connective tissue grow from both the annular vessel and the major arterial circle to form the pupillary membrane, a system of radial vascular loops over the surface of the iris and lens. The pupillary arcades disappear centrally but remain peripherally as the minor circle of the iris. They provide vessels of the mature iris. Because the tissues that demarcate the anterior chamber angle are repositioned during development, the major arterial circle of the iris is ultimately located in the ciliary body.

At the fourth month of gestation, spindle-shaped mesenchymal cells arise from the hyaloid artery at the optic disc. These cells infiltrate the inner layers of the retina as solid cords of undifferentiated cells. Lumina develop, initially as slitlike openings behind the advancing edge of the invading mesenchymal cells. Retinal vascularization proceeds centripetally, and a boundary zone consisting of undifferentiated cells distinguishes the avascular and vascular retina. Endothelial cells differentiate first; adjacent cells are joined by zonulae occludentes and gap junctions.

Vascularization of the nasal retina is complete before that of the temporal retina because of the shorter distance from the optic disc to the nasal ora serrata. By the fifth month, patent vessels have extended superiorly and inferiorly on the temporal aspect of the retina, sparing the region of the putative macula. Small blood vessels begin to develop in the ganglion cell layer of the foveal slope at the sixth month. The adult pattern of arterioles, veins, and capillaries is established through a process of remodeling and retraction of the primitive capillary network. Although capillaries reach the ora serrata by the eighth month, the mature pattern of vascularization is not achieved until 3 months after birth.

The hyaloid system and the tunica vasculosa lentis atrophy in the third trimester. Occasionally, either system may persist after birth (Fig 4-15).

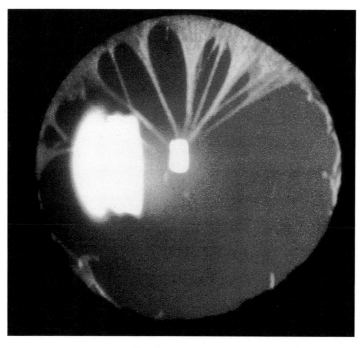

Figure 4-15 Persistent pupillary membrane.

Penfold PL, Provis JM, Madigan MC, van Driel D, Billson FA. Angiogenesis in normal human retinal development: the involvement of astrocytes and macrophages. *Graefes Arch Clin Exp Ophthalmol.* 1990;228(3):255–263.

Periocular Tissues and Eyelids

The frontonasal and maxillary processes of neural crest cells occupy the space that surrounds the optic cups by the fourth week of gestation. The bones, cartilage, fat, and connective tissues of the orbit develop from these cells. All bones of the orbit are membranous except the sphenoid, which is initially cartilaginous. Ossification begins during the third month of gestation, and fusion occurs between the sixth and seventh months.

The extraocular muscles arise from myotomic cells of the preotic mesodermal somites that have shifted cranially. These cells become located within the neural crest mesenchyme, which is situated on the dorsal and caudal aspects of the developing eye. Although the extraocular muscles were once thought to begin developing at the primitive muscle cone that surrounds the optic nerve in the fifth week of gestation, recent evidence suggests that the muscles arise in situ. Myoblasts with myofibrils and immature Z bands are distinguishable by the fifth week of gestation. At approximately 7 weeks, the dorsomedial aspect of the superior rectus muscle gives rise to the levator muscle, which grows laterally and over the superior rectus toward the eyelid. The tendons of the extraocular muscles fuse with the sclera in the vicinity of the equator late in the third month.

The upper eyelid first develops as a proliferation of surface ectoderm in the region of the future outer canthus at 4–5 weeks' gestation. During the second month, both the upper and the lower eyelids are discernible as undifferentiated skin folds that surround mesenchyme of neural crest origin (Fig 4-16). Later, mesodermal mesenchyme infiltrates the eyelids and differentiates into the palpebral musculature. The eyelid folds grow toward each other as well as laterally. Starting near the inner canthus, the margins of the folds fuse at approximately 10 weeks' gestation. As the folds adhere to each other, evolution of cilia and glands continues. The orbicularis muscle condenses in the fold in week 12. The eyelid adhesions gradually break down late in the fifth month, coincident with the secretion of sebum from the sebaceous glands and cornification of the surface epithelium.

The lacrimal gland begins to develop between the sixth and seventh weeks of gestation. Solid cords of epithelial cells proliferate from the basal cell layer of the conjunctiva in the temporal region of the fornix. Neural crest–derived mesenchymal cells aggregate at the tips of the cords and differentiate into acini. Ducts of the gland are formed at approximately 3 months by vacuolation of the cord cells and the development of lumina. Lacrimal gland (reflex) tear production does not begin until 20 or more days after birth. Hence, newborn infants cry without tears.

Between the third and sixth months of gestation, eyelid appendages and pilosebaceous units develop from invaginations of epithelial cells into the underlying mesenchyme.

Realignment of the Globe

Initially, the axes of the 2 optic cups and the optic stalks form an angle of 180°. At 3 months' gestation, this angle has decreased to 105°. With continued enlargement; remodeling; and repositioning of the head, face, and brain throughout gestation, the eyes become oriented in their anterior position. At birth, the axes form an angle of 71°. However, the adult orientation of 68° is not achieved until the age of 3 years.

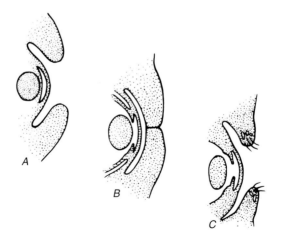

Figure 4-16 Development of the eyelids. *A,* Seventh week: upper and lower eyelid folds grow over the eye. *B,* Eyelids fuse during the eighth week; fusion starts along the nasal margin. *C,* From the fifth to the seventh month, as cilia and glandular structures develop, eyelids gradually open.

Congenital Anomalies

Congenital anomalies are defects present at birth. They result both from genetic influences and from a variety of local and systemic environmental effects. A teratogen is an agent that produces or increases the incidence of congenital malformation. Because exposure to a teratogen can occur at any stage of embryonic development, its effects differ according to the time, duration, and intensity of exposure.

A teratogen acting in the first trimester on primordial cells produces severe damage to the ocular primordium and its derivative tissues. Because cellular development continues after organogenesis, genetic influences or environmental effects at a later time may lead to dysfunction without gross structural abnormalities.

For more discussion of congenital anomalies, see BCSC Section 8, *External Disease and Cornea.*

Genetic Influences

Mutations in homeobox genes are known to produce congenital ocular abnormalities. Often, the mutation results from the deletion or insertion of a single nucleotide that causes a frameshift in the coding region. Several congenital ocular anomalies have been matched to specific mutations—for example, aniridia, posterior embryotoxon, Peters anomaly, Axenfeld anomaly, and congenital cataract are produced by mutations in *PAX6* (see the Human PAX6 Allelic Variant Database Web Site, http://pax6.hgu.mrc.ac.uk, for more information); oculorenal syndrome and coloboma of the optic nerve, by *PAX2* mutations; and cyclopia and holoprosencephaly, by Sonic hedgehog mutations. A mutation in different homeobox genes may produce the same clinical manifestations (eg, a mutation in *RIEG1* also results in Peters anomaly), or a different mutation in the same gene may produce a similar but distinct phenotype (eg, a mutation in *RIEG1* causes Rieger anomaly). Future investigations will identify additional roles for homeobox genes in normal development and their aberrant expression in abnormal ocular development.

Borges AS, Susanna R Jr, Carani JC, et al. Genetic analysis of PITX2 and FOXC1 in Rieger syndrome patients from Brazil. *J Glaucoma.* 2002;11(1):51–56.

Kumar JP, Moses K. Expression of evolutionarily conserved eye specification genes during Drosophila embryogenesis. *Dev Genes Evol.* 2001;211(8-9):406–414.

Nongenetic Teratogens

Nongenetic teratogens include

- toxins
- maternal infections
- nutritional deficiencies
- radiation
- drugs
- developmental failures
- traumatic insult

Early studies showed that an excess or deficiency of vitamin A during development causes eye abnormalities such as coloboma and lens defects. However, it is now apparent that the acid form of this vitamin—retinoic acid—is critical not only to early ocular development but also to the induction of congenital anomalies. Exposure of the developing human embryo to excess amounts of retinoic acid causes malformation of the retina and optic nerve by affecting the expression of homeobox genes such as *PAX2, MSH-C,* and Sonic hedgehog.

Hyatt GA, Dowling JE. Retinoic acid. A key molecule for eye and photoreceptor development. *Invest Ophthalmol Vis Sci.* 1997;38(8):1471–1475.

Prenatal exposure to alcohol results in a distinct pattern of delayed growth, mental retardation, and abnormal behavior patterns, as well as multiple congenital malformations, that is recognized as *fetal alcohol syndrome (FAS)* (Fig 4-17). Various ocular abnormalities include anomalies of the adnexa (strabismus, blepharoptosis, epicanthus) and intraocular defects (cataract, glaucoma, coloboma of uvea, persistent fetal vasculature, dysmorphogenesis of the retina, and optic nerve hypoplasia).

The majority of children with FAS have optic nerve hypoplasia, which, in experimental models, results from reduced densities of ganglion cells and their axons as well as from damage to glial cells and myelin sheaths in the optic nerve.

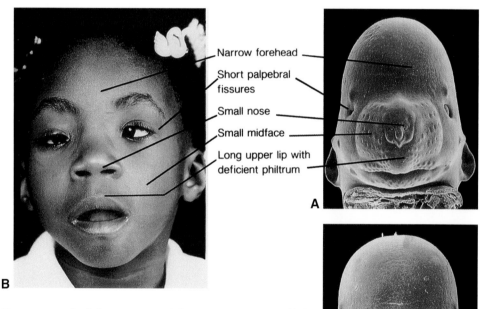

Narrow forehead

Short palpebral fissures

Small nose

Small midface

Long upper lip with deficient philtrum

A

B

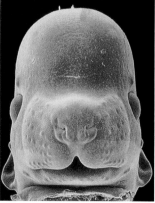

C

Figure 4-17 **A,** A fetus removed from a mouse, to which alcohol (ethanol) had been administered early in pregnancy (gastrulation stage), shows numerous facial characteristics similar to those of a child with fetal alcohol syndrome **(B). C,** A control mouse fetus. *(Parts A and C reproduced with permission from Kathleen Sulik, PhD. In: Serafin D, Georgiade NG. Pediatric Plastic Surgery. St Louis: Mosby; 1984. Part B courtesy of Marilyn Miller, MD.)*

The mouse model of FAS shows that the teratogenic effect of alcohol starts with the insult to the optic primordia during the gastrula stage. A small optic vesicle results in a deficient lens vesicle, which manifests as microphakia. Delay in lens detachment from surface ectoderm leads to myriad anterior segment anomalies that resemble Peters and Axenfeld anomalies. Such conditions are explained by impairment of the migration of the neural crest cells that should have formed the corneal stroma, endothelium, and iris. Together, they cause microphthalmos with a secondary persistence of primary vitreous.

Persistence of the embryonic fissure, which leads to a failure in maintaining intraocular pressure, is one explanation for microphthalmos and coloboma formation. In the mouse model, these malformations appear to be primary events caused by faulty induction produced by the early insult of alcohol on the gastrula forebrain, which gives rise to the evaginating optic primordia.

Hug TE, Fitzgerald KM, Cibis GW. Clinical and electroretinographic findings in fetal alcohol syndrome. *J AAPOS*. 2000;4(4):200–204.

PART III

Genetics

Introduction

Genetics is the study of human variability. Although genetics is a relatively new science compared to such disciplines as anatomy and physiology, its significance in the overall understanding of human life cannot be overstated. Genetic knowledge can enhance our understanding of the processes of cellular function, embryology, and development, as well as our concepts of what is and is not a genetic disease. Many researchers think that as much as 90% of medical disease either has a major genetic component or involves genetic factors that may significantly influence the disease.

The discovery of previously unknown genes has opened new areas of understanding of physiology at the cellular or tissue level, one important example of which is the discovery of *homeotic selector genes* (eg, the *HOX* and *PAX* gene families) that regulate, guide, and coordinate early embryologic development and differentiation. (These genes, also called *homeobox genes,* are discussed in Part II, Embryology, as well.) Another example is the identification of the genes that appear to be transcribed as initiating events in the process of *apoptosis,* or programmed cell death, which itself appears critical for normal embryogenesis.

Genetic disorders affect about 5% of the liveborn infants in the United States. Approximately 50% of childhood blindness has a genetic cause. At the beginning of this millennium, more than 10,000 human gene loci were known by mendelian phenotypes and/ or cellular and molecular genetic methods. In about 10%–15% of known genetic diseases, clinical findings are limited to the eye; a similar percentage includes systemic disorders with ocular manifestations.

Terminology

Not knowing the vocabulary of genetics and molecular biology is one of the greatest impediments to understanding these fields. Readers are strongly encouraged to read the glossary before proceeding through the chapters, paying particular attention to those terms with which they are unfamiliar.

Glossary

Acceptor splice site The junction between the 3′, or downstream, end of an intron and the 5′, or upstream, end of the next exon. The consensus sequence is $\frac{T}{G}N\frac{C}{T}AG/G$ for the intron–exon boundary, where N is a purine (G or A). See *donor splice site* and *splice junction site.*

Acrocentric Type of chromosome in which the centromere is located near one end—for example, chromosomes 13, 14, 15, 21, and 22.

Allele Alternative form of a gene or DNA sequence that may occupy a given locus on a pair of chromosomes. Clinical traits, gene products, and disorders are said to be *allelic* if they are determined to be at the same locus and *nonallelic* if they are determined to reside at different loci.

Allele-specific oligonucleotide (ASO) A synthetic segment of DNA approximately 20 nucleotides in length. When hybridized to an unknown DNA sample, the ASO will bind to and thus identify the complementary sequence or specific string of base pairs. Used in detecting disease mutation.

Allelic association See *linkage disequilibrium.*

Allelic heterogeneity When different alleles at the same locus are capable of producing an abnormal phenotype.

Alu repeat sequence A common short interspersed element (SINE), 300 base pairs long, that occurs 500,000 times scattered throughout the genome. Often involved in errors of duplication or in mutational events. Unique to primates.

Amber codon The primitive stop codon TAG, which is thought to become the consensus sequence for the exon–intron and intron–exon boundaries (or *splice junction sites*) with loss of the thymine. See *stop codon.*

Aneuploidy An abnormal number of chromosomes.

Anticipation The occurrence of a dominantly inherited disease at an earlier age (often with greater severity) in subsequent generations. Now known to occur with expansion of a trinucleotide repeat sequence. Seen, for example, in fragile-X syndrome, myotonic dystrophy, and Huntington disease.

Antioncogene See *tumor-suppressor genes.*

Antisense strand of DNA That strand of double-stranded DNA that serves as template for RNA transcription. Also called the *noncoding,* or *transcribed,* strand. See *sense strand of DNA.*

Apoptosis The process by which internal or external messages trigger expression of specific genes and their products, resulting in the initiation of a series of cellular events that involve fragmentation of the cell nucleus, dissolution of cellular structure, and orderly cell death. Unlike traumatic cell death, apoptosis results in the death of individual cells rather than clusters of cells and does not lead to the release of inflammatory intracellular products. Also called *programmed cell death (PCD).*

Ascertainment The method of selecting families for inclusion in a genetic study.

Assortative mating Mating between individuals with preference for or against a specific genotype; that is, nonrandom mating.

Autosome Any chromosome other than the sex (X or Y) chromosomes. The normal human has 22 pairs of autosomes.

BAC A *b*acterial *a*rtificial *c*hromosome used as a cloning vector. BACs can be used to clone up to 150 kilobases (kb) of DNA.

Bacteriophage A virus containing DNA or RNA whose host is bacteria. Bacteriophage can be used for the transduction or insertion of fragments of DNA into bacteria for cloning purposes.

Barr body Inactive X chromosome seen in the nucleus of some female somatic cells.

Base pair (bp) Two complementary nitrogen bases that are paired in double-stranded DNA. Used as a unit of physical distance or length of a sequence of nucleotides.

Carrier An individual who has a pair of genes consisting of 1 normal and 1 abnormal, or *mutant,* gene. Usually, such individuals are by definition phenotypically "normal," although in certain disorders biochemical evidence of a deficient or defective gene product may be present. Occasionally, carriers of an X-linked disorder may show partial expression of a genetic trait.

CCAAT box Approximately 75–80 bp upstream from the transcription initiation site of many genes is this sequence of nucleotides that is thought to play a role in promoter function.

cDNA clone A host cell that has a vector containing a fragment of complementary DNA (cDNA) from another organism.

Centimorgan (cM) A measure of the crossover frequency between linked genes. One centimorgan equals 1% recombination and represents a physical distance of approximately 1 million bp.

Centromere The constricted region of the chromosome. It is associated with spindle fibers during mitosis and meiosis and is important in the movement of chromosomes to the poles of the dividing cell.

Chorionic villus sampling (CVS) Transcervical procedure in which chorionic villi are retrieved with a flexible suction catheter and used in studies to establish a prenatal diagnosis.

Chromatid One of the duplicate arms (also called *sister chromatids*) of chromosomes that are created after DNA replication during mitosis or the first division of meiosis.

Chromatin The complex of DNA and proteins that is present in chromosomes.

Clinical heterogeneity Different mutations at the same locus producing different phenotypes. Examples include macular dystrophy and retinitis pigmentosa from differing mutations of peripherin/*RDS* and Crouzon, Pfeiffer, and Apert syndromes from mutations of *FGFR2*.

Cloning vector Any DNA molecule capable of autonomous replication within a host cell into which DNA can be inserted for amplification. Cloning vectors can be derived from plasmids, bacteriophages, viruses, and yeast. Examples of cloning vectors include YAC (yeast artificial chromosome), BAC (bacterial artificial chromosome), and PAC (P1 artificial chromosome).

Codominance Simultaneous expression of both alleles of a heterozygous locus (eg, ABO blood groups).

Codon The basic unit of the genetic code. The DNA molecule is a chain of nucleotide bases that is "read" in units of 3 bases *(triplets),* which will translate (through messenger RNA) to an amino acid. Thus, each triplet codon specifies a single amino acid.

Complementary DNA (cDNA) DNA created by the action of reverse transcriptase from messenger RNA. cDNA does not have introns, as does genomic DNA.

Compound heterozygote Gene locus having 2 different, abnormal alleles.

Congenital Present at birth. The term has no implications about the origin of the congenital feature.

Consanguinity Mating between blood relatives, or a genetic relationship by descent from a common ancestor.

Consensus sequence The most common or idealized sequence of base pairs (or encoded amino acids) for a given region of a gene. See *acceptor splice site* for an example.

Conservation A genetic sequence or nucleotide position is said to be conserved or show conservation if a similar sequence is present among different species at one gene or related genes of similar sequence.

Contig A set of overlapping clones, each containing a fragment of a specific region or DNA sequence, that collectively covers the region without an interruption.

Cosmid A self-replicating vector (hybrid bacteriophage) used for cloning of DNA fragments into bacteria. Cosmids accommodate a DNA sequence of approximately 40 kb and are useful for creating gene libraries.

Crossing over A process in which homologous chromosomes (chromatids) exchange segments by breakage and by the physical exchange of segments, followed by repair of the breaks. Crossing over is a regular event in meiosis but occurs only rarely in mitosis. Also termed *recombination.*

Degeneracy of the code The genetic code is termed *degenerate* because most of the 20 amino acids are encoded by more than 1 of the 64 possible triplet codons.

Digenic inheritance Simultaneous inheritance of 2 nonallelic mutant genes, giving rise to a genetic disorder wherein inheritance of only 1 of the 2 is insufficient to cause disease. An example is retinitis pigmentosa caused by simultaneous inheritance in the heterozygous state of otherwise tolerable mutations of both the *ROM1* and peripherin/*RDS* genes. The simplest form of polygenic inheritance.

Diploid The number of chromosomes in most somatic cells, which in humans is 46. The diploid number is twice the haploid number, which is the number of chromosomes in gametes.

DNA Deoxyribonucleic acid, the nucleic acid of chromosomes.

Dominant An allele that is expressed in the phenotype when inherited along with a normal allele. See *recessive*.

Dominant medical disorder A distinctive disease state that occurs in a (dominant) heterozygous genotype. Classically, normal dominant traits give the same phenotype in both the heterozygous and the homozygous states. Homozygotes for dominant disease-producing alleles are rare and are usually more severely affected than heterozygotes.

Dominant negative An autosomal dominant mutation that disrupts the function of the normal or wild-type allele in the heterozygous state, giving a phenotype approaching that of the homozygous mutant.

Donor splice site The junction between the 3′ end of an exon and the 5′ end of the next intron. The consensus sequence is $\frac{C}{A}$AG/GT$\frac{A}{G}$AGT for the exon–intron boundary. See *acceptor splice site* and *splice junction site*.

Endonuclease A phosphodiester-cleaving enzyme, usually derived from bacteria, that cuts nucleic acids at internal positions. Restriction endonucleases cut at specific recognition sites determined by the occurrence of a specific sequence of 4, 5, or 6 bp. Endonuclease specificity may also be confined to substrate conformation, nucleic acid species (DNA, RNA), and the presence of modified nucleotides.

Enhancer Any sequence of DNA upstream or downstream of the coding region that acts in *cis* (ie, on the same chromosome) to increase (or, as a negative enhancer, decrease) the rate of transcription of a nearby gene. Enhancers may display tissue specificity and act over considerable distances.

Eukaryote Organisms with their DNA located within a nucleus (includes all multicellular and higher unicellular organisms). See *prokaryote*.

Exon Any segment of a gene that is represented in the mature mRNA product. See *intron*.

Expressed-sequence tag (EST) A partial sequence of a gene that uniquely identifies the gene's message. These tags are useful, through reverse transcriptase polymerase chain reaction (RT-PCR), for determining the expression of genes.

Expressivity The variation in clinical manifestation among individuals with a particular genotype, usually a dominant medical disorder. The variability may be a difference in either age of onset (manifestation) or severity. See *penetrance*.

Fragile sites Reproducible sites of secondary constrictions, gaps, or breaks in chromatids. Fragile sites are transmitted as mendelian codominant traits and are usually not associated with abnormal phenotype. The most notable exceptions are the association of fragile X chromosomes with X-linked mental retardation and postpubertal macro-orchidism (fragile-X syndrome). See *trinucleotide repeat expansion.*

Frameshift mutation (framing error, frameshift) Any mutation, usually a deletion or insertion of a nucleotide or a number of nucleotides not divisible by 3, that results in a loss of the normal sequences of triplets, causing the new sequence to code for entirely different amino acids from the original. The mutation usually leads to the eventual chance formation of a *stop codon.*

Gene The segment of DNA and its associated regulatory elements coding for a single trait, usually a single polypeptide or mRNA. The definition was expanded to include any expressed sequence of nucleotides that has functional significance, including DNA sequences that govern the punctuation (promoter) or regulation (enhancer) of transcription.

Genetic Related to or produced by a gene.

Genocopy Different nonallelic genotypes that result in a similar phenotype (often a medical disorder).

Genome The sum total of the genetic material of a cell or of an organism.

Genomic clone A host cell that has a vector containing a fragment of genomic DNA from another organism.

Genotype The genetic constitution of an organism. Also used to denote the specific set of 2 alleles inherited at a locus.

Germinal mosaicism The occurrence of 2 populations of gametes in an individual, one population with a normal allele and the other with a disease-producing mutant gene. Of "new" cases of some autosomal dominant diseases (eg, osteogenesis imperfecta), 5%–10% are thought to result from germinal mosaicism; offspring of the affected parent are at significant risk for the same disease.

Haploid Half the number of chromosomes in most somatic cells, equal to the number of chromosomes in gametes. In humans, the haploid number is 23. Also used to denote the state in which only 1 of a pair or set of chromosomes is present. See *diploid.*

Haploid insufficiency (haploinsufficiency) The condition of dominant genetic disease caused by reduction in gene product to levels that are insufficient to produce the desired function of the protein. For example, aniridia and Waardenburg syndrome result from insufficiency of the single functional copy of the *PAX6* and *PAX3* genes, respectively, to activate transcription of the genes that they normally control.

Haplotype The combination of linked polymorphisms or marker alleles for a given region of DNA on a single chromosome.

Hemizygous (hemizygote) Having only 1 allele at a locus; usually refers to X-linked loci in males, who normally have only 1 set of X-linked genes. An individual who is missing an entire chromosome or a segment of one chromosome is considered hemizygous for the genes on the homologous chromosome.

Hereditary Genetically transmitted or capable of being genetically transmitted from parent to offspring. Not quite synonymous with *heritable,* which implies the ability to be transmitted to the next generation but does not intrinsically connote inheritance from the last generation. See *genetic.*

Heterogeneity (genetic heterogeneity) The production of a phenotype (or apparently similar phenotypes) by different genetic entities. Refers to genetic disorders that are found to be 2 or more fundamentally distinct entities. See *genocopy.*

Heteronuclear RNA (hnRNA) The mRNA from the initiator codon to the stop codon. Approximately 25% of these represent immature RNAs prior to splicing out of the introns. The function of the other 75% is unknown. Also called *heterogeneous nuclear RNA.*

Heteroplasmy The presence of 2 or more different populations of mitochondria within a cell, each population carrying a different allele (or the presence or absence of a mutation) at a given locus.

Heterozygous (heterozygote) Having 2 unlike alleles at a particular locus. See *hemizygous, homozygous.*

Homeobox A conserved 180 bp sequence of DNA, first detected within homeotic selector genes, that helps determine the cell's fate.

Homeotic selector genes Genes that appear to regulate the activity or expression of other genes, eventually guiding the embryonic development of cells into body segments, body parts, and specialized organ systems. Examples are the *HOX* and *PAX* families of developmental genes. The *HOX* family represents 38 homeobox genes that are linearly arranged in 4 independent complexes termed *HOX1, HOX2, HOX3,* and *HOX4.* These gene clusters reside on chromosomes 7, 17, 12, and 2, respectively. Whereas *HOX* genes are involved in early body plan organization, *PAX* genes are involved in somewhat later organ and body part development. See the discussion of homeobox genes in Chapter 4, Ocular Development.

Homologous chromosomes The 2 members of a matched pair of (sister) chromosomes, 1 derived from each parent, that have the same gene loci, but not necessarily the same alleles, in the same order.

Homoplasmy The presence of a single population of mitochondria within a cell, each carrying the same allele (or the same presence or absence of a mutation) at a given locus.

Homozygous (homozygote) Having 2 like or identical alleles at a particular locus in diploid genome. The term is sometimes misused to refer to *compound heterozygote* (see above).

Host cell In the context of recombinant genetics, the organism (usually a bacterium such as *Escherichia coli*) into which is inserted the vector (usually a plasmid or bacteriophage) containing the foreign DNA. Hosts are used to propagate the vector and, hence, the cloned DNA segment.

Hybridization The bonding (by Watson-Crick base-pairing) of single-stranded DNA or RNA into double-stranded DNA or RNA. The ability of stretches of DNA or RNA to hybridize with each other is highly dependent on the similarity or identity of the base-pair sequence.

Imprinting The reversible marking or inactivation of an allele by inheritance (through either the maternal or the paternal lineage), which may significantly alter gene expression. The imprinting is reversed if the gene is passed through subsequent generations through the opposite parental line. This phenomenon occurs in Prader-Willi and Angelman syndromes; it may also occur with mutations of the Wilms tumor gene. One mechanism of imprinting is thought to involve methylation of 5′ elements of the gene.

Initiator codon The triplet code that, when coded into mRNA, initiates translation of the mRNA by causing binding of a special type of transfer RNA called *initiator tRNA*. In prokaryotes (bacteria), either AUG or GUG can act as an initiator codon. In eukaryotes, AUG is the only initiator codon, and it codes for methionine.

Intervening sequence Intron.

Intron A segment of DNA that is transcribed into RNA but is ultimately removed from the transcript by splicing together the sequences on either side of it (exons).

Isochromosome An abnormal chromosome created by deletion of 1 arm and duplication of the other arm, such that the chromosome has 2 equal-length arms of the same loci sequence extending in opposite directions from the centromere.

Karyotype A photographic record or a computer printout of an individual's chromosome set arranged in a standard pattern in pairs by size, shape, band pattern, and other identifiable physical features.

Kilobase (kb) 1000 bp of DNA or 1000 bases of single-stranded RNA.

Liability With reference to polygenic or multifactorial inheritance, the graded continuum of increasing susceptibility to a disease or trait.

Library A complete set of clones presumably including all genetic material of interest from an organism, tissue, or specific cell type at a specified stage of development. A *genomic library* contains cloned DNA fragments from the entire genome; a cDNA library contains fragments of cloned DNAs generated by reverse transcription from mRNA. Genomic libraries are useful sources to search for genes, whereas cDNA libraries give information about expression within the source cell or tissue.

Linkage A concept that refers to loci rather than to the alleles that reside on those loci. Exists when the loci of 2 genes or DNA sequences are physically close enough to each other on the same chromosome that alleles at the 2 loci do not assort independently at meiosis but tend to be inherited together.

Linkage disequilibrium The state in which alleles that reside at loci close together in the genome remain inherited together through many generations because the close physical distance makes crossover between the loci extremely unlikely. Thus, alleles that are in linkage disequilibrium are present in subpopulations of individuals (eg, those with a given disease) in greater-than-expected frequencies. Also called *allelic association*.

Locus The physical site on a chromosome occupied by a particular gene; term is often colloquially used interchangeably with *gene*.

Locus heterogeneity Term applies when a similar phenotype is produced by mutations at different loci, for example, X-linked retinitis pigmentosa resulting from *RP2* at Xp11 and *RP3* at Xp21.

LOD score (*l*ogarithm of *od*ds, or log of the likelihood ratio) A statistical method that tests whether a set of linkage data indicates that 2 loci are linked or unlinked. The LOD score is the logarithm to the base 10 of the odds favoring linkage. By convention, an LOD score of 3 (1000:1 odds in favor of linkage) is generally accepted as proof of linkage.

Lyonization Inactivation of genes on either the maternally or the paternally derived X chromosome in somatic cells, occurring at about the time of implantation. First proposed by Mary Lyon.

Meiosis The special form of cell division that occurs in germ cells by which gametes of haploid chromosomal number are created. Each of the chromatids, which are clearly visible by prophase, contains a long double helix of DNA associated with histones and other chromosomal proteins. At anaphase, the chromatids separate at the centromere and migrate to each half of the dividing cell; thus, each daughter cell receives an identical set of chromatids (which become the chromosomes for that cell). During the first, or *reduction,* division of meiosis, the chromatids of homologous chromosomes undergo crossover (during the diplotene phase), and the number of chromosomes is reduced to the haploid number by the separation of homologous chromosomes (with duplicate chromatids) to each daughter cell. During the second division of meiosis, the sister chromatids separate to form the haploid set of chromosomes of each gamete.

Mendelian disorder (single-gene disorder) A trait or medical disorder that follows patterns of inheritance suggesting the state is determined by a gene at a single locus.

Microsatellite (eg, dinucleotide or trinucleotide repeats) Tandemly repeated segments scattered throughout the genome of varying numbers of 2 to 4 nucleotides in a row. For example, a stretch of consecutive CA combinations of bases (NNNCACACACACACA CACACACANNN or $[CA]_{10}$, where N is any base) in a DNA strand. The highly variable nature of the number of repeats provides information useful as markers for establishing linkage to disease loci. See *satellite DNA* and *short tandem repeats*.

Minisatellite Array of repeated, nested segments of the same sequence of multiple triplet codons, each segment (consensus repeat unit) varying between 14 and 100 bp. Minisatellites are extraordinarily polymorphic and extremely useful as markers for establishing linkage, because they are often situated upstream or downstream from genes. The repeats are inherently unstable and can undergo mutation at a rate of up to 10%. Defects of some minisatellites are associated with cancer and insulin-dependent diabetes mellitus. Other terms used are *variable number of tandem repeats (VNTR)* and *variable tandem repeats (VTR)*. See *satellite DNA*.

Missense mutation A mutation, often the change of a single nucleotide, that results in the substitution of 1 amino acid for another in the final gene product.

Mitosis The ordinary form of cell division, which results in daughter cells identical in chromosomal number to the parent cell.

Mosaic An individual or tissue with at least 2 cell lines of different genotype or distinctive chromosomal constitution that develop after the formation of the zygote.

Multifactorial inheritance The combined operation of several unspecified genetic and environmental factors in the inheritance of a particular trait or disease. See *polygenic inheritance.*

Mutation Any alteration of a gene or genetic material from its "natural" state, regardless of whether the change has a positive, neutral, or negative effect.

Nitrogen bases Nitrogen-containing compounds, either the *purines* guanine and adenine or the *pyrimidines* cytosine, thymine, and uracil. These bases are abbreviated as G, A, C, T, and U, respectively.

Nondisjunction Failure of 2 chromosomes to separate during meiosis or mitosis.

Nonsense mutation Any mutation that either results directly in formation of a stop codon or creates a stop codon in the downstream sequence after a frameshift mutation through creation of a frameshift.

Northern blot Imprint of an electrophoretic gel that separates fragments of mRNA according to their size and mobility. The fragments are identified by hybridization to cDNA probes.

Nucleoside The combination of a nitrogen-containing base and a 5-carbon sugar. The 5 nucleosides are adenosine (A), guanosine (G), cytidine (C), uridine (U), and thymidine (T). Note that the abbreviations are the same as those for the nitrogen bases that characterize the nucleoside.

Nucleosome The primary unit of chromatin, consisting of a 146-bp sequence of DNA wrapped twice around a core composed of 8 histone molecules.

Nucleotide The combination of a nitrogen-containing base, a 5-carbon sugar, and 1 or more phosphate groups. The nucleotides are designated by 3 capital letters as follows:

adenosine monophosphate (AMP), deoxyadenosine monophosphate (dAMP), uridine diphosphate (UDP), adenosine triphosphate (ATP), etc. Although nucleotides are linked together by phosphodiester linkage into long sequences known as *nucleic acids,* they also perform other important functions, such as carrying chemical energy (ATP), combining with other groups to form coenzymes (coenzyme A, or CoA), and acting as intracellular signaling molecules (cyclic AMP, or cAMP).

Oncogene A defective gene that is capable of transforming cells to a neoplastic phenotype characterized by loss of growth control and/or tumorigenesis in a suitable host or site. In many cases, cancer is caused by the growth-stimulating effects of increased expression, protein activation, or aberrant regulation of transcription factors required for normal growth. Certain oncogenes are produced by chromosomal translocations of normal transcription factor genes to other regions adjacent to more abundantly expressed genes, causing inappropriate excessive expression. See *tumor-suppressor genes.*

Open reading frame (ORF) Any part of the genome that could be translated into a protein sequence because of the absence of stop codons. An exon is an example of an ORF. See *exon.*

Origin of replication The site(s) on a chromosome where replication is initiated and proceeds bidirectionally. The site of binding of the origin replication complex (ORC). Also called the *replication origin.*

Origin replication complex (ORC) A series of proteins involved in DNA synthesis and replication that bind to the origin of replication as one of the initiating events of DNA replication.

p arm The short arm of a chromosome in relation to the centromere. From *petit.*

Penetrance The proportion of individuals of a given genotype who show any evidence of an associated phenotype. Usually refers to the proportion of individuals heterozygous for a dominant disease who show any evidence of the disease. Nonpenetrance is the lack of phenotypic evidence of the genotype. See *expressivity.*

Pharmacogenetics The area of biochemical genetics concerned with genetically controlled variations in drug responses.

Phenocopy The occurrence of a particular clinical phenotype (often a medical disorder) as a result of nonmutagenic environmental factors (eg, exposure to a drug or virus), when the more usual basis for the phenotype is an altered genotype.

Phenotype The total observable nature of an individual, resulting from interaction of the genotype with the environment (in medicine, often a disease phenotype).

Plasmid Circular extrachromosomal DNA molecules in bacteria that can independently reproduce in a host. Plasmids were detected because of their ability to transfer antibiotic resistance genes to bacteria. They can be used as vectors in recombinant DNA research.

Pleiotropism Multiple end effects (in different organ systems) arising from a single (mutant) gene or gene pair.

Polygenic inheritance Determined by the operation of an unspecified number of genes with additive effects. See *multifactorial inheritance.*

Polymerase chain reaction (PCR) A procedure whereby segments of DNA or RNA can be amplified without resorting to the conventional techniques of molecular cloning by use of flanking oligonucleotides called *primers* and repeated cycles of amplification with DNA polymerase. The steps involve

- heating to separate the molecules into single-stranded DNA
- repeated annealing to the complementary target DNA sequences or primers specifically designed to delimit the beginning and ending of the target segment
- extension of the primer sequences with the enzyme DNA polymerase, creating double-stranded DNA
- separation of the products into single-stranded DNA

In effect, the amount of DNA is doubled with each cycle. Often, 30 or more cycles are used to obtain sufficient amplification for further testing.

Polymorphism Two or more alleles with a frequency greater than 1% in a given population.

Posttranslational modification Changes or modifications of gene products after translation, including removal of amino acids from the end of the peptide, addition or removal of sugars, and addition of lipid side chains or phosphate groups to specific sites in the protein. Often, such changes are essential for proper protein localization or function.

Proband The affected person whose disorder, or concern about a disorder, brings a family or pedigree to be genetically evaluated. Also called the *propositus* (male), *proposita* (female), or *index case.*

Prokaryote Single-cellular organisms, such as bacteria, that lack a nucleus and have their DNA located within the cytoplasm. See *eukaryote.*

Promoter That sequence of nucleotides upstream (5′) from the coding sequence of a gene that determines the site of binding of RNA polymerase and, hence, initiation of transcription. Different promoters for the same gene may exist and can result in alternately spliced gene products and tissue-specific expression. The promoter may contain the consensus DNA sequence TATA$\frac{A}{T}$A$\frac{A}{T}$ (the so-called TATA box) approximately 25–30 bp (5′) upstream from the transcription start site.

Proposita, propositus Same as *proband,* above.

Proto-oncogene A normal gene that is involved in cell division or proliferation. Abnormalities in expression or regulation can cause the gene to become activated to an oncogene, which can lead to cancer. Several proto-oncogenes are involved in intracellular signal transduction—the process by which external messages influence the machinery that governs growth and differentiation.

Pseudodominance The appearance of vertical transmission of a recessive genetic disorder from one generation to the next, usually through the mating of an affected homozygote with a heterozygote, which produces affected offspring.

Pseudogene A defective copy of a gene. It often lacks introns and is rarely, if ever, expressed. Some pseudogenes are thought to have arisen by reverse transcription of mRNA that has had the introns spliced out. Others, such as globin pseudogenes, have arisen from silencing of a tandem duplicate. Since they are released from conservation (the maintenance of essential DNA sequences necessary for function) through selection, pseudogenes (compared to the original functional gene) often contain numerous base-pair changes and other mutational events.

Purine Nitrogen-containing base: adenine (A) and guanine (G) in DNA or RNA.

Pyrimidine Nitrogen-containing base: thymine (T) and cytosine (C) in DNA or uracil (U) in RNA.

q arm The long arm of a chromosome. See *p arm*.

Recessive Classically, a gene that results in a phenotype only in the homozygous state. See *dominant*.

Recessive medical disorder A disease state whose occurrence requires a homozygous (or compound heterozygous) genotype—that is, a double dose of the mutant allele. Heterozygotes are essentially normal.

Recombinant An individual who has a combination of genes on a single chromosome unlike that in either parent. Usually applied to linkage analysis, wherein *recombinant* refers to a haplotype (a set of alleles on a specific chromosome) that is not present in either parent because of a recombination crossover.

Recombinant DNA DNA that has been cut out of a single organism, reinserted into the DNA of a vector (plasmid or phage), and then reimplanted into a host cell. Also, any act of altering DNA for further use.

Recombination The formation of a new set of alleles on a single chromosome unlike that in either parent; due to crossover during meiosis.

Relatives, first-degree Individuals who share on average half of their genetic material with the proband: parents, siblings, offspring.

Relatives, second-degree Individuals who share on average one fourth of their genetic material with the proband: grandparents, aunts and uncles, nieces and nephews, grandchildren.

Replication Creation of a new linear DNA copy by the enzyme DNA polymerase, proceeding from the 5′ side of bound primer to the 3′ end of the DNA sequence. Replication of DNA occurs during chromosomal duplication.

Replication slippage An error of DNA replication or copying. Because of the similarity of repeated base-pair sequences, 1 or more repeats are skipped over and not represented in the copied DNA sequence.

Replicative segregation The process by which, through partitioning of copies of mtDNA to each daughter cell during division, some cells receive a preponderance of normal or mutant copies. Replicative segregation tends to result in conversion of heteroplasmy to homoplasmy with associated development of disease within the affected tissue, if the tissue becomes homoplasmic for the mutant mtDNA. This phenomenon explains the development of new organ system involvement in multisystem mitochondrial diseases.

Restriction fragment length polymorphisms (RFLPs) RFLPs represent the variation in the length of genomic DNA fragments created by the loss or gain of an endonuclease restriction site. They can be used to map genes or link specific physical or genetic traits.

Retrotransposition The insertion of a *retroposon* (a segment of DNA created by reverse transcription from an RNA template) into the genome. Because of the staggered cut made in the target DNA by the endonuclease involved in the recombination event, a short duplication (3–12 bp) of the target site sequence is created at the ends of the transposed element. Because the transposable element may contain transcriptional initiation and/or termination signals, this process is one mechanism by which fusion genes, such as those causing certain forms of leukemia or cancer, can arise.

Reverse transcription The process, performed by the enzyme reverse transcriptase, whereby mRNA is converted back to DNA. If the introns have already been spliced out of the precursor mRNA, the product of this process is cDNA.

Satellite DNA Nuclear DNA that migrates at separate positions or bands from the bulk of DNA during CsCI gradient centrifugation. Satellite DNAs are long segments of DNA that consist of short DNA sequences repeated hundreds or thousands of times at a stretch in the genome. Satellite DNAs form the ends and centers of chromosomes. Telomeric DNA is a form of satellite DNA.

Segregation The separation of pairs of alleles at meiosis.

Sense strand of DNA The strand of double-stranded DNA that corresponds in its 5′ to 3′ sequence to the expressed mRNA. Also called the *coding,* or *nontranslated, strand.*

Sequence-tagged sites (STSs) Short unique sequences of DNA, usually 200–500 bp, scattered throughout the genome that serve as landmarks for the physical mapping of genes. The presence of a specific STS in any sample can be determined by the polymerase chain reaction. If the STS is detected, the sample has genomic material from the known region of that STS. Currently, the average distance between STSs is 100 kb.

Sex linked Genes on the X or Y (sex) chromosomes. The term is often used improperly to mean X linked.

Short tandem repeats (STRs) Sequences of repeated copies of 2–5 bp that occur every 10 kb in the human genome. The variation in number of copies within a given STR is highly polymorphic and thus useful for gene mapping. See *microsatellite* and *minisatellite.*

Simplex A term used to denote that only a single individual is affected within a given family. Thus, a single male or female with a genetic disease would be called a *simplex case.* This term implies no inheritance type. The term *isolated* is also sometimes used.

Smallest region of overlap (SRO) The minimum chromosomal or nucleotide sequence that is deleted among all individuals who have a phenotype thought to be the result of a particular chromosomal deletion. This deleted region is presumed to contain the gene or genes that cause the phenotype.

Southern blot Imprint of an electrophoretic gel that separates fragments of DNA according to their size.

Splice junction site The DNA region that demarcates the boundaries between exons and introns. The specific sequence determines whether the site acts as a 5′ donor or a 3′ acceptor site during splicing. Single base-pair changes or mutations that involve splice junction sites may result in skipping of the following exon or incorporation of part of the adjacent intron into the mature mRNA. See *acceptor splice site* and *donor splice site* for the consensus sequences.

Spliceosome Multicomponent ribosomal ribonuclear protein complex (40S to 60S) that is involved in the removal of introns from heteronuclear, or *precursor messenger,* RNAs.

Splicing That process by which the introns are removed from the precursor mRNA and the exons are joined together as mature mRNA prior to translation. Takes place within spliceosomes.

Sporadic A trait that occurs in a single member of a kindred with no other family members affected. The term has been used by some geneticists to imply that the trait is nongenetic.

Stop codon (termination codon) The DNA triplet that causes translation to end when the translation is coded into mRNA. The DNA stop codons are TAG, TAA, and TGA. Expressed as mRNA, these are UAG, UAA, and UGA.

Synteny The presence of genes on the same chromosome, even if linkage cannot be demonstrated. Also used to denote homologous chromosomal locations between species.

TATA box A promoter element approximately 25–30 bp (5′) upstream from the transcription start site that contains the consensus sequence $\text{TATA}\frac{A}{T}\text{A}\frac{A}{T}$. The TATA box is recognized by transcription factors that bind to the region, and it is critical in the initiation of transcription.

Telomeric DNA A type of highly repetitive satellite DNA that forms the tips of chromosomes and prevents them from fraying or joining. It decreases in size as a concomitant of aging. Defects in the maintenance of telomeres may play a role in cancer formation.

Threshold In polygenic or multifactorial inheritance, a relatively sharp qualitative difference beyond which individuals are considered to be affected. The threshold is presumed to have been reached by the cumulative effects of the polygenic and multifactorial influences.

Transcription The synthesis as catalyzed by a DNA-dependent RNA polymerase of a single-stranded RNA molecule from the antisense strand of a double-stranded DNA template in the cell nucleus.

Translation The process by which a polypeptide is synthesized from a sequence of specific mRNA.

Translocation The transfer of a part of 1 chromosome to a nonhomologous chromosome.

Trinucleotide repeat expansion (contraction) The process by which long sequences of multiple triplet codons (see *minisatellite*) are lengthened or shortened in the process of gene replication. The process of expansion of trinucleotide repeats over consecutive generations results in the genetic phenomenon of *anticipation*. The underlying mechanisms for expansion (or contraction) appear to be replication slippage and unequal crossing over in the region of the repeats. Most disorders involving trinucleotide repeats are dominant in inheritance (eg, fragile-X syndrome, myotonic dystrophy, Huntington disease, Kennedy disease), but one is autosomal recessive (Friedreich ataxia).

Tumor-suppressor genes Genes that must be present in one fully functional copy in order to keep cells from uncontrolled proliferation. Two "hits" (inactivations) of the gene, one for each allele, must occur in a given cell for tumor formation to occur. Examples include the genes for retinoblastoma, Wilms tumor, tuberous sclerosis, p53, ataxia-telangiectasia, and von Hippel–Lindau disease. Also called *antioncogenes*. See *oncogene*.

Unequal crossing over An error in the events of chromosomal duplication and cell division occurring during meiosis and, rarely, during mitosis. Probably because of similar sequences or repeated segments, chromosomal exchange occurs between nonhomologous regions of the chromosome, resulting in duplication and deletion of genetic material in the daughter cells.

Uniparental disomy The conveyance to a child of 2 copies of an abnormal gene or chromosome by only 1 parent (the other parent makes no contribution). The child can be affected with autosomal recessive disease even if only 1 of the parents is a carrier for the abnormal gene. This occurrence has been reported in cystic fibrosis and in Prader-Willi and Angelman syndromes.

Untranslated region (UTR) The regions upstream (5′ UTR) and downstream (3′ UTR) of the open reading frame of a gene. The 5′ UTR contains the promoter and part or all of the regulatory regions of the gene. The 3′ UTR presumably also serves important functions in regulation and mRNA stability.

Vector A viral, bacteriophage, or plasmid DNA molecule into which a stretch of genomic DNA or cDNA or a specific gene can be inserted. The λ-bacteriophage can accept segments of DNA up to 25 kb long. Cosmid vectors can accommodate a segment 40 kb long. BAC (bacterial artificial chromosome) and YAC (yeast artificial chromosome) vectors can accept much larger fragments of DNA.

Western blot Imprint of an electrophoretic gel that separates proteins according to their size and mobility. The proteins are usually identified by immunologic methods.

Wild type A normal phenotype of an organism. Also, a normal allele as compared to a mutant allele.

X linked Term that refers to genes on the X chromosome.

Y linked Term that refers to genes on the Y chromosome.

Yeast artificial chromosome (YAC) Used as a cloning vector. YACs can be used to clone very large segments of DNA (up to 1000 kb).

CHAPTER 5

Molecular Genetics

This chapter provides a review of molecular genetics (with emphasis on clinical applications in ophthalmology), an overview of the techniques for manipulating deoxyribonucleic acid (DNA) in the laboratory, and an appreciation of the power and implications of molecular investigations for the study of inherited diseases.

Gene Structure

A *gene* is the coding sequence for a protein, ribosomal RNA (rRNA), or other gene product, and associated regulatory sequences. Following the initiation codon (start sequence) is the structural *open reading frame (ORF)*, which is composed of *exons* (sequences that code for amino acids that will be present in the final protein) and *introns* (sequences that are spliced out during the processing of mRNA). Following the last exon is the *3′ untranslated region (3′ UTR)*. The function of this region is partly regulatory. Thus, for example, a mutation within the 3′ UTR of the gene for the enzyme myotonin kinase is thought to cause myotonic dystrophy.

The development of introns in higher organisms may have had evolutionary benefits. Introns have allowed eukaryotes to evolve beyond the limits of genes seen in single-celled organisms, and they may have other roles as well. The compartmentalization of coding segments into exons may have allowed for more rapid evolution of proteins by allowing for alternative processing of precursor RNA (alternative splicing) and for rearrangements of exons during gene duplication (exon shuffling).

Some introns contain complete separate genes, and some of these may cause disease or influence the expression of other genes. Expansion of unstable repeats within introns can cause abnormal splicing and result in genetic disease.

"Junk" DNA

Approximately 97% of the base sequences in human DNA have been considered "biologically meaningless," in that they do not encode proteins or RNAs or have any other known function. It is possible, however, that important roles for this so-called *junk DNA* will emerge when the structure and function of the genome, chromosomes, nucleus, and nuclear proteins are fully understood. It has been suggested, for example, that RNA transcribed from junk DNA may directly influence the transcription of other sequences and participate in normal genome repair and regulation. When defective, junk DNA may lead to cancer. Some of the repetitive sequences of nontranscribed DNA form *telomeric DNA*, which is essential for the correct formation and maintenance of chromosomes. Indeed, loss of telomeric DNA correlates with cell senescence and carcinogenesis. Therefore, sequences within junk DNA may influence the transcription or otherwise regulate the expression of numerous other genes.

Much of junk DNA is composed of highly repetitive sequences, some of which include *satellites, minisatellites, microsatellites, short interspersed elements (SINEs),* and *long interspersed elements (LINEs).* The most frequently appearing of the repetitive DNAs is the 300-base-pair (bp) *Alu* sequence, named for the restriction enzyme used to identify it. The Alu sequence is a SINE that occurs 500,000 times in the human genome. Alu sequences are distributed through retroposition (Alu → Alu RNA → Alu cDNA → insertion) and may cause disease if one inserts within and disrupts a gene. This process accounts for one cause of neurofibromatosis 1 (von Recklinghausen disease). An important LINE is the L1 repeat sequence, composed of about 10,000 copies, each 1–6 kilobases (kb) in length. The L1 repeat sequence has also been implicated as a cause of mutations.

Gene Transcription

Genes control cellular activity through 2 processes:

1. transcription *(expression)*, in which DNA molecules give rise to RNA molecules, followed by translation in most cases
2. *translation,* in which RNA directs the synthesis of proteins. Translation occurs at ribosomes, where mRNA induces tRNA-mediated recruitment of amino acids to "build" a protein. A fuller discussion of translation is beyond the scope of this chapter.

Transcription Factors and Regulation

Transcription factors contain DNA-binding domains that typically include a helical unit (α-helix) within or near positively charged amino acids. Four classes of structural protein motifs characterize 80% of transcription factors (Fig 5-1):

1. helix-turn-helix (HTH)
2. zinc finger
3. leucine zipper
4. helix-loop-helix (HLH)

Many ophthalmic diseases result from transcription-factor mutations. *PAX2* mutations cause colobomas of the optic nerve and renal hypoplasia. *PAX3* mutations cause Waardenburg syndrome with dystopia canthorum (types WS1 and WS3). *PAX6* mutations are the basis of virtually all cases of aniridia, occasional cases of Peters anomaly, and several other rarer phenotypes, specifically autosomal dominant keratitis and dominant foveal hypoplasia.

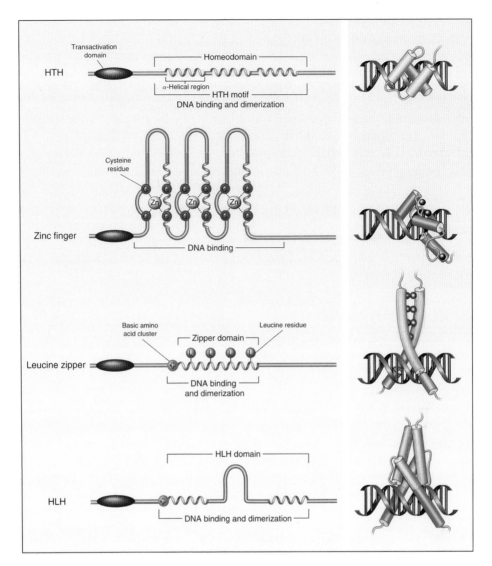

Figure 5-1 The general protein structures of the 4 major classes of transcription factors are shown on the left. The structures include a transactivation domain linked to a DNA-binding domain and, in certain cases, a dimerization domain. The types of transcription factors take their names from the characteristic motifs involved in DNA binding and protein dimerization and are shown on the right, interacting with the DNA. The cylinders represent α-helical regions, and the areas that contact DNA directly are *green*. C = cysteine, *HLH* = helix-loop-helix, *HTH* = helix-turn-helix, *L* = leucine, *Zn* = zinc. The *plus sign* indicates a positive charge. *(Reproduced with permission from Papavassiliou AG. Molecular medicine: transcription factors. N Engl J Med. 1995;332(1):46.)*

Hanson IM, Fletcher JM, Jordan T, et al. Mutations at the PAX6 locus are found in heterogeneous anterior segment malformations including Peters' anomaly. *Nat Genet.* 1994;6(2):168–173.

Latchman DS. Transcription-factor mutations and disease. *N Engl J Med.* 1996;334(1):28–33.

Mirzayans F, Pearce WG, MacDonald IM, Walter MA. Mutation of the PAX6 gene in patients with autosomal dominant keratitis. *Am J Hum Genet.* 1995;57(3):539–548.

Papavassiliou AG. Molecular medicine: transcription factors. *N Engl J Med.* 1995;332(1):45–47.

Tassabehji M, Read AP, Newton VE, et al. Waardenburg's syndrome patients have mutations in the human homologue of the Pax-3 paired box gene. *Nature.* 1992;355(6361):635–636.

Intron Excision

The modified mRNA undergoes excision of the introns by a highly organized process called *splicing,* which leaves the mRNA composed of only exons, or coding segments. The exons can then undergo translation in the ribosomes. Splicing takes place in specialized structures composed of RNA and proteins called *spliceosomes.* The exact process of splicing is complex but involves intermediate steps that look like a lariat. Splicing must recognize precisely the beginning and end of each coding sequence, and errors of splicing can lead to genetic disease. Approximately 15% of point mutations that cause human disease do so by the generation of splicing errors that result in aberrations such as exon skipping, intron retention, or use of a cryptic splice site. Mutations in proteins important in splicing can cause retinitis pigmentosa.

Alternative Splicing and Isoforms

Alternative splicing is the creation of multiple pre-mRNA sequences from the same gene by the action of different promoters. These promoters cause the transcription of the gene to skip certain exons. The protein products of alternative splicing are often called *isoforms.* The promoters are usually tissue-specific, so different tissues express different isoforms. The gene for dystrophin is an example of alternative splicing: full-length dystrophin is the major isoform expressed in muscle; shorter isoforms predominate in the retina, peripheral nerve, and central nervous system. Another example of alternative splicing's relevance underlies the basis of the cornea's avascularity. Vascular endothelial growth factor (VEGF) receptor-1 is a key blood vessel receptor that binds and transduces a signal from the primary mediator of angiogenesis, VEGF. In the cornea, high levels of an alternatively spliced isoform, soluble VEGFR-1 are expressed. As this is the soluble form, it is present in the extracellular matrix and serves as an endogenous VEGF trap or decoy receptor. Without it, the cornea becomes vulnerable to vascular invasion.

Ambati BK, Nozaki M, Singh N, et al. Corneal avascularity is due to soluble VEGF receptor-1. *Nature.* 2006;443(7114):993–997.

Methylation

Regions of DNA that are undergoing transcription lack 5-methyl cytidine residues, which normally account for 1%–5% of total DNA. Evidence suggests a close correlation between methylation and gene inactivation. Regulation of DNA methylation may be responsible for imprinting control.

X-Inactivation

A major occurrence in early development of the human embryo is the random inactivation of 1 of the 2 X chromosomes in the female, resulting in the lack of expression of the majority of genes on that chromosome. The time of *X-inactivation* is not precisely known but is thought to vary over a period of several cell divisions during the blastocyst–gastrula transition. X-inactivation is also known as *lyonization,* after its discoverer, Mary Lyon. Lyonization affects the severity of the phenotype of several X-linked retinal conditions, such as retinitis pigmentosa and incontinentia pigmenti.

Lee JT, Jaenisch R. The (epi)genetic control of mammalian X-chromosome inactivation. *Curr Opin Genet Dev.* 1997;7(2):274–280.

Lyon MF. The William Allan memorial award address: X-chromosome inactivation and the location and expression of X-linked genes. *Am J Hum Genet.* 1988;42(1):8–16.

Imprinting

Genetic imprinting, also called *allele-specific marking,* is a heritable yet reversible process by which a gene is modified, depending on which parent provides it. The mechanism is unclear but appears to operate at the chromatin organization level and involves hetero-chromatization and methylation of CpG sites. Examples of genes that can be imprinted include the Wilms tumor–suppressor gene and the human *SNRPN* (small nuclear ribonu-cleoprotein polypeptide N) gene.

Prader-Willi and Angelman syndromes are examples of diseases resulting from ab-normalities of imprinting. Approximately 70%–80% of patients with Prader-Willi syn-drome harbor a deletion of the paternally derived chromosome 15q11-q13, resulting in the loss of this region's normal contribution from the paternal line. About 70%–80% of patients with Angelman syndrome also have a deletion of 15q11-q13 but from the ma-ternally derived chromosome, resulting in loss of the maternal contribution. Uniparen-tal disomy, wherein both 15 chromosomes are inherited from the same parent, can also cause each syndrome. Again, the 2 chromosome 15s in uniparental disomy are maternal in Prader-Willi syndrome and paternal in Angelman syndrome. The *SNRPN* gene maps to 15q11-q13 but appears to be expressed only from the paternally inherited allele.

DNA Damage and Repair

DNA is constantly sustaining damage from mutagens such as ultraviolet light, chemicals, and spontaneous deamination. Each cell loses 10,000 bases per day from spontaneous DNA breakdown related to normal body temperature alone. This process may involve hydrolytic loss of purine bases or deamination of cytosine to uracil and, less frequently, adenine to hypoxanthine. Oxidation, alkylation, generation of free radicals, and other common metabolic reactions can also injure DNA. In the absence of repair, these muta-tions would accumulate and result in tumor formation. Damaged DNA is estimated to cause approximately 80%–90% of cancers in humans.

Damaged DNA sites are repaired chiefly by 2 mechanisms: *excision repair* and *mis-match repair.* The processes of replication, transcription, mismatch repair, excision repair, and gene expression are closely coordinated by cross-acting systems. Enzymes that cut or patch segments of DNA during crossing over at meiosis are also involved in DNA repair. Molecules that unwind double-stranded DNA (called *helicases*) are involved in replica-tion, transcription, and DNA excision repair.

The *antioncogene p53* appears to play an extremely important role as the "guardian of the genome" by preventing cells from proliferating if their DNA is irreparably damaged. Levels of p53 increase after ultraviolet or ionizing radiation. p53 inhibits DNA replication directly and binds with 1 of the RNA polymerase transcription factors, TFIIH. If the degree of damage is slight, increased production of p53 induces reversible cell arrest until DNA repair can take place. If DNA damage is too great or irreversible, p53 production is massively increased and apoptosis occurs, probably through stimulation of the expression of the *BAX* gene, whose product promotes apoptosis. Loss of p53 causes cells to fail to arrest in response to DNA damage, and these cells do not enter apoptosis. Thus, mutations of p53 predispose to tumorigenesis.

The gene mutated in ataxia-telangiectasia (Louis-Bar syndrome), a protein kinase called *ATM,* also appears to be integrally involved in DNA repair, possibly by informing the cell of radiation damage. The ATM gene product associates with synaptonemal complexes, promotes chromosomal synapsis, and is required for meiosis. People with ataxia-telangiectasia have a threefold greater risk of cancer.

Xeroderma pigmentosa is a severe condition in which DNA repair enzyme functions are crippled. Patients with this condition typically have diffuse pigmented anomalies on their sun-exposed skin surfaces and are at high risk for squamous cell carcinoma of the ocular surface.

Latchman DS. Transcription-factor mutations and disease. *N Engl J Med.* 1996;334(1):28–33.

Levine AJ. p53, the cellular gatekeeper for growth and division. *Cell.* 1997;88(3):323–331.

Yu CE, Oshima J, Fu YH, et al. Positional cloning of the Werner's syndrome gene. *Science.* 1996;272(5259):258–262.

Mutations and Disease

Requirements for Identifying a Disease-producing Mutation

The major requirements for a given DNA mutation to be verified as disease-producing are the following:

- The mutation does not occur in the normal population (the variation cannot be more frequent than the disease).
- It produces a DNA sequence that alters protein function or expression.
- The presence of the variation cosegregates with disease in family members according to the inheritance type (the significance of cosegregation in a given family depends on the number of possible chances for noncosegregation).

Mutations

Mutations can involve a change in a single base pair; simple deletion or insertion of DNA material; or more complex rearrangements such as inversions, duplications, or translocations. Deletion, insertion, or duplication of any number of base pairs in other than groups of 3 creates frameshifts of the entire DNA sequence downstream, resulting in the eventual formation of a stop codon and truncation of the message.

Mutations that result in no active gene product being produced are called *null mutations*. Null mutations include missense or nonsense mutations that (1) produce either a stop mutation directly or a frameshift with creation of a premature stop codon downstream or (2) cause the loss or gain of a donor or acceptance splice junction site, resulting in the loss of exons or inappropriate incorporation of introns into the spliced mRNA.

Mutations can also lead to a gain of function that may be beneficial (leading to evolution) or detrimental (leading to disease). An example of a beneficial gain in function is the emergence, among bacteria, of antibiotic resistance. An example of a detrimental gain of function is a receptor protein that binds too tightly with its target protein, creating loss of normal physiologic function. Most autosomal dominant disorders are of this type.

Single base-pair mutations may code for the same amino acid or a tolerable change in the amino acid sequence, leading to harmless polymorphisms or DNA variations that are in turn inherited. These are called *conserved base-pair mutations.*

Polymorphisms

A *polymorphism* is any variation in DNA sequence that occurs, by convention, at a frequency of 1% or greater in the normal population. Key polymorphisms that have been associated with disease include the *TIGR/myocilin* gene with glaucoma, and the *HTRA1* gene with neovascular macular degeneration.

Cancer Genes

Cancer can result from any of a number of genetic mechanisms, including the activation of oncogenes and the loss of tumor-suppressor genes. The product of proto-oncogenes is often involved in signal transduction of external messages to the intracellular machinery that governs normal cell growth and differentiation (Fig 5-2). As such, the DNA sequences of proto-oncogenes are highly conserved in nature between such different organisms as humans and yeast. Proto-oncogenes can be activated to oncogenes by loss or disruption of normal regulation.

Oncogenes

Oncogenes were first detected in retroviruses, which had acquired them from their host in order to take control of cell growth. Such oncogenes are often identified by names that refer to the viral source, one example being *ras* (*rat* sarcoma virus). They are found to be activated not only in virus-induced malignancies but in common nonviral cancers in humans. Oncogenes behave the same way that autosomal dominant traits behave, and only 1 mutant allele is needed for tumor formation, presumably by a dominant negative effect on regulation of signal transduction.

Tumor-suppressor genes

Tumor-suppressor genes, also called *antioncogenes,* are genes that must be present in one functional copy to prevent uncontrolled cell proliferation. Although some may represent genes whose products participate in checkpoints for the cell cycle, one characteristic of tumor-suppressor genes is the diversity of their normal functions. Some examples of

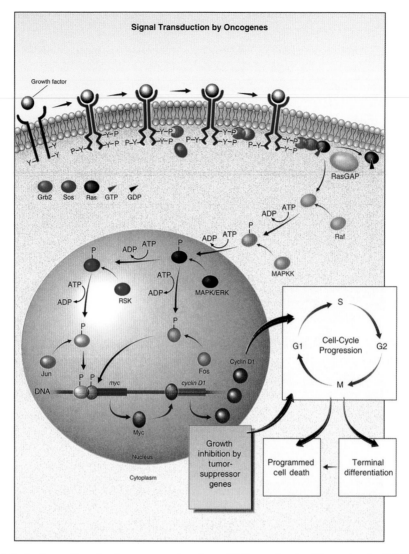

Figure 5-2 In the cell cycle, the progression from DNA synthesis *(S)* to mitosis *(M)* includes phases before *(GI)* and after *(G2)* the replication of DNA. On receiving signals to differentiate, cells leave the cycle and enter the pathway of terminal differentiation. Under certain circumstances, cells may enter the pathway to programmed cell death (apoptosis). Signal transduction begins with the binding of a growth factor to its transmembrane receptor *(upper left)*. Usually, the next step is the dimerization of the receptor. The receptor subunits then phosphorylate one another on tyrosine residues *(Y)*. The phosphotyrosines *(P)* create docking sites on the receptor for many proteins, some of which undergo phosphorylation; others recruit multicomponent complexes to the plasma membrane. One such interaction, shown here, is the activation of the Ras GTPase. In the cascade of phosphorylation initiated by the activation of Ras, the Raf kinase phosphorylates another kinase (mitogen-activated protein kinase kinase, or *MAPKK*), which in turn phosphorylates a third kinase, the mitogen-activated protein kinase, or *MAPK*. MAPK directly activates transcription factors and ribosomal S6 protein kinase *(RSK)*, which also phosphorylates transcription factors. MAPK probably represents at least 2 related proteins. Two transcription proteins, *Fos* and *Jun,* are shown. They join to form a fully active transcription factor. The phosphorylation of Fos by MAPK and of Jun by RSK causes them to bind to specific DNA sequences near the *MYC* gene, thereby initiating transcription of the gene. The Myc protein itself is a transcription factor with several binding partners (not shown). The binding of Myc to its specific recognition sites on DNA activates another set of genes. Cyclin D1 initiates the progression cells through G1 to the S-phase. *GDP* = guanosine diphosphate, *GTP* = guanosine triphosphate. *(Reproduced with permission from Krontiris TG. Oncogenes. N Engl J Med. 1995;333(5):304.)*

tumor-suppressor genes include the genes for retinoblastoma, Wilms tumor, neurofibromatosis types 1 and 2, tuberous sclerosis, ataxia-telangiectasia, and von Hippel–Lindau disease. All of these examples (except ataxia-telangiectasia) behave as autosomal dominant traits, but the mechanism of tumor formation is very different for tumor-suppressor genes than it is for oncogenes. If 1 allele is already defective because of a hereditary mutation, the other allele must also be lost for tumor formation to occur (also known as the "2-hit hypothesis"). This loss of the second allele is termed *loss of heterozygosity,* and it can occur from a second mutation, gene deletion, chromosomal loss, or mitotic recombination.

Krontiris TG. Oncogenes. *N Engl J Med.* 1995;333(5):303–306.

Mitochondrial Disease

A significant number of disorders associated with the eye or visual system involve mitochondrial deletions and mutations. Mitochondrial diseases should be considered whenever the inheritance pattern of a trait suggests maternal transmission. Although the inheritance pattern might superficially resemble that of an X-linked trait, maternal transmission differs in that all of the offspring of affected females—both daughters and sons—can inherit the trait, but only the daughters can pass it on.

The phenotype and severity of mitochondrial disease appear to depend on the nature of the mutation, the presence or degree of heteroplasmy (coexistence of more than 1 species of mitochondrial DNA [mtDNA]—ie, wild type and mutant), and the oxidative needs of the tissues involved. Spontaneous deletions and mutations of mtDNA accumulate with age, and the effect of this accumulation is to decrease the efficiency and function of the electron transport system, reducing the availability of ATP. When energy production becomes insufficient to maintain the function of cells or tissue, disease occurs. There appears to be an important interaction between age and tissue threshold of oxidative phosphorylation need and the expression of inherited mutations of mtDNA.

With each cell division, the number of mutant mtDNA copies that are partitioned to a given daughter cell is random, unlike with mendelian inheritance characteristics. After a number of cell divisions, some cells, purely by chance, receive more normal or more mutant copies of mtDNA, resulting in a drift toward homoplasmy in subsequent cell lines. This process is called *replicative segregation.* With mtDNA deletions, preferential replication of the smaller deleted molecules causes an increase of deleted copy over time. The trend toward homoplasmy helps explain why disease worsens with age and why organ systems not previously involved in multisystem mitochondrial disease become involved.

Mitochondrial diseases can be subdivided into these categories (Fig 5-3):

- disorders resulting from large rearrangements of mtDNA (deletions and insertions), such as chronic progressive external ophthalmoplegia (CPEO), Kearns-Sayre syndrome, and Pearson marrow-pancreas syndrome
- mutations of mtDNA-encoded rRNA, such as maternally inherited sensorineural deafness and aminoglycoside-induced deafness
- mutations of mtDNA-encoded tRNA, such as the syndromes of MELAS, myoclonic epilepsy with ragged red fibers (MERRF), adult-onset diabetes and deafness, and (in about 30% of cases) CPEO

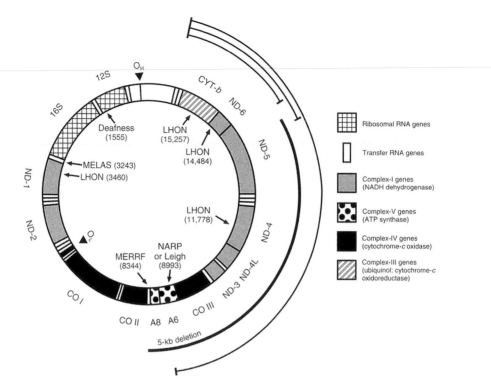

Figure 5-3 Diagram of human mitochondrial DNA and the most common associated pathogenetic mutations. Point mutations in structural and protein-coding genes are shown inside the circle, with the clinical phenotype indicated and the nucleotide position of the mutation shown in parentheses. The position of the most common single deletion, which is 5 kb long, and the multiple deletions are indicated by the arcs outside the circle. *A6, A8* = ATPase subunits; *CO I, CO II, CO III* = cytochrome-*c* oxidase subunits; *CYT-b* = apocytochrome-*b* subunit; *Leigh* = maternally inherited Leigh disease; *LHON* = Leber hereditary optic neuropathy; *MELAS* = syndrome of mitochondrial encephalomyopathy, lactic acidosis, and strokelike episodes; *MERRF* = myoclonic epilepsy with ragged red fibers; *NARP* = neuropathy, ataxia, and retinitis pigmentosa; *ND-1, ND-2, ND-3, ND-4L, ND-4, ND-5, ND-6* = NADH dehydrogenase subunits; O_H = origin of heavy-stranded DNA replication; O_L = origin of light-stranded DNA replication; *12S and 16S* = ribosomal RNA subunits. The large open space at the top, which includes O_H, is the noncoding D (displacement) loop. *(Reproduced with permission from Johns DR. Seminars of medicine of the Beth Israel Hospital, Boston. Mitochondrial DNA and disease. N Engl J Med. 1995;333(10):641.)*

- missense and nonsense mutations such as Leber hereditary optic neuropathy (LHON) and neuropathy, ataxia, and retinitis pigmentosa (NARP)

Chronic Progressive External Ophthalmoplegia

CPEO is a disorder involving progressive ptosis and paralysis of eye muscles associated with a ragged red myopathy, usually as a result of deletion of a portion of the mitochondrial genome. Patients with CPEO commonly have pigmentary retinopathy that does not create significant visual disability. Infrequently, they may have more marked retinal or other system involvement, the so-called *CPEO-plus syndromes*. In Kearns-Sayre syndrome, CPEO is associated with heart block and severe retinitis pigmentosa (RP) with marked visual impairment. Pearson marrow-pancreas syndrome results from a large de-letion of mtDNA and presents in younger patients with an entirely different phenotype involving sideroblastic anemia and pancreatic exocrine dysfunction. However, in patients afflicted during their later years, Pearson marrow-pancreas syndrome can present with a phenotype resembling Kearns-Sayre syndrome.

Although roughly 50% of patients with CPEO have demonstrable mtDNA deletions, virtually all patients with Kearns-Sayre syndrome have large deletions. As many as 30% of patients with CPEO who do not harbor demonstrable mtDNA deletions may have a point mutation at nucleotide position 3243, the same mutation in the tRNA for leucine that in other people is associated with MELAS syndrome. For all of the syndromes associated with deletions, such as Kearns-Sayre and CPEO, detection of the deletion usually requires study of the muscle tissue.

Leber Hereditary Optic Neuropathy

The most important ophthalmic disease of mitochondria is *Leber hereditary optic neu-ropathy (LHON),* which is more prevalent in males than in females but does not fit a classic X-linked pattern of transmission. The trait is not transmitted to the offspring of af-fected males, but virtually every daughter and son of a female patient with LHON inherits the trait. In approximately 50% of cases, LHON development is correlated with a single base change (G to A at nucleotide position 11778 in the *ND-4* gene) in human mtDNA involved in the synthesis of NADH dehydrogenase. In addition to optic atrophy, patients can exhibit peripapillary microangiopathy and cardiac abnormalities, especially Wolff-Parkinson-White syndrome. LHON can also occur from other so-called primary muta-tions at nucleotide positions 3460 of *ND-1,* 14484 of *ND-6,* 14459 of *ND-6,* and (more controversially) 15257 of cytochrome-*b.* At least 12 secondary mutations have been as-sociated with LHON, often when multiple mutations are present in an individual's mito-chondria. Some authors think that these secondary mutations cause disease by additive detrimental effects on the electron transport system of oxidative phosphorylation. Most of these secondary mutations appear in the general population. Debate persists on whether each mutation alone is truly pathogenic.

The likelihood of improvement with time in the recovery of visual acuity appears to differ among the separate mutations associated with LHON. Mutation at nucleotide position 11778 is associated with the least, and mutation at nucleotide position 14484 is associated with the greatest, likelihood of recovery. The mutation at 14459 of *ND-6* ap-pears to be associated with 2 very different clinical phenotypes, one LHON and the other a severe, early-onset progressive dystonia with pseudobulbar syndrome, short stature, and reduced intelligence. The 2 phenotypes may reflect different proportions or distribution of mutant mtDNA.

Neuropathy, Ataxia, and Retinitis Pigmentosa

NARP is associated with a single base-pair mutation at nucleotide position 8993 in the *ATPase-6* gene. The NARP phenotype occurs when the percentage of mutant mtDNA is less than 80%, whereas the same mutation present at much higher proportions (greater than 95%) can cause Leigh syndrome, a severe neurodegenerative disease of infancy and early childhood. The 8993 mutation is demonstrable in fibroblasts and lymphoblasts.

Other Mitochondrial Diseases

Aminoglycoside-induced deafness and streptomycin ototoxicity are instances wherein antibiotic administration, often only a modest dose, is associated with severe hearing loss. This susceptibility to ototoxicity is a maternally inherited trait. Aminoglycosides (kanamycin, gentamicin, tobramycin, and neomycin) "target" the evolutionarily related bacterial ribosome. The mechanism of action is thought to include interference with the production of ATP in the mitochondria of hair cells in the cochlea.

Brown MD, Wallace DC. Molecular basis of mitochondrial DNA disease. *J Bioenerg Biomembr.* 1994;26(3):273–289.

Johns DR. Seminars in medicine of the Beth Israel Hospital, Boston. Mitochondrial DNA and disease. *N Engl J Med.* 1995;333(10):638–644.

Nikoskelainen EK, Savontaus ML, Wanne OP, Katila MJ, Nummelin KU. Leber's hereditary optic neuroretinopathy, a maternally inherited disease. A genealogic study in four pedigrees. *Arch Ophthalmol.* 1987;105(5):665–671.

Phillips CI, Gosden CM. Leber's hereditary optic neuropathy and Kearns-Sayre syndrome: mitochondrial DNA mutations. *Surv Ophthalmol.* 1991;35(6):463–472.

The Search for Genes in Specific Diseases

A variety of methods have been used to assign individual genes to specific chromosomes, to link individual genes to one another, and to link diseases to specific genes.

Synteny

The presence of genes on the same chromosome, even if the genes are too far apart to demonstrate linkage, is called *synteny*. Genes that are X-linked, such as red-green color blindness, choroideremia, and hemophilia, are by definition syntenic. The term is also used to denote homologous chromosomal regions between species. For example, the mouse gene for opsin is localized to the distal half of mouse chromosome 1, which is syntenic or homologous to human chromosome 3q.

Both the value and the limitations of the study of genetic disease in other animals can be seen in the following example: the mouse's role in the discovery of the gene for a form of Usher syndrome type I *(USH1B)* (profound congenital deafness, vestibular dysfunction, and RP). A mouse mutant for deafness, *shaker-1 (sh1),* had been mapped to a conserved linkage region on mouse chromosome 7, and *USH1B* was linked to human chromosome 11q13, suggesting that the 2 might result from similar or homologous genes. The *shaker-1* gene was isolated in 1995 by positional cloning and the mutated gene identified as *myosin VIIa.* The human counterpart to this gene, *MYO7A,* was quickly identified as the gene mutated also in *USH1B.* The subsequent twist to the story is that, because of differences in tissue-specific expression, the mouse mutant has deafness and vestibular dysfunction but not RP. Thus, animal models may help to find genes that cause human disease, but the expression of mutations in the homologous genes may have important species differences.

el-Amraoui A, Sahly I, Picaud S, Sahel J, Abitbol M, Petit C. Human Usher IB/mouse shaker-1: the retinal phenotype discrepancy explained by the presence/absence of myosin VIIA in the photoreceptor cells. *Hum Mol Genet.* 1996;5(8):1171–1178.

Gibson F, Walsh J, Mburu P, et al. A type VII myosin encoded by the mouse deafness gene shaker-1. *Nature.* 1995;374(6517):62–64.

Meisler MH. The role of the laboratory mouse in the human genome project. *Am J Hum Genet.* 1996;59(4):764–771.

Weil D, Blanchard S, Kaplan J, et al. Defective myosin VIIA gene responsible for Usher syndrome type 1B. *Nature.* 1995;374(6517):60–61.

Cytogenetic Markers (Morphologically Variant Chromosomes)

If a specific chromosomal structure is abnormal or even normally variant, its transmission through a family with a hereditary disease, as mapped by a pedigree, may allow the assumption that the mutant gene and the variant chromosome are comigrating. Thus, the mutant gene is physically located on the variant chromosome—that is, a cytogenetic marker.

Gene Dosage

If a portion of a chromosome containing a specific gene is physically deleted, the amount of the gene product will be determined only by the remaining homologue. For example, 50% of normal levels of esterase D may be found in the serum of people with an interstitial deletion of part of the long arm of chromosome 13. When several such persons were also found to have retinoblastoma, it was suggested that both the esterase and the retinoblastoma genes are located in the missing segment. By contrast, duplication mapping requires finding 150% of normal activity of a given gene product, together with either a chromosomal trisomy or triplication of a specific chromosomal segment.

Association

Certain combinations of traits may occur for reasons other than the physical relationship of genes. For example, blood group O and peptic ulcer are found together in the same person more often than would be expected from their individual frequencies in the population. This finding occurs not because the *ABO* gene and another gene for peptic ulcer are located on the same chromosome but because people with type O blood have a physiologic peculiarity that predisposes them to peptic ulcerations. In another example, retinal detachment occurs more frequently in patients with Marfan syndrome and homocystinuria than in the general population. Rather than resulting from the concurrent action of 2 linked genes, this association is the result of *pleiotropism,* the multiple effects of a single gene.

Linkage

Even if no information is known about the nature or function of a gene for a disease, linkage studies may be able to localize the gene to a given chromosome or specific marker.

In 1937, Bell and Haldane recognized the first linkage between 2 diseases on a human chromosome: congenital color deficiency and hemophilia on the X chromosome. Subsequent investigations have led to the chromosomal mapping of a large number of different human ocular diseases.

Gene assignments

As of March 15, 2004, OMIM *(Online Mendelian Inheritance in Man: www.ncbi.nlm.nih .gov/omim)* listed over 15,000 established human gene loci. Every chromosome has numerous defined genes. Human gene mapping has 2 major applications. The first is identification of the gene for a specific genetic disease by its linkage to a known marker. For example, suppose gene A causes a hereditary disease and gene B is a known enzyme or polymorphic marker closely linked to A. Even though no biochemical test exists for A, a tight linkage to B would allow a reasonable probability of identifying the disease for prenatal diagnosis and sometimes for carrier detection. The second impact of linkage is understanding the cause of the phenotypic malformations in specific chromosomal diseases. For example, the phenotype of Down syndrome may result from triplication of only the distal long arm of chromosome 21 through a chromosome rearrangement rather than trisomy of the entire chromosome.

Mets MB, Maumenee IH. The eye and the chromosome. *Surv Ophthalmol.* 1983;28(1):20–32.

Markers: restriction fragment length polymorphisms

Polymorphisms detectable by the presence or absence of a specific restriction endonuclease cleavage site are called *restriction fragment length polymorphisms (RFLPs).* The differences between 2 chromosomes in DNA genetic material fragment size between restriction endonuclease cleavage sites are inherited and become useful markers for following various genetically determined disorders.

Identification of RFLPs begins when DNA is isolated from peripheral blood lymphocytes. The DNA fragments are then produced when the DNA is cut with restriction endonucleases. Each restriction endonuclease recognizes a highly specific sequence of 4–9 bases and cuts double-stranded DNA wherever this sequence occurs. Change of a single base within the recognition sequence results in the loss of that cleavage site and a change in the corresponding DNA fragment length. A single base-pair change elsewhere may create a new recognition cleavage site where none had existed. A variation in DNA sequence involving a single base pair occurs with a frequency of approximately 1 per 200–500 bp. The variable-length fragments, determined by the spacing of the restriction enzyme recognition sites, are then separated by agarose gel electrophoresis. The gel will contain millions of DNA fragments.

To identify a certain fragment that might be linked to a specific genetic locus (ie, a defective gene), a radioactively labeled DNA probe is hybridized with the DNA fragments generated by the restriction endonucleases. The various probes represent cloned DNA sequences, which are complementary (homologous in base-pair sequence) to a part of the DNA fragment containing the RFLPs. Any fragments containing part or all of the radioactively labeled sequence can be identified by radioactive or nonradioactive detection methods (Fig 5-4).

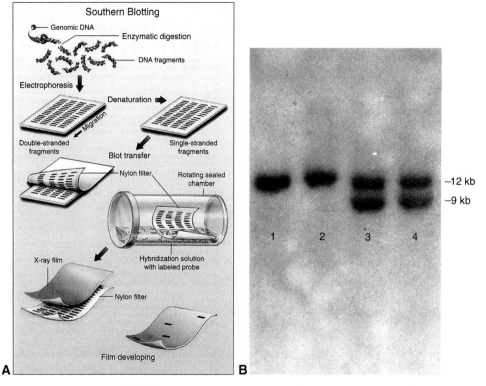

Figure 5-4 A, Analysis of DNA by gel electrophoresis and Southern blotting. In Southern blotting, genomic DNA is cut with restriction enzymes into fragments before being separated according to size by gel electrophoresis. The 4 lanes on the gel represent the digestion of the DNA with 4 different restriction enzymes. After electrophoresis, the nucleic acids in the gel are transferred directly onto a charged nylon filter to which they are tightly bound. Thus, the filter contains a precise replica of the nucleic acid distribution in the gel. The filter is then hybridized in a rotating sealed chamber with a DNA or RNA probe specific for the target of interest (in this case, sequences in a microbial pathogen). Probes have traditionally been radioactively labeled with nucleotides containing phosphorus-32; however, use of nonradiolabeled probes is becoming more common. After the probe has hybridized to its target sequence, the nonhybridized probe is washed away and the filter is exposed to x-ray film. A DNA sequence complementary to the probe is seen as a dark band on the developed film. The position of the hybridized target sequence in each lane is unique to the restriction enzyme used to digest the DNA. **B,** Autoradiograph of a Southern blot with radiolabeled probe L1.28 after the DNA was cut with enzyme Taq1, separated by size on an agarose gel, and then transferred to a nylon filter. Four female carriers of X-linked retinitis pigmentosa are depicted. Note that 2 females, numbers 1 and 2, have only a 12-kb band, whereas carriers 3 and 4 have both 12-kb and 9-kb bands. *(Part A reproduced with permission from Naber SP. Molecular pathology—diagnosis of infectious disease.* N Engl J Med. *1994;331(18):1212.)*

RFLPs have been used to map the gene locus implicated in numerous diseases. In many cases, the gene in question has been identified by positional cloning or candidate screening; the latter is discussed later in this chapter.

It is possible to detect linkage by observing the frequency with which a polymorphic marker is inherited with a disease trait, provided that the disease locus is within 20–30 centimorgans (cM) of the *marker* site. The physical distance represented by 1 cM

(0.01 recombination fraction) is approximately 1 million bp (1000 kb) and corresponds to a 1% chance that recombination will result from a single meiosis. When a genetic probe is sufficiently close to a disease gene, both are rarely separated by meiotic recombination. The frequency of separation by chromosomal exchange at meiosis is their *recombination frequency.* Linked markers should be no more than 20 cM apart. For perspective, the average chromosome contains about 150 cM; there are about 3300 cM in the entire human genome, which corresponds to 3×10^9 bp.

Botstein D, White RL, Skolnick M, Davis RW. Construction of a genetic linkage map in man using restriction fragment length polymorphisms. *Am J Hum Genet.* 1980;32(3):314–331.

When determining linkage between a diseased gene and a marker, geneticists compare different models by calculating likelihood ratios. When the likelihood ratio is 1000:1 that the odds of 1 model are greater than those of another, the first is accepted over the second. The log of the likelihood ratio (*logarithm of odds* score, or *LOD score*) is usually reported. An LOD score of 1–2 is of potential interest in terms of linkage; 2–3 is suggestive; and greater than 3 is generally considered proof of linkage. Although an LOD score of 3 gives a probability ratio of 1000:1 in favor of linkage versus independent assortment, this score does not indicate a type I error as low as 0.001, but, in fact, it indicates an error that is close to 0.05, the standard significance level used in statistics. (BCSC Section 1, *Update on General Medicine,* explains these concepts in depth in Chapter 16, Using Statistics in Practice and Work.)

Markers: microsatellites, minisatellites, and satellites

Within the genome exist variable lengths of repetitive DNA composed of multiple units that may each be 1–5 bp in length *(microsatellites),* 14–100 bp in length *(minisatellites),* or over 100 bp in length *(satellites).* One class of such repeats is also called *short tandem repeats (STRs)*; these are tandemly repeated blocks of 2–5 nucleotides. The variability in the number of repeats produces polymorphisms that are useful for linkage studies (Fig 5-5). STRs have moderate to high mutation rates. The instability of certain minisatellites can lead to cancer and acquired diseases such as insulin-dependent (type 1) diabetes mellitus.

Housman D. Human DNA polymorphism. *N Engl J Med.* 1995;332(5):318–320.
Litt M, Luty JA. A hypervariable microsatellite revealed by in vitro amplification of a dinucleotide repeat within the cardiac muscle actin gene. *Am J Hum Genet.* 1989;44(3):397–401.

Candidate Gene Approaches

Candidate gene screening

The process of candidate gene screening involves screening for mutations of genes that are abundantly expressed within a tissue and are either important for function or specifically expressed only in that tissue. Sometimes, the candidate gene is one that recapitulates the human disease in transgenic animals. Examples of candidate gene screening discoveries include the findings of mutations of peripherin/*RDS* in autosomal dominant RP and

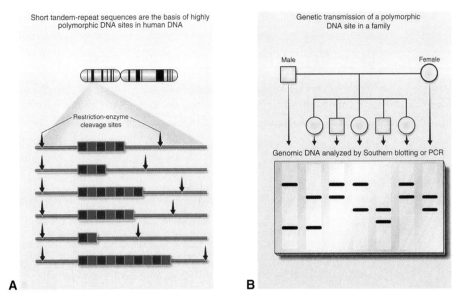

Short tandem-repeat sequences are the basis of highly polymorphic DNA sites in human DNA

Restriction-enzyme cleavage sites

A

Genetic transmission of a polymorphic DNA site in a family

Male

Female

Genomic DNA analyzed by Southern blotting or PCR

B

Figure 5-5 **A,** Variable-length sequences in human DNA can be created by variations in the number of copies of a tandem-repeat DNA sequence. Each line in the figure represents a copy of a human DNA sequence. The copies are identical in sequence except for the tandemly repeated DNA sequence indicated by the boxes. The number of copies of the tandemly repeated DNA sequence is indicated by the number of boxes. The size of the DNA fragment that includes the tandem-repeat sequence is measured between 2 fixed points. In Southern blotting, the sites of restriction-enzyme digestion are the fixed points that determine the ends of the DNA fragment. **B,** A family in which a highly polymorphic marker is used for genetic analysis. The 2 copies of the DNA fragment from the offspring can be distinguished from the 2 copies of the fragment from the father, making the inheritance pattern from each parent clear for this chromosomal site. Detection may be carried out by Southern blotting or polymerase chain reaction (PCR), depending on the size of the tandem-repeat sequence. *(Reproduced with permission from Housman D. Human DNA polymorphism.* N Engl J Med. *1995;332(5):319.)*

macular dystrophies and the finding of mutations of the rod *cyclic guanosine monophosphate (cGMP)* β-subunit of rod phosphodiesterase and the cGMP-gated cation channel in autosomal recessive RP.

Dryja TP, Finn JT, Peng YW, McGee TL, Berson EL, Yan KW. Mutations in the gene encoding the alpha subunit of the rod cGMP-gated channel in autosomal recessive retinitis pigmentosa. *Proc Natl Acad Sci U S A.* 1995;92(22):10177–10181.

Kajiwara K, Sandberg MA, Berson EL, Dryja TP. A null mutation in the human peripherin/RDS gene in a family with autosomal dominant retinitis punctata albescens. *Nat Genet.* 1993;3(3):208–212.

McLaughlin ME, Sandberg MA, Berson EL, Dryja TP. Recessive mutations in the gene encoding the beta-subunit of rod phosphodiesterase in patients with retinitis pigmentosa. *Nat Genet.* 1993;4(2):130–134.

Nichols BE, Sheffield VC, Vandenburgh K, Drack AV, Kimura AE, Stone EM. Butterfly-shaped pigment dystrophy of the fovea caused by a point mutation in codon 167 of the *RDS* gene. *Nat Genet.* 1993;3(3):202–207.

Positional candidate gene screening

Whenever linkage studies localize a gene to a given chromosomal region, genes already known to reside in the same region become candidate genes for that disease. Following are some examples of disease localization that resulted from linkage to a given region, which in turn led to finding the disease-causing gene by screening for mutations of genes in the region: autosomal dominant RP from rhodopsin mutations (3q); Sorsby fundus dystrophy from *TIMP3* mutations (22q); and Oguchi disease from point deletions within the arrestin gene (2q).

Dryja TP, McGee TL, Reichel E, et al. A point mutation of the rhodopsin gene in one form of retinitis pigmentosa. *Nature.* 1990;343(6256):364–366.

Fuchs S, Nakazawa M, Maw M, Tamai M, Oguchi Y, Gal A. A homozygous 1-base pair deletion in the arrestin gene is a frequent cause of Oguchi disease in Japanese. *Nat Genet.* 1995;10(3):360–362.

Weber BH, Vogt G, Pruett RC, Stöhr H, Felbor U. Mutations in the tissue inhibitor of metalloproteinases-3 (TIMP3) in patients with Sorsby's fundus dystrophy. *Nat Genet.* 1994;8(4):352–356.

Mutation Screening

DNA Libraries

DNA libraries exist as a means of collecting and organizing genes of interest for future study. Libraries can be made from either genomic DNA or complementary DNA (cDNA). *Genomic DNA libraries* are created by cleaving whole DNA from an organism, tissue, or cell type with restriction enzymes that produce fragments of DNA. These fragments can be cloned into vectors and plated onto media. The specific clones are identified with probes derived from the original sequence or gene of interest and then isolated and grown as needed (Fig 5-6). *cDNA libraries* are created by using reverse transcriptase to generate complementary DNA from mRNA expressed by the cell or tissue to be studied. Recent technology allows many cDNA sequences or expressed sequence tags (ESTs) to be placed on a microscopic glass slide. Literally thousands of cDNAs can be screened using this microarray technique.

Single-stranded Conformational Polymorphism

With the *single-stranded conformational polymorphism (SSCP)* technique for mutation detection, single-stranded DNA is electrophoresed under nondenaturing conditions, allowing the molecules to fold on themselves according to their inherent similarity of sequences. Molecules of differing sizes and sequences fold differently and migrate at different rates of speed on the gel. Mutations that alter amino acid residues often change the way in which single-stranded DNA folds upon itself, creating different tertiary configurations that can be separated from the normal sequence by differences in mobility on gel electrophoresis.

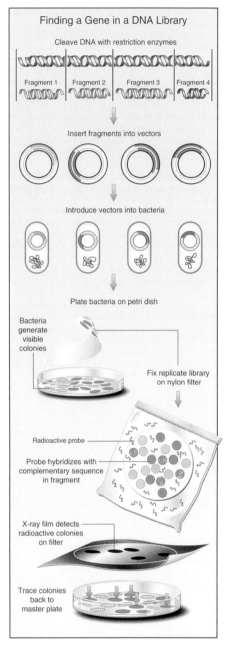

Finding a Gene in a DNA Library

Cleave DNA with restriction enzymes

Fragment 1   Fragment 2   Fragment 3   Fragment 4

Insert fragments into vectors

Introduce vectors into bacteria

Plate bacteria on petri dish

Bacteria generate visible colonies

Fix replicate library on nylon filter

Radioactive probe

Probe hybridizes with complementary sequence in fragment

X-ray film detects radioactive colonies on filter

Trace colonies back to master plate

Figure 5-6 The first step in making a library of DNA sequences is to cut DNA into fragments with restriction enzymes. These DNA fragments, when inserted into vectors, form recombinant molecules with the DNA of the vector (a plasmid vector is shown, but viral vectors are also used). Bacteria carrying the vectors can replicate on an agar-coated Petri dish, where they grow to form colonies. Each colony originates from a single bacterial cell and thus contains a single type of recombinant DNA fragment. A nylon filter put on the surface of the Petri dish picks up a portion of each colony. Chemical treatment of the filter lyses the bacterial cells, denaturing the DNA and fixing it in place. A radioactive probe for a known sequence of nucleotides can reveal the desired fragment on the filter. The filter, with the replicate library of the colonies on its surface, is incubated in a plastic bag (or glass dish) with a solution containing the radioactive DNA probe; after the unbound probe is washed away, an x-ray film can locate the radioactive colonies *(black ovals)*. The position of the signals on the film serves as a map with which to locate the corresponding colonies on the original master plate. Once identified, these colonies can then be amplified in culture to produce large quantities of the desired recombinant DNA molecule.
(Reproduced with permission from Rosenthal N. Stalking the gene—DNA libraries. N Engl J Med. 1994;331(9):599.)

Denaturing Gradient Gel Electrophoresis

With *denaturing gradient gel electrophoresis (DGGE)*, double-stranded DNA samples are electrophoresed against a gradient of denaturing agent such as urea. Molecules of differing size and composition reach differing points on the gel before they become denatured. Mutations affect the point in the gel for which a given DNA molecule will denature and hence alter the migration patterns. The sensitivity of DGGE in detecting mutations is improved if a 40-bp sequence rich in guanine and cytosine (a GC clamp) is added to 1 primer before polymerase chain reaction (PCR). Identification of a polymorphism detected by DGGE can be determined by direct DNA sequencing of the PCR-amplified exonic product.

Direct Sequencing

One of the most important advances in molecular genetics has been the development of techniques for rapid sequencing of DNA. Currently, it is far cheaper to sequence a stretch of DNA than to sequence and characterize the amino acid peptide that it produces.

Although other mutation screening techniques exist, sequencing of DNA is the surest and most direct. Sequencing of cDNA derived from mRNA provides a quick look at the reading frames (exons) of the gene, whereas sequencing of genomic DNA is more time-consuming because of the presence of introns between the exons. The intron–exon boundaries must be known and multiple PCR assays set up in order to screen not only the exons and their splice-site junctions but also upstream and downstream regions that may be important for gene activation and regulation.

The 2 DNA sequencing techniques used today are the *enzymatic* (or *Sanger*) *method*, which can be implemented manually or semiautomatically, and *automated sequencing*, which (for high-volume laboratories) is faster and less prone to errors of reading. Figure 5-7 illustrates these procedures.

Rosenthal N. Molecular medicine: fine structure of a gene—DNA sequencing. *N Engl J Med.* 1995;332(9):589–591.

Use of Restriction Endonucleases

If a point mutation destroys or creates a restriction site, screening for this mutation can be accomplished quickly through the use of the particular enzyme that recognizes the changed restriction site. Figure 5-8 illustrates the detection of mutations using restriction enzymes, oligonucleotide hybridization, PCR, and Southern blot analysis.

Allele-specific Oligonucleotides

An *allele-specific oligonucleotide (ASO)* is a synthetic probe made of a sequence of nucleotides. It is constructed so that it uses hybridization to recognize a specific DNA sequence in order to detect a specific point mutation. Often, diagnostic testing is done with 2 separate ASOs, 1 that recognizes the specific base-pair change of a given genetic mutation and another that recognizes the normal allelic sequence. ASOs are commonly used for diagnosing point mutations that occur frequently or for testing multiple members of a large family with a previously identified genetic disorder.

Gene Therapy

Gene therapy holds much promise, but the field remains in its infancy. The potential for cure is not matched by either technology or understanding. No clinical ophthalmic applications yet exist. Key challenges remain in characterizing linkages of genes to major

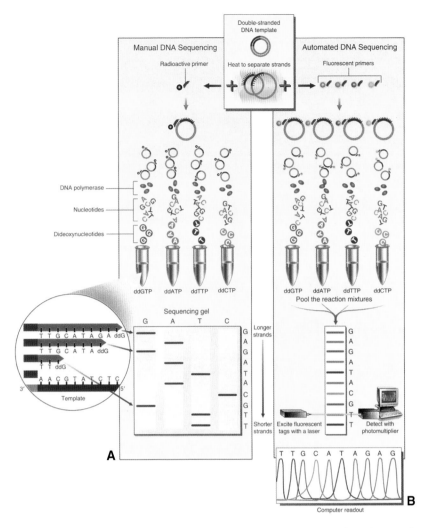

Figure 5-7 **A,** A double-stranded fragment of DNA whose sequence is unknown is cloned into a plasmid, which is then heated to separate the 2 strands. A primer with a sequence complementary to a short plasmid sequence near the junctional site is added and hybridizes to 1 of the 2 template strands. In manual sequencing, the DNA primer has a radioactive tag (alternatively, 1 of the nucleotide precursors is radioactive). The plasmid-primer hybrid is added to 4 tubes, each containing DNA polymerase, all 4 nucleotides, and a single dideoxynucleotide-dideoxyguanosine triphosphate *(ddGTP)*, dideoxyadenosine triphosphate *(ddATP)*, dideoxythymidine triphosphate *(ddTTP)*, or dideoxycytidine triphosphate *(ddCTP)*. DNA polymerase extends the DNA primer, which incorporates nucleotides (and occasionally dideoxynucleotides) into the growing DNA chains. The incorporation of dideoxynucleotides prevents further elongation of the chain (the *circular inset* shows the elongation products in the ddGTP sample). Electrophoresis of the 4 reactions on a very thin gel separates the radioactive fragments according to size. Autoradiography reveals these fragments as bands. Each band corresponds to a nucleotide in the DNA sequence. **B,** Automated sequencing uses a DNA primer labeled with 4 different fluorescent tags. Each fluorescent primer hybridizes to the template DNA and undergoes the same synthesis reactions as in manual sequencing. After elongation of the primer, samples containing the 4 kinds of newly synthesized fragments are pooled and undergo electrophoresis in a single lane of a gel. A laser beam directed near the bottom of the gel excites each fragment, which emits a specific fluorescent signal as it passes through the beam. A photomultiplier senses the specific wavelength of each signal, which corresponds to the dideoxynucleotide incorporated in the elongation reaction. A computer stores and translates the signals as a nucleotide sequence. *(Reproduced with permission from Rosenthal N. Fine structure of a gene—DNA sequencing. N Engl J Med. 1995;332(9):590.)*

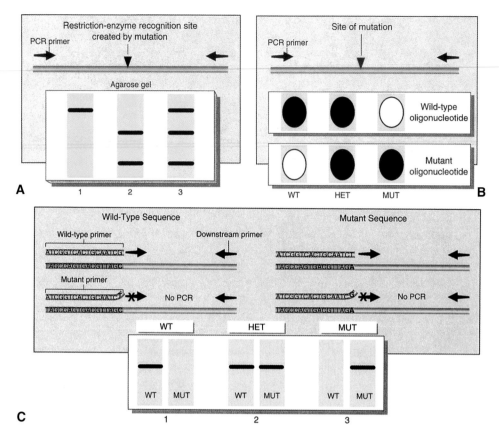

Figure 5-8   A, The detection of a point mutation by digestion of DNA with a restriction enzyme. The mutation creates a new recognition site. The region surrounding the mutation is amplified by the polymerase chain reaction *(PCR),* and the resulting PCR product is incubated with the restriction enzyme and then analyzed by agarose gel electrophoresis. *Lane 1* shows DNA from a person without the mutation; only 1 band appears because the enzyme does not cut the DNA. *Lane 2* shows DNA from a person homozygous for the mutation; 2 bands represent the 2 fragments obtained after enzyme digestion. *Lane 3* shows DNA from a heterozygote, with 1 uncut fragment and 2 cut fragments. **B,** A mutation detected by oligonucleotide hybridization. The segment of DNA is amplified by PCR, divided into aliquots, and spotted onto separate filter membranes, which are hybridized with a labeled oligonucleotide corresponding to the wild-type or mutant sequence. The amplified segment of DNA from a person with the wild-type sequence *(WT)* hybridizes only with the wild-type oligonucleotide, whereas the DNA from a person homozygous for the mutant sequence *(MUT)* hybridizes only with the mutant oligonucleotide. DNA from a heterozygote *(HET)* hybridizes with both oligonucleotides. **C,** The detection of a mutation by PCR. The mutant sequence differs from the wild-type sequence by the substitution of an A for a C. To search for the 2 kinds of sequences by PCR, 2 primers are necessary. A separate reaction is carried out with each, together with a common downstream primer. With a wild-type gene, the primer corresponding to the wild-type sequence yields a PCR product. Similarly, the mutant primer produces a product with the mutant sequence. However, with the wild-type primer and the mutant sequence, or the mutant primer and the wild-type sequence, there is no PCR product. The agarose gel pattern shows that DNA from a person homozygous for the wild-type allele reacts only with the wild-type primer; DNA from a person homozygous for the mutant sequence reacts only with the mutant primer; and DNA from a heterozygote yields PCR products with both primers.

(continued)

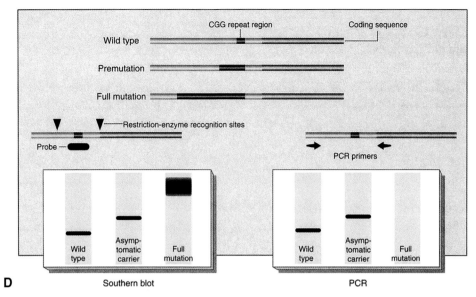

D   Southern blot   PCR

Figure 5-8   **D,** Detection of a triplet-repeat mutation by Southern blot analysis or PCR. In the fragile-X syndrome, a CGG repeat occurs near the 5′ end of the gene. The number of repeats ranges from 5 to 50 in the general population and from approximately 50 to 200 in those with the fragile-X syndrome. The abnormality is detected as follows: DNA is treated with a restriction enzyme that cuts at recognition sites flanking the CGG repeat. Hybridization on a Southern blot *(left)* with labeled DNA from the region of the gene reveals a single band in a normal male subject (wild type). An asymptomatic male carrier will have a band of higher molecular weight, and a subject with a full mutation will have a very large, diffuse band because of the instability of the full-mutation allele. The normal and asymptomatic-carrier alleles can also be detected by PCR *(right)*. The full-mutation allele cannot be amplified by PCR because it is too large. *(Reproduced with permission from Korf B. Molecular diagnosis (2). N Engl J Med. 1995;332(22):1500–1501.)*

diseases (especially chronic diseases that, although common, are likely multifactorial), understanding the pathogenic relevance of identified linked genes, and developing proper delivery systems for curative gene constructs (viruses, the main long-term gene therapy vehicle, are plagued by inflammation and the risk of oncogenesis).

Replacement of Absent Gene Product in X-Linked and Recessive Disease

For genetic diseases wherein the mutant allele produces either no message or an ineffective gene product (a so-called *null allele*), correction of the disorder may be possible by simple replacement of the gene in the deficient cells or tissues. It is theoretically possible to transfer normal genes into human cells that harbor either null or mutant genes not producing a stable, translated product. Vectors used to carry the genetic material into the cells include adenoviruses, retroviruses (especially adeno-associated viruses [AAV]), and plasmid–liposome complexes. AAV vector gene therapy has been successful in curing many disorders in animal models, such as the RPE65 mutation that causes RP in the Briard dog.

Plasmid–liposome complexes may have advantages as vectors because they can be used for nondividing cells and may be less likely to incite inflammation or immune responses.

However, as vectors, these complexes are inefficient and may not produce sufficient expression of the wanted product. Strategies are being developed to direct the new genetic material into the nucleus, with the possibility of subsequent incorporation into the genome to perpetuate expression of the new gene.

Blau HM, Springer ML. Gene therapy—a novel form of drug delivery. *N Engl J Med.* 1995; 333(18):1204–1207.

Crystal RG. Transfer of genes to humans: early lessons and obstacles to success. *Science.* 1995;270(5235):404–410.

Hangai M, Kaneda Y, Tanihara H, Honda Y. In vivo gene transfer into the retina mediated by a novel liposome system. *Invest Ophthalmol Vis Sci.* 1996;37(13):2678–2685.

Strategies for Dominant Diseases

Dominant diseases are caused by production of a gene product that is either insufficient *(haploid insufficiency)* or conducive to disease *(dominant-negative effect).* Theoretically, haploid insufficiency should be treatable by gene replacement as outlined previously for X-linked or recessive disease. (For dominant disorders produced by defective developmental genes, this correction would have to occur in early uterine development.)

Disorders resulting from a dominant-negative effect require a different approach. Thus, strategies for treatment of dominant disease differ, depending on whether a functional gene product is produced. Some genes code for RNAs that can bind to mRNA from another gene and block their ability to be translated. Greater understanding of these genes may allow for creation of either drugs or new gene-encoded RNAs that can block the translation of mRNA for defective alleles, thus allowing only the normal allele to be expressed.

Another approach is the use of oligonucleotides that are designed to bind with mRNA from mutant alleles, stopping the mRNA from being translated by ribosomes (Fig 5-9) or ribozymes, molecules that specifically degrade the mRNA. Although many problems need to be worked out for such therapy to be effective, this approach holds promise for autosomal dominant disorders wherein disease is caused by expression of the mutant gene product.

One approach to the treatment of autosomal dominant diseases is to target the translated strand of the mutant allele by antisense DNA, a sequence of DNA designed to anneal to and block the processing or translation of the abnormal mRNA. Another approach involves ribozymes, RNA molecules that have the ability to cleave certain RNAs. A third approach utilizes *small interference RNAs (siRNAs),* also known as *short interfering RNAs,* to bind to mRNAs and lead to the eventual degradation of specific mRNAs. The use of siRNAs as potential therapeutic agents has become increasingly popular in the last few years, and siRNAs have proven to be a powerful means by which to study the function of novel gene products. However, siRNAs suffer from difficulty in achieving intracellular delivery and from cell–surface TLR3 receptor stimulation, which can induce immune or antiangiogenic processes as a generic class property.

Askari FK, McDonnell WM. Antisense-oligonucleotide therapy. *N Engl J Med.* 1996;334(5): 316–318.

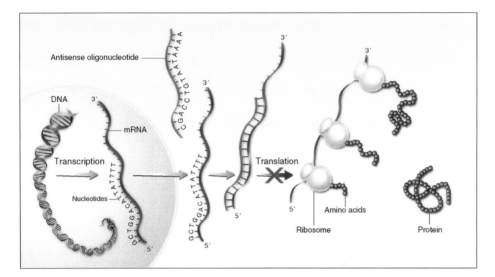

Figure 5-9 Blockade of translation by antisense oligonucleotides. Normal gene transcription of DNA into mRNA is followed by translation of mRNA into protein. Antisense oligonucleotides complementary to a portion of mRNA bind mRNA, preventing translation—either by the steric effect of the binding process itself or (possibly) by inducing degradation of the mRNA by RNase. *(Reproduced with permission from Askari FK, McDonnell WM. Antisense-oligonucleotide therapy.* N Engl J Med. *1996;334(5):316.)*

Della NG. Molecular biology in ophthalmology. A review of principles and recent advances. *Arch Ophthalmol.* 1996;114(4):457–463.

Kleinman M, Yamada K, Takeda A, et al. Sequence- and target-independent angiogenesis suppression by siRNA via TLR3. *Nature.* 2008;452(7187):591–597.

CHAPTER 6

Clinical Genetics

It is important for a clinician not only to diagnose a disease state accurately and minimize its effects in the patient but to ensure that the siblings and parents are evaluated for milder or earlier forms of the disease. Any family with a genetic disorder should receive genetic counseling as a primary care responsibility. However, only the ophthalmologist will be sensitive to the wide variability of traits affecting the visual system and to the subtleties of carrier-state detection (both by direct evaluation and with indirect diagnostic technology). The ophthalmologist is an important member of the team that can appropriately counsel the patient and family about the ocular effects of a given genetic disorder and its attendant risks and burdens.

Terminology: Hereditary, Genetic, Familial, Congenital

Hereditary indicates that a disease or trait under consideration results directly from an individual's particular genetic composition (or *genome*) and that it can be passed from one generation to another. *Genetic* denotes that the disorder is caused by a defect of genes, whether acquired or inherited. In some instances (eg, with large deletions of mitochondrial DNA [mtDNA] associated with chronic progressive ophthalmoplegia), the disease is clearly genetic, but it is not passed to subsequent generations and is therefore not hereditary. These deletions associated with ocular myopathies presumably arise in the oocyte or during early embryologic development. Thus, the terms *hereditary* and *genetic* are not exactly synonymous but are sometimes used to convey similar concepts. A hereditary or a genetic disorder may or may not be congenital.

A condition is *familial* if it occurs in more than 1 member of a family. It may, of course, be hereditary but need not be. A familial disorder can be caused by common exposure to infectious agents (eg, tuberculosis), traumatizing materials (eg, radiation), deficient or excess food intake (eg, vitamin deficiencies or obesity), or environmental agents such as asbestos or coal dust.

The term *congenital* refers to characteristics that are present at birth. These may be hereditary or familial, or they may occur as an isolated event, often as the result of an infection (eg, rubella, toxoplasmosis, or cytomegalic inclusion disease). The presence of such characteristics *at birth* is the defining factor. Findings suggesting but not establishing that a congenital anomaly may be genetic include a phenotype similar to that from known genetic disorders (eg, aniridia) or a tendency toward bilaterality (eg, bilateral colobomas) and symmetry. However, some nongenetic congenital disorders, such as cataracts from rubella, can be bilateral. Moreover, not all hereditary disorders are bilateral or symmetric—for example, optic nerve coloboma in only 1 eye has been observed in multiple generations and presumably in this case is an autosomal dominant trait.

Although numerous hereditary disorders are expressed at the time of birth, the complex interrelationships between genomic expression and factors such as the environment may alter the time of onset and the extent to which a disorder is manifested. For example, the overt clinical onset of signs for diabetes mellitus—a condition with a heritable tendency mediated by multiple genes—in individual monozygotic twins can differ appreciably with each twin's level of carbohydrate intake or other factors. In addition, although the enzyme deficiency responsible for galactosemia is clearly inherited, the expression of systemic disease as well as cataract formation can be avoided by the removal of galactose from the diet.

A condition known to be genetic and hereditary may appear in only 1 individual of a family (eg, retinitis pigmentosa [RP]). Such an individual is said to have a *simplex,* or *isolated,* form of a genetic disease. A genetically determined trait may be isolated in the pedigree for several reasons:

- The pedigree is small.
- The full expression of the disease has not been sought or has not manifested in other relatives.
- The disorder represents a new genetic mutation.
- The disorder is recessive, and the investigation to determine whether the parents are carriers has been inadequate.
- The disorder is caused by chromosomal changes.

Clinically similar disorders may be inherited in several different ways—for example, RP can occur as an autosomal dominant, autosomal recessive, or X-linked trait or result from a mitochondrial mutation. These various genetic forms represent distinct gene defects with different alterations in gene structure and different biochemical pathogeneses, each of which has similar clinical phenotypic expressions. Clarification of genetic heterogeneity is important, because only with the proper diagnosis and inheritance pattern identification can appropriate genetic counseling and prognosis be offered.

Some genetic disorders originally thought to be a single and unique entity are found, on close scrutiny, to be 2 or more fundamentally distinct entities. Further clarification of the inheritance pattern or biochemical analysis permits separation of initially similar disorders. Such has been the case for Marfan syndrome and homocystinuria. Although both disorders cause unusual body habitus and ectopia lentis, the presence of dominant inheritance, aortic aneurysms, and valvular heart disease in Marfan syndrome distinguishes it from the recessive pattern and thromboembolic disease of homocystinuria.

Genetic heterogeneity is a general term that applies to the phenotypic similarity that may be produced by 2 or more fundamentally distinct genetic entities; this term implies that the genes are nonallelic. The term *locus heterogeneity* has been used when linkage studies have shown that different families with similar phenotypes map at different loci; hence, the phenotype can be caused by mutations of different genes. When different alleles at the same locus are capable of producing an abnormal phenotype, the term *allelic heterogeneity* can be applied. With *clinical heterogeneity,* different mutations at the same locus can produce different phenotypes.

Once the location on a chromosome is determined for a particular disease gene and once the gene's molecular structure is identified, most examples of genetic heterogeneity cease to be a problem for diagnosis or classification. However, clinical, allelic, and locus heterogeneity can remain perplexing issues. For example, mutations of the Norrie disease gene, *NDP,* usually result in the typical phenotype of pseudoglioma from exudative retinal detachments, but some mutations of *NDP* have been associated with X-linked exudative vitreoretinopathy. Mutations of the proto-oncogene *RET* can give rise to medullary thyroid carcinoma, multiple endocrine neoplasia 2A and 2B, and Hirschsprung disease. Such examples give added meaning to the term *heterogeneity.* Ultimately, greater understanding of these and other disorders at the molecular and cellular levels results in more reliable patient management and improved classification of genetic disease.

> Mulvihill JJ. Craniofacial syndromes: no such thing as a single gene disease. *Nat Genet.* 1995;9(2): 101–103.
> van Heyningen V. Genetics. One gene—four syndromes. *Nature.* 1994;367(6461):319–320.

Genes and Chromosomes

In 1909, the Danish biologist Wilhelm Johannsen coined the word *genes,* from the Greek for "giving birth to," as a name for segments of the DNA molecule containing individual units of hereditary information. Genes are the basic units of inheritance, and they include the length of nucleotides that codes for a single trait or a single polypeptide chain and its associated regulatory regions. Human genes vary greatly in size, from approximately 500 base pairs (bp) to more than 2 million bp. However, more than 98% range from less than 10 kilo base pairs (kb; 1 kb = 1000 bp) to 500 kb in size. Many are considerably larger than 50 kb. Whereas a single human cell contains enough DNA for 6 million genes, about 50,000–100,000 genes are found among the 23 pairs of known chromosomes. The function of the remaining 95% of the genetic material is unknown.

The relative sequence of the genes, which are arranged linearly along the chromosome, is called the *genetic map.* The physical position or region on the chromosome occupied by a single gene is known as a *locus.* The physical contiguity of various gene loci becomes the vehicle for close association of genes with one another *(linkage)* and their clustering in groups that characteristically move together or separately *(segregation)* from one generation to the next.

Each normal human somatic cell has 46 chromosomes composed of 23 homologous pairs. Each member of a homologous pair carries matched, although not necessarily identical, genes in the same sequence. One member of each chromosome pair is inherited from the father, the other from the mother. Each normal sperm or ovum contains 23 chromosomes, one representative from each pair; thus, each parent transmits half of his or her genetic information to each child. Of the 46 chromosomes, 44 are called *autosomes* because they provide information on somatic characteristics. (The X and Y chromosomes provide such information as well; eg, genes on the Y chromosome influence teeth and height.)

The 2 *sex chromosomes* differ in males and females. Whereas males have an X chromosome and a Y chromosome, females have 2 X chromosomes. Unique to phenotypically normal males, the Y chromosome determines development of the testes and other male secondary sexual characteristics.

Bishop JE, Waldholz M. Genome: the story of the most astonishing scientific adventure of our time—the attempt to map all the genes in the human body. New York: Simon & Schuster; 1990.

Hartl DL, Jones EW, eds. *Genetics: Analysis of Genes and Genomes.* 7th ed. Sudbury, MA: Jones & Bartlett; 2009.

Rimoin DL, Connor JM, Pyeritz RL, Korf BR, eds. *Emery and Rimoin's Principles and Practice of Medical Genetics.* 5th ed. Philadelphia: Churchill Livingstone; 2007.

Alleles

Alternative forms of a particular gene at the same locus on each of an identical pair of chromosomes are called *alleles* (Greek for "reciprocals"). If both members of a pair of alleles for a given autosomal locus are identical (ie, the DNA sequence is the same), the individual is *homozygous* (a *homozygote*); if the allelic genes are distinct from each other (ie, the DNA sequence differs), the individual is *heterozygous* (a *heterozygote*). Different gene defects can cause dramatically different phenotypes and still be allelic. For example, sickle cell disease (SS hemoglobinopathy) caused by homozygosity of 1 mutant gene is significantly different from the phenotypic expression of SC hemoglobinopathy, yet the *Hb S* gene and the *Hb C* gene are allelic. The term *polyallelism* refers to the many possible variants or mutations of a single gene. Mutant proteins that correspond to mutant alleles frequently have been shown to possess slightly different biochemical properties. Among the mucopolysaccharidoses, for example, the enzyme alpha-L-iduronidase is defective in both Hurler disease and Scheie syndrome. Because these are mutations of the same gene, they are abnormalities of the same enzyme and thus allelic. However, the clinical severity of these 2 disorders (age of onset; age of detection; and severity of affliction of skeleton, liver, spleen, and cornea) is entirely different, presumably because the function of the mutant enzyme is less altered by the Scheie syndrome mutation. Because the enzyme is a protein composed of hundreds of amino acids, a mutation resulting in a base substitution within a certain codon might cause a change in 1 or more amino acids in a portion of the enzyme remote from its active site, thus reducing its effect on the enzyme's function. However, the substitution of 1 amino acid at a critical location in the enzyme's active site might abolish most or all of its enzymatic activity. Several examples of allelic disorders appear among the mucopolysaccharidoses.

The phenotype of the usual heterozygote is determined by 1 mutant allele and 1 "normal" allele. However, the genotype of a compound heterozygote comprises 2 different mutant alleles, each at the same locus. The genetic Hurler-Scheie compound heterozygote is biochemically proven and clinically manifests features intermediate between the homozygotes of the 2 alleles. Whenever detailed biochemical analysis is possible, the products of the 2 alleles manifest slightly different properties (such as rates of enzyme activity or electrophoretic migration). Among other autosomal recessive diseases, a spectrum of phenotypes can be caused by a diversity of mutant alleles occurring in various paired combinations. Most recessive diseases (as well as dominant disorders) do not permit more than speculation on this alternative in the clinical setting.

In contrast, and as noted earlier, some genetic disorders originally thought to be single and unique may, on close scrutiny, reveal 2 or more fundamentally distinct entities. Occasionally, this genetic heterogeneity is seen with diseases that are inherited in the same manner, such as tyrosinase-negative and tyrosinase-positive oculocutaneous albinism. Because these 2 conditions are phenotypically similar and each is inherited as an autosomal recessive trait, it was assumed for some time that they were allelic. When a tyrosinase-negative person bears children with a tyrosinase-positive person, the offspring appear clinically normal. This observation excludes the possibility that these 2 conditions are allelic: each condition occurs only when an offspring is heterozygous for the gene causing the condition. Separate gene loci (the tyrosinase gene and the *P* gene) are now known to cause oculocutaneous albinism. The offspring of such matings of individuals with phenotypically similar but genotypically different disorders are called *double heterozygotes* because they are heterozygous for each of the 2 loci.

Because a female has 2 X chromosomes, she may be either homozygous or heterozygous with respect to X-linked genes. A male is said to be *hemizygous* for X-linked genes because he has only a single X chromosome, and the Y chromosome has little comparable material. A person is also termed *hemizygous* for a given genetic locus when the second allele is missing, either through loss of an entire chromosome or through rearrangements resulting in deletion of any segment of 1 of a pair of chromosomes.

Mitosis

A cell may undergo 2 types of cell division—mitosis and meiosis. *Mitosis* gives rise to the multiple generations of genetically identical cells needed for the growth and maintenance of the organism. When mitosis is about to occur, the cell accurately duplicates all of its chromosomes. The replicated chromosomes then separate into 2 identical groups that migrate apart and eventually reach opposite sides of the cell. The cell and its contents then divide, forming 2 genetically identical daughter cells, each with the same diploid chromosome number and genetic information as the parent cell.

Meiosis

In contrast to mitosis, *meiosis* leads to the production of cells that have only 1 member of each chromosome pair (Fig 6-1). The specialized cells that arise from meiosis and participate in sexual reproduction are called *gametes*. The male gamete is a sperm, the female gamete, an ovum. During meiosis, a modified sequence of divisions systematically reduces the number of chromosomes in each cell by one half to the *haploid* number. Consequently, each gamete contains 23 chromosomes, 1 representative of each pair. This assortment occurs randomly, except that 1 representative of each pair of chromosomes is incorporated into each sperm or egg.

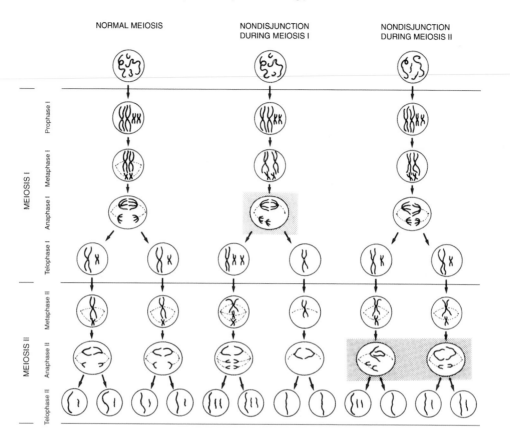

NORMAL MEIOSIS   NONDISJUNCTION DURING MEIOSIS I   NONDISJUNCTION DURING MEIOSIS II

Figure 6-1 Normal meiosis and chromosomal nondisjunction occurring at different phases of meiosis. Nondisjunction is discussed in the text.

At conception, a sperm and an ovum unite, forming a *zygote*, a single cell that contains 46 chromosomes. Because both parents contribute equally to the genetic makeup of their offspring, new and often advantageous gene combinations may emerge.

Segregation

Two allelic genes, which occupy the same gene locus on 2 homologous chromosomes, separate with the division of the 2 chromosomes during meiosis, and each goes to a different gamete. Thus, the genes are said to *segregate,* a property limited to allelic genes, which cannot occur together in a single offspring of the bearer. For example, if a parent is a compound heterozygote for both hemoglobin S and hemoglobin C, which occupy the same genetic locus on homologous chromosomes, none of the offspring will inherit both hemoglobins from that parent; each will inherit either 1 or the other.

Independent Assortment

Genes on different *(nonhomologous)* chromosomes may or may not separate together during meiotic cell division. This random process, called *independent assortment,* states that nonallelic genes assort independently of one another. Because *crossing over* (exchange of chromosomal material between the members of a pair of homologous chromosomes) can occur in meiosis, 2 nonallelic genes originally on opposite members of the chromosomal pair may end up together on either of the 2 or remain separated, depending on their original positions and on the sites of genetic interchange. Thus, the gametes of an individual with 2 nonallelic dominant traits, or *syntenic traits,* located on the same chromosome could produce 4 possible offspring. A child may inherit

- both traits if the separate alleles remain on the same chromosome and the child inherits this chromosome
- neither trait if the genes remain on 1 chromosome but the child inherits the opposite chromosome with neither allele
- only 1 of the 2 alleles if crossing over occurred between the loci, and the child received the chromosome with that particular allele

This scheme for nonallelic traits depends on the independent assortment of chromosomes in the first division of meiosis. Approximately 50 crossovers (1–3 per chromosome) occur during an average meiotic division.

Linkage

Linkage is the major exception or modification to the law of independent assortment. Nonallelic genes located reasonably close together on the same chromosome tend to be transmitted together, from generation to generation, more frequently than chance alone would allow for; thus, they are said to be linked. The closer together the 2 loci, the less likely they are to be affected by crossovers. Linear physical proximity along a chromosome cannot be considered an automatic guarantor of linkage, however. In fact, certain sites on each chromosome may be more vulnerable to homologous crossing over than others.

Jorde LB, Carey JC, Bamshad MJ, White RL. *Medical Genetics.* Updated ed. for 2006–2007. 3rd ed. Philadelphia: Elsevier Mosby; 2006.

Chromosomal Analysis

Cytogenetics is a branch of genetics concerned with the study of chromosomes and their properties. Chromosomal defects are changes in the chromosome number or structure that damage sensitive genetic functions and lead to developmental or reproductive disorders. These defects usually result from (1) a disruption of the mechanisms controlling chromosome movement during cell division or (2) alterations of chromosome structure that lead to changes in the number or arrangement of genes or to abnormal chromosomal behavior.

Chromosomal abnormalities occur in approximately 1 of 200 term pregnancies and in 1%–2% of all pregnancies involving parents over the age of 35 years. About 7% of perinatal deaths and some 40%–50% of retrievable spontaneous abortuses have significant chromosomal aberrations. Virtually any change in chromosome number during early development profoundly affects the formation of tissues and organs and the viability of the entire organism. Most major chromosomal disorders are characterized by both developmental and mental retardation, as well as a variety of somatic abnormalities.

Indications

The usual indications for chromosome analysis are listed in Table 6-1. Ophthalmologists should be aware of the value of constitutional and tumor karyotypes in infants with retinoblastoma, especially if the tumor represents a new genetic mutation. Chromosome analysis is also suggested in patients with isolated (nonfamilial) aniridia (which is often associated with Wilms tumor) and other systemic malformations and in patients who survive a neoplastic syndrome and experience a second neoplasm.

A chromosomally abnormal state in a previous child warrants consideration of amniocentesis or chorionic villus sampling for prenatal diagnosis in subsequent pregnancies to avoid the risk of recurrence. Amniocentesis can be undertaken at approximately the 16th week of pregnancy.

Preparation

Karyotype

The systematic display of chromosomes from a single somatic cell is called a *karyotype*. Chromosome preparations can be made from any tissue whose cells will divide in culture. The tissue most commonly used is peripheral venous blood, although bone marrow, skin fibroblasts, and cells from amniotic fluid or chorionic villi are useful under specific circumstances. In special situations, chromosome analyses can be obtained directly from rapidly dividing neoplastic tissues, as has been done with fresh cells from retinoblastoma and Wilms tumor.

The blood of healthy individuals without leukemia contains no dividing cells. Therefore, T lymphocytes in a small sample (often less than 5 mL) of fresh heparinized blood are

---

Table 6-1 Some Indications for Chromosome Analysis

Clinical diagnosis in newborns: multiple malformations, especially involving more than 1 organ system, with or without intrauterine growth retardation; perinatal death

Clinical diagnosis at any age: mental retardation with or without congenital malformations, in the absence of unequivocal identifiable cause; gonadal ambiguity; infertility, amenorrhea, or reproductive dysfunction; ocular malformations associated with any malformations of other organ systems with no known cause

Multiple miscarriages: spontaneous abortions or stillbirths without apparent cause, even in clinically normal parents

Studies of malignancy: constitutional and tumor karyotypes, especially leukemia, retinoblastoma, aniridia–Wilms tumor, and other embryonal malignancies; specific syndromes with high risks of malignancy-ataxia-telangiectasia, Bloom syndrome, Fanconi anemia; tumor karyotypes on all second tumors in neoplasia syndromes

Prenatal diagnosis: in advanced maternal age, known translocation carrier state, X-linked carrier state for sexing; previous child with chromosomal abnormalities; and as part of either amniocentesis or chorionic villus sampling

---

stimulated to divide by adding phytohemagglutinin to a culture medium. After approximately 72 hours, as the dividing cells approach metaphase, a drug that has colchicine-like effects is added to prevent formation of the mitotic spindle apparatus.

Fluorescence in situ hybridization and chromosome arm painting

With the *fluorescence in situ hybridization (FISH)* technique, DNA fragments from genes of interest are first tagged with a fluorescent compound and then annealed or hybridized to chromosomes. The regions of interest are stained to determine whether duplication, deletion, or rearrangement has occurred. Such fluorescent molecular probes can detect and often quantify the presence of specific DNA sequences on a chromosome and can find microscopic abnormalities that would be indiscernible by conventional cytogenetic methods.

Probes have been developed from microdissections of chromosomal regions and FISH that label entire arms of chromosomes and each of the individual chromosomes (multicolor spectral karyotyping and combinatorial multifluor FISH). With 2-color FISH, both arms of each chromosome can be simultaneously labeled (Fig 6-2). These probes are valuable for detecting and understanding the mechanisms of complex chromosomal rearrangement (Fig 6-3), such as can occur in cancer. *Chromosome arm painting (CAP)* is also being used to generate information on the 3-dimensional organization of chromatin domains within the nucleus in interphase.

Guan X-Y, Zhang H, Bittner M, Jiang Y, Meltzer P, Treat J. Chromosome arm painting probes. *Nat Genet.* 1996;12(11):10–11.

Schröck E, du Manoir S, Veldman T, et al. Multicolor spectral karyotyping of human chromosomes. *Science.* 1996;273(5274):494–497.

Speicher MR, Gwyn Ballard S, Ward DC. Karyotyping human chromosomes by combinatorial multi-fluor FISH. *Nat Genet.* 1996;12(4):368–375.

Aneuploidy of Autosomes

Aneuploidy denotes an abnormal number of chromosomes in nongametic cells. The presence of 3 homologous chromosomes in a cell rather than the normal pair is termed *trisomy. Monosomy* is the presence of only 1 member of any pair of autosomes or only 1 sex chromosome. The absence of a single autosome is almost always lethal to the embryo; an extra autosome is often catastrophic to surviving embryos. Aneuploidy of sex chromosomes (such as X, XXX, XXY, and XYY) is less disastrous. Monosomies and trisomies are generally caused by mechanical accidents that increase or decrease the number of chromosomes in the gametes. The most common type of accident, meiotic *nondisjunction,* results from a disruption of chromosome movement during meiosis (see Fig 6-1). *Polyploidy* describes a cell that contains an exact multiple of the normal diploid number, such as 3n(69) or 4n(92).

de Grouchy J, Turleau C. *Clinical Atlas of Human Chromosomes.* 2nd ed. New York: Wiley; 1984.

Jorde LB, Carey JC, Bamshad MJ, White RL. *Medical Genetics.* Updated ed. for 2006–2007. 3rd ed. Philadelphia: Elsevier Mosby; 2006.

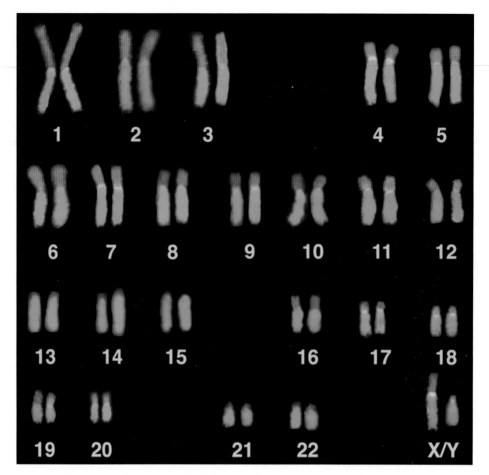

Figure 6-2 Composite karyotype of all human chromosomes hybridized with chromosome arm painting. Metaphase chromosomes were hybridized with corresponding short arm *(red)* and long arm *(green)* painting probes simultaneously, and a composite karyotype was generated. Short-arm probes were not generated for the acrocentric chromosomes 13, 14, 15, 21, and 22. Minimal regions of overlap *(yellow)* between long-arm and short-arm probes were identified for chromosomes 2, 3, 4, 7, 9, 11, 17, 18, 20, X, and Y. The size distribution of PCR-amplified microdissected DNA fragments of each individual arm were analyzed by running PCR products on 1% agarose gels. All PCR products showed a smear ranging from 200 to 600 bp with no apparent dominant bands. After PCR amplification, microdissected DNA fragments from all 19 short arms were labeled with SpectrumOrange fluorescent label (Abbott Laboratories, Des Plaines, IL) for DNA probes. The short arms of the acrocentrics were not dissected so that cross-hybridization between repetitive sequences localized on the short arms of the acrocentric chromosomes would be avoided. Microdissected DNA fragments from all long arms were labeled with biotin and detected with fluorescein-conjugated avidin (Vector Labs, Burlingame, CA). *(Reproduced with permission from Guan X-Y, Zhang H, Bittner M, Jiang Y, Meltzer P, Treat J. Chromosome arm painting probes. Nat Genet. 1996;12(11):10.)*

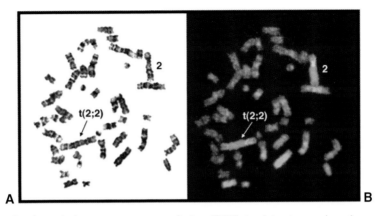

Figure 6-3 Application of chromosome arm painting (CAP) to detect complex chromosome rearrangements. A cell line with complex, defined chromosome rearrangements was identified for hybridization (human lymphoma cell line SU-DHL-4). **A,** G-banded metaphase from SU-DHL-4. **B,** The identical metaphase hybridized with CAPs 2p *(red)* and 2q *(green)*. A normal 2 and a rearranged chromosome 2[t(2;2)(q37;p13)] *(arrow)* were observed. *(Reproduced with permission from Guan X-Y, Zhang H, Bittner M, Jiang Y, Meltzer P, Treat J. Chromosome arm painting probes. Nat Genet. 1996;12(11):11.)*

Trisomy 21 syndrome

Trisomy 21 syndrome, or *Down syndrome,* is the most common chromosomal syndrome in humans, with an overall incidence of 1:800 live births. It was also the first chromosomal disease defined in humans. Clinical features of this syndrome have been well known since the British physician John Langdon Down originally described them in 1866.

The frequency of Down syndrome clearly increases with age of the mother, from about 1:1400 live births (to mothers aged 20–24 years) to approximately 1:40 live births (to mothers aged 44 years). Yet the frequency of Down syndrome is greater (1:1250) for mothers between 15 and 19 years of age than it is in the next-higher age range. Above age 50, the frequency is 1:11 live births. The eponym *Down syndrome* summarizes a clinical description of certain distinctive if variable phenotypic features, whereas the karyotype describes the chromosomal constitution of the cells and tissue studied.

The chromosomal basis of this disorder was first demonstrated by French geneticist Jerome Lejeune and coworkers in 1959. Approximately 95% of children with this disorder have an extra chromosome 21 as a result of meiotic nondisjunction. Either parent may contribute the third chromosome 21, but the most important risk factor in having a child with Down syndrome is maternal age. When it has been possible to determine where the meiotic error took place, more than 80% occurred in the first meiosis, and more than 95% occurred with maternal rather than paternal meiosis.

Approximately 5% of patients with Down syndrome have a *translocation* resulting from the attachment of the long arm of chromosome 21 with the long arm of one of the other acrocentric chromosomes, usually 14 or 22. These translocations cause pairing problems during meiosis, and the translocated fragment of chromosome 21 appears in one of the daughter cells along with a normal 21. As in nondisjunction, the fragment becomes trisomic on fertilization. Trisomy of only the distal third of chromosome 21q is sufficient to cause the disorder. Genes that lie within the q22 band of chromosome 21 appear to be specifically responsible for the pathogenesis of Down syndrome.

The increased incidence of this disorder with maternal age is principally the result of a greater likelihood of nondisjunction, because translocation errors are not related to maternal age. The extra chromosome is of paternal origin in fewer than 5% of affected individuals. A major positive correlation between advanced paternal age and an increased incidence of Down syndrome has not been established. The empirical recurrence risks to parents who have had 1 child with trisomy 21 are approximately 1%, although this number is higher among older women.

Patients with Down syndrome exhibit the following features:

- mental retardation
- short stature
- poor muscular control (hypotonia)
- brachycephaly with a broad, flat occiput
- hypoplasia of the middle phalanx of the fifth finger
- wide space between the first and second toes
- small ears
- various forms of congenital heart disease, including ventricular and atrial septal defects (40%) and, occasionally, duodenal atresia and tracheoesophageal fistulas
- infertility
- dental hypoplasia
- characteristic dermatoglyphic findings

A single palmar crease occurs in about 50% of those with Down syndrome but in only 1% of the general population. Approximately half of the infants and young children with this disorder have unspecified hearing loss. The most common ocular findings of Down syndrome are presented in Table 6-2.

Additional medical complications in patients with Down syndrome include an increased susceptibility to infection and a 20-fold to 50-fold increase in the risk of leukemia. The shortened life span in patients affected by Down syndrome is partly secondary to

---

Table 6-2 Ocular Findings in Down Syndrome (Trisomy 21)

Almond-shaped palpebral fissures
Upslanting (mongoloid) palpebral fissures
Prominent epicanthal folds
Blepharitis, usually chronic, with cicatricial ectropion
Strabismus, usually esotropic
Nystagmus (typically horizontal)
Aberrant retinal vessels (at disc)
Iris stromal hypoplasia
Brushfield spots
Keratoconus
Cataract
Myopia
Optic atrophy

these related medical problems. Studies of autopsy material from affected patients show that virtually all patients with Down syndrome over the age of 35 years develop abnormal microscopic senile plaques and neurofibrillary tangles in the brain, similar to those in Alzheimer disease. Down syndrome patients also appear to be at significantly increased risk for the cognitive symptoms of Alzheimer disease. It has been shown that the amyloid-β precursor protein (a major component of the neurofibrillary plaques that accumulate in the brain of people with Alzheimer disease) is identical to the protein that accumulates in apparently identical lesions in people with Down syndrome who are older than 35 years. The relationship of the gene for amyloid precursor protein and the form of Alzheimer disease in Down patients is unknown.

Catalano RA. Down syndrome. *Surv Ophthalmol.* 1990;34(5):385–398.

de Grouchy J, Turleau C. *Clinical Atlas of Human Chromosomes.* 2nd ed. New York: Wiley; 1984: 338–349.

Patterson D. The causes of Down syndrome. *Sci Am.* 1987;257(2):52–60.

Mosaicism

Occasionally, an individual or a tissue contains 2 or more cell lines with distinctly different chromosomal constitutions. Such individuals or tissues are termed *mosaics.* Sometimes the peripheral blood, which is the usual source for chromosomal analysis, contains populations of cells with completely different chromosomal constitutions. One population of cells may be so infrequent that a second tissue, such as skin fibroblasts, must be analyzed to demonstrate the mosaicism. It is not known if mosaicism occurs in all human tissues.

Cytogenetic defects arise because of abnormal chromosomal distribution during the early stages of embryonic development. These embryos possess 2 or more chromosomally different cell populations. Mosaicism usually results either from *mitotic nondisjunction,* in which 1 replicated chromosome fails to separate in the dividing cell; or from *anaphase lag,* in which normal separation occurs, but 1 member of the replicated pair fails to migrate and is lost.

The clinical effects of mosaicism are difficult to predict because the distribution of abnormal cells in the embryo is determined by the timing of the error and other variables. If mitotic nondisjunction immediately follows conception, the zygote divides into 2 abnormal cells, 1 trisomic and 1 monosomic. The monosomic cells rarely survive and may decrease in number or even disappear entirely over time. Mitotic nondisjunction may occur when the embryo is composed of a small population of cells. Thus, 3 populations of cells are established, 1 normal and 2 abnormal, although some abnormal cell lines may be "discarded" or lost during development. If mitotic nondisjunction occurs at a more advanced stage of development, resulting abnormal populations constitute a minority of the embryo's cells, and mosaicism may have little or no measurable effect on development.

A small population of aneuploid mosaic cells may not have a direct effect on development. However, when cells of this type occur in the reproductive tissues of otherwise normal people, some of the gametes may carry extra chromosomes or be missing some entirely. Consequently, mosaic parents tend to be at high risk for chromosomally abnormal children.

The most common example of autosomal mosaicism is *trisomy 21 mosaicism*. Some patients with trisomy 21 mosaicism have the typical features of Down syndrome; others show no abnormalities in appearance or intelligence. The critical variable seems to be the frequency and the embryologic distribution of the trisomic cells during early development, which does not necessarily correlate with the percentage of trisomic cells in any one tissue, such as peripheral blood.

Several types of sex chromosome mosaicism may occur. Again, the physical effects tend to vary, probably reflecting the quantity and distribution of the abnormal cells during development. For example, the cell population that lacks 1 of the X chromosomes can arise in a female embryo, leading to 45,X/46,XX mosaicism. In some cases, these patients develop normally; in other cases, some or all of the features of Turner syndrome appear. Similarly, the Y chromosome may be lost in some cells of a developing male embryo. This produces 45,X/46,XY mosaicism. X/XY mosaics may develop as normal males, as females with the features of Turner syndrome, or as individuals with physical characteristics intermediate between the sexes (*intersexes*, or *pseudohermaphrodites*).

Etiology of Chromosomal Aberrations

Long arm 13 deletion (13q14) syndrome: retinoblastoma

Retinoblastoma is one of several heritable childhood malignancies. Ocular tumors, which are usually noted before the age of 4 years, affect between 1 in 15,000 and 1 in 34,000 live births in the United States. The disease exhibits both hereditary occurrence (approximately 30%–40%), in which tumors tend to be bilateral and multicentric; and sporadic occurrence, in which unilateral and solitary tumors are the rule. Only about 10% of patients with hereditary retinoblastoma have a family history of the disease; the remaining 90% have a new mutation in their germ cells.

Retinoblastoma does not develop in approximately 10% of all obligate carriers of a germline mutation. In addition, a karyotypically visible deletion of part of the long arm of chromosome 13 occurs in 3%–7% of all cases of retinoblastoma. The larger this deletion, the more severe the phenotypic syndrome, which includes mental and developmental retardation, microcephaly, hand and foot anomalies, and ambiguous genitalia (Table 6-3).

Although the hereditary pattern in familial retinoblastoma is that of an autosomal dominant mutation, the defect is recessive at the cellular level. The predisposition to retinoblastoma is caused by hemizygosity of the Rb locus within human chromosome band 13q14. The Rb locus is a member of a class of genes called *recessive tumor-suppressor genes*. The alleles normally present at these loci help to prevent tumor formation. At least 1 active normal allele is needed to prevent the cell from losing control of proliferation. Patients who inherit a defective allele from 1 parent are at greater risk for losing the other allele through a number of mechanisms. Thus, tumor formation in retinoblastoma is caused by the loss of function of both normal alleles. Homozygous deletions within the 13q14 region have been noted in retinoblastomas derived from enucleated eyes.

The first step in tumorigenesis is a recessive mutation of 1 of the homologous alleles at the retinoblastoma locus by inheritance, germinal mutation, or somatic mutation. Hereditary retinoblastomas arise from a single additional somatic event in a cell that carries an inherited mutation, whereas sporadic cases require 2 somatic events. In approximately

Table 6-3 Systemic Findings in the Long Arm (13q14) Deletion Syndrome

"Failure to thrive" growth retardation
Mental retardation
Microcephaly
Trigonencephaly; scalp defect
Micrognathia
Large, malformed, low-set ears
Cleft of highly arched palate
Facial asymmetry
Congenital heart disease
Pelvic girdle anomalies
Anal atresia
Cryptorchidism, bifid scrotum
Hypospadias or epispadias, underdeveloped labia
Hypoplastic thumbs
Short incurved fourth and/or fifth finger
Foot anomalies (clubfoot, short great toe, syndactyly of the fourth and fifth toes)
Associated esterase D deficiency

50% of tumors, homozygosity for such a recessive mutation results from the mitotic loss of a portion of chromosome 13, including the 13q14 band. The resulting homozygosity for recessive mutant alleles at this locus allows the genesis of the tumor. Retinoblastoma, therefore, seemingly represents a malignancy caused by defective gene regulation rather than the presence of a dominant mutant oncogene. Those who inherit a mutant allele at this locus have a high incidence of nonocular second tumors thought to be caused by the same mutation. Almost half of these tumors are osteosarcomas.

Cavenee WK, Dryja TP, Phillips RA, et al. Expression of recessive alleles by chromosomal mechanisms in retinoblastoma. *Nature.* 1983;305(5937):779–784.

Dryja TP, Rapaport JM, Joyce JM, Petersen RA. Molecular detection of deletions involving band q14 of chromosome 13 in retinoblastomas. *Proc Natl Acad Sci USA.* 1986;83(19):7391–7394.

Friend SH, Bernards R, Rogelj S, et al. A human DNA segment with properties of the gene that predisposes to retinoblastoma and osteosarcoma. *Nature.* 1986;323(6089):643–646.

Friend SH, Dryja TP, Weinberg RA. Oncogenes and tumor-suppressing genes. *N Engl J Med.* 1988;318(10):618–622.

Godbout R, Dryja TP, Squire J, Gallie BL, Phillips RA. Somatic inactivation of genes on chromosome 13 is a common event in retinoblastoma. *Nature.* 1983;304(5925):451–453.

Lohmann DR, Brandt B, Oehlschläger U, et al. Molecular analysis and predictive testing in retinoblastoma. *Ophthalmic Genet.* 1995;16(4):135–142.

Wiggs J, Nordenskjöld M, Yandell D, et al. Prediction of the risk of hereditary retinoblastoma, using DNA polymorphisms within the retinoblastoma gene. *N Engl J Med.* 1988;318(3): 151–157.

Short arm 11 deletion (11p13) syndrome: aniridia

Aniridia (AN2) occurs from a defect of a gene that encodes a transcription factor needed for development of the eye. This developmental gene, *PAX6*, is located at 11p13. Aniridia is a panophthalmic disorder characterized by the following:

- subnormal visual acuity
- congenital nystagmus

- strabismus
- corneal pannus
- cataracts
- ectopia lentis
- glaucoma
- optic nerve hypoplasia
- foveal or macular hypoplasia
- iris absence or severe hypoplasia

Although almost all cases of aniridia result from *PAX6* mutations, a rare autosomal recessive disorder called *Gillespie syndrome* (MIM 206700) also produces partial aniridia, cerebellar ataxia, mental deficiency, and congenital cataracts.

Aniridia (often with cataract and glaucoma) can also occur sporadically in association with Wilms tumor, other genitourinary anomalies, and mental retardation, the so-called *WAGR syndrome.* This complex of findings is called a *contiguous gene-deletion syndrome* because it results from a deletion involving nearby genes. Most of the affected patients have a karyotypically visible interstitial deletion of a segment of chromosome 11p13. This region also includes the gene for the enzyme catalase, and an adjacent locus (11p12) contains the gene for lactic dehydrogenase, *LDH-A*. Patients with aniridia that is not clearly part of an autosomal dominant trait and those with coincident systemic malformations should undergo chromosomal analysis and observation for possible Wilms tumor.

When working with a new patient with aniridia, the ophthalmologist should conduct a careful biomicroscopic examination of the patient's parents for the variable expression of autosomal dominant aniridia. For female infants with isolated aniridia, a high-resolution banded chromosomal analysis is essential, as the genital variation caused by 11p deletion can be extraordinarily subtle. If a male infant with isolated aniridia has no genital aberrations, a chromosomal analysis is desirable although probably not mandatory (because of the more severe expression of 11p deletions in males). In older children without other anomalies or developmental delay, a baseline intravenous pyelogram and periodic urinalysis (for microscopic hematuria) are recommended. Intravenous pyelography is probably a more sensitive procedure than either echography or computed tomography for the embryonal malignancy associated with this chromosomal deletion.

The *PAX6* gene product is a transcription factor that is required for the normal development of the eye. Mutations of *PAX6* have also been reported in Peters anomaly, autosomal dominant keratitis, and dominant foveal hypoplasia. The mechanism for disruption of normal embryology and the degenerative disease in aniridia and other *PAX6* disorders appears to be *haploinsufficiency*, the inability of a single active allele to activate transduction of the developmental genes that are regulated by the *PAX6* gene product. In this way, aniridia is different from retinoblastoma and Wilms tumor, which result from an absence of both functional alleles at each of the homologous gene loci.

de Grouchy J, Turleau C. *Clinical Atlas of Human Chromosomes.* 2nd ed. New York: Wiley; 1984: 208–209.

Fearon ER, Vogelstein B, Feinberg AP. Somatic deletion and duplication of genes on chromosome 11 in Wilms' tumours. *Nature.* 1984;309(5964):176–178.

Littlefield JW. Genes, chromosomes, and cancer. *J Pediatr.* 1984;104(4):489–494.

Solomon E. Recessive mutation in aetiology of Wilms' tumour. *Nature.* 1984;309(5964): 111–112.

Mutations

Change in the structure or sequence of a gene is called a *mutation.* A mutation can occur more or less randomly anywhere along the DNA sequence of a gene and may result when one nucleotide is substituted for another (sometimes called a *point mutation*). A mutation that occurs in a noncoding portion of the gene may or may not be of clinical consequence. Similarly, a mutation may structurally alter a protein but in a manner that does not notably compromise its function. A new mutation that compromises function appears in a given gene as the gene is transmitted from parent to offspring at a frequency of approximately 1 in a million. Mutations are more likely within certain genes than in others. Aniridia has a mutation rate (mutations/locus/generation) of 2.5–5.0×10^{-6}; retinoblastoma's rate is 5.0–12.0×10^{-6}. Two examples of disorders with even higher mutation rates are von Recklinghausen neurofibromatosis 1 and Duchenne muscular dystrophy, each with an estimated mutation rate of approximately 0.4–1.0×10^{-4}.

A classic example of a simple point mutation is sickle cell anemia, which affects approximately 1 in 600 African Americans. This disorder results from a mutant gene that defines the sequence of amino acids in the β-polypeptide chain of adult hemoglobin. In sickle cell hemoglobin, the valine is substituted for glutamic acid at the sixth position in the β-polypeptide chain. This substitution is caused by an abnormal specific base, where adenine is substituted for thymine. This seemingly small alteration causes a profound reduction of solubility when hemoglobin is deoxygenated: red blood cells tend to become deformed into a characteristic sickle shape when the partial pressure of oxygen is low.

More gross mutations may involve deletion, translocation, insertion, or internal duplication of a portion of the DNA. Some mutations cause either destruction of the offspring or sterility. Others are less harmful or are potentially beneficial and become established in subsequent generations. Mutations can occur spontaneously for reasons that are not understood. They may also be produced by a variety of environmental agents called *mutagens,* such as radiation, viruses, and certain chemicals.

Mutations may arise in somatic as well as germinal cells, but these are not transmitted to subsequent generations. Somatic mutations in humans are difficult to identify, but some account for the inception of certain forms of neoplasia (eg, retinoblastoma).

Jorde LB, Carey JC, Bamshad MJ, White RL. *Medical Genetics.* Updated ed. for 2006–2007. 3rd ed. Philadelphia: Elsevier Mosby; 2006.

Polymorphisms

Many mutations have either little or no deleterious effect on the organism. A *polymorphism* is defined as the occurrence of 2 or more alleles at a specific locus with a frequency greater than 1% each. At least one third of all structural genes may exist in polymorphic forms. For example, at least 400 variants of hemoglobin are known, many with essentially no detectable phenotypic abnormalities. Similarly, several dozen functional and electrophoretic variants of glucose-6-phosphate dehydrogenase exist; again, many have no significant effect on the biochemical function of the affected individual. Finding additional polymorphisms will be important for the completion of gene mapping and for linkage to human diseases.

Genome, Genotype, Phenotype

The *genome* is the sum total of the genetic material within a cell or of an organism—thus, the total genetic endowment. By contrast, the *genotype* defines the genetic constitution, and thus biological capacity, with regard to a specific locus (eg, individual blood groups or a specific single enzyme). *Phenotype* indicates the total observable or manifest physical, physiologic, biochemical, or molecular characteristics of an individual, which are determined by the genotype but can be modified by the environment.

A clinical picture produced entirely by environmental factors that nevertheless closely resembles, or is even identical with, a phenotype is known as a *phenocopy*. Thus, for example, the pigmentary retinopathy of congenital rubella has occasionally been confused with a hereditary dystrophic disorder of the retinal pigment epithelium (RPE). Similarly, chloroquine-induced changes in the corneal epithelium resemble those seen as cornea verticillata in the X-linked dystrophic disorder Fabry disease.

Single-Gene Disorders

Approximately 4500 different diseases are known to be caused by a defect in a single gene. As a group, these disorders are called *monogenic,* or *mendelian, diseases.* They most often show 1 of 3 patterns of inheritance: autosomal dominant, autosomal recessive, or X-linked. Disorders of mtDNA are inherited in a fourth manner, termed *maternal inheritance.* These mtDNA disorders obey galtonian rather than mendelian inheritance characteristics.

Variability

Variability is an intrinsic property of human genetic disease that reflects the quantitative and qualitative differences in phenotype among individuals with the "same" mutant allele. Even within the homogeneous population of a single family with a genetic disease, each affected individual may manifest the disease to a different degree, with different features, or at a different age. Steinert myotonic dystrophy, for example, presents its features of motor myotonia, characteristic cataracts, gonadal atrophy, and presenile baldness with a wide variation in severity and age of detection. Even within a single family, the cataracts may begin to affect vision any time from the second to the seventh decade of life.

Such variability of clinical manifestation led to the concept of *anticipation,* the phenomenon of apparently earlier and more severe onset of a disease in successive generations within a family. Before 1990, most geneticists thought that anticipation was not a biological phenomenon but an artifact of ascertainment. With the relatively recent discovery of triplet or trinucleotide tandem-repeat expansion diseases, anticipation has been shown to reflect the increased length of trinucleotide tandem repeats from 1 generation to the next. Myotonic dystrophy, fragile-X syndrome, Huntington disease, and a form of spinobulbar muscular atrophy called *Kennedy disease* are some of the diseases whose discovery contributed to the rejuvenation of the concept of anticipation.

Some human variability may result from the intrinsic differences in genetic background of every human being. Other recognizable or presumptive influences on the variable intra- or interfamilial phenotype of the same gene include the following:

- sex influences or limitations
- maternal factors such as intrauterine environment and even cytoplasmic (eg, mitochondrial) inheritance factors
- modifying loci
- genetic heterogeneity, including both isoalleles and genocopies
- gene alterations induced either by position effects with other genes or by somatic mutations

Obviously, nongenetic factors extrinsic to a cell, tissue, or organism such as diet, temperature, and drugs may effect major changes in gene expression, either as phenocopies or through ecologic parameters.

Penetrance

The presence or absence of any effect of a gene is called *penetrance*. If a gene generates any evidence of phenotypic features, no matter how minimal, it is termed *penetrant;* if it is not expressed at any level of detection, it is termed *nonpenetrant.* Thus, penetrance is an all-or-nothing concept, statistically representing the fraction of individuals carrying a given gene that manifests any evidence of the specific trait. In families with an autosomal dominant mutant gene that has 100% penetrance of the phenotype, an average of 50% of the offspring will inherit the gene and show evidence of the disease.

Even though penetrance has an exact statistical definition, its clinical ascertainment is affected by diagnostic awareness and the methods of physical examination. For example, many mild cases of Marfan syndrome would be missed without careful biomicroscopy of the fully dilated pupil and echocardiography of the heart valves and great vessels. Similarly, if the criteria for identification of the retinoblastoma gene include indirect ophthalmoscopy and scleral depression, some "nonpenetrant" parents or siblings in families with "dominantly inherited" retinoblastoma may be found to have a spontaneously involuted tumor, which clearly identifies them as bearers of the gene. In another example, some family members who have a gene for Best macular dystrophy will be identified not by clinical ophthalmoscopic examination but only by electro-oculographic testing. Therefore, in examining a potential bearer of a gene, the examiner must carefully search for any manifestations of the gene's effects in all susceptible tissues before dismissing someone as a "skipped generation."

Expressivity

The presence of a defective gene does not necessarily imply a complete expression of every potential manifestation. The variety of ways and levels of severity in which a particular genetic trait manifests its presence among different affected individuals is called *expressivity.*

In von Recklinghausen disease, for example, an affected child may have only café-au-lait spots. The affected parent may have Lisch nodules of the iris, extensive punctiform and pedunculated neurofibromas of the skin, a huge plexiform neurofibroma of 1 lower extremity, and a glioma of the anterior visual pathway. It is extremely rare that all affected members in the same family have uniform textbook presentations of the disorder.

Differences in the age of onset of manifestation are one way that expressivity commonly varies in dominant disorders. In von Recklinghausen disease, for example, the affected child may have only café-au-lait spots at birth, develop iris Lisch nodules that gradually increase in number and size at about age 5–10 years, develop punctiform neurofibromas of the skin in early adolescence, experience subareolar neurofibromas post-puberty (females), and experience visual impairment from the effect of an optic glioma in the late teens. Although all of these features are phenotypic components of the mutant gene, each feature has a characteristic age of onset and a natural history of growth and effect within the umbrella of the total disease.

Pleiotropism

Alteration within a single mutant gene may have consequences in various tissues in a given individual. The presentation of multiple phenotypic abnormalities produced by a single mutant gene is termed *pleiotropism*. For example, in Marfan syndrome, ectopia lentis is coupled with arachnodactyly, aortic aneurysms, and long extremities. Optic atrophy is found in association with juvenile diabetes mellitus, diabetes insipidus, and moderate perceptive hearing impairment in an autosomal recessive syndrome known as the *DIDMOAD* (*d*iabetes *i*nsipidus, *d*iabetes *m*ellitus, *o*ptic *a*trophy, and neural *d*eafness) *syndrome*. Neurosensory hearing loss can also be associated with hereditary hematuric nephritis, lenticular changes (anterior lenticonus, spherophakia, cataracts), arcus juvenilis, and whitish yellow retinal lesions in the dominantly inherited Alport syndrome. Similarly, the Bardet-Biedl syndrome comprises pigmentary retinopathy, obesity, genital hypoplasia, mental debility, and polydactyly. In each of these disorders, a single mutant gene is responsible for dysfunction in multiple systems.

Frequently, however, a disease is mistakenly termed "pleiotropic" when several different disorders with the same inheritance pattern and similar clinical manifestations are actually present. Thus, Leber congenital amaurosis has been attributed to a single pleiotropic gene. Based on the symmetry of the phenotype of affected siblings in individual families, however, the more likely conclusion is that the clinical disease is heterogeneous and is indeed caused by several genes (not necessarily allelic), each of which is autosomal recessive.

Racial and Ethnic Concentration of Genetic Disorders

Most genetic diseases occur without regard to the affected individual's racial or ethnic background. Some, however, are concentrated in certain population groups.

Tay-Sachs disease, with its characteristic macular cherry-red spot, occurs predominantly in persons of Eastern European Jewish (Ashkenazi) ancestry, especially those whose ancestors lived in northeastern Poland and southern Lithuania. An estimated rate of 1 in 30 for carriers of this disorder in the Jewish population of New York City compares with an estimated carrier rate of 1 in 300 in non-Jewish Americans. Although the reported incidence of this disorder among Ashkenazi Jewish newborns is 1 in 6000, the actual incidence among this population may be closer to 1 in 3600 births. Approximately 50 new cases occur each year in the United States. In addition, familial dysautonomia *(Riley-Day syndrome)* with hypolacrima, corneal hypoesthesia, exodeviation, and methacholine-induced miosis also occurs more frequently in persons of Ashkenazi ancestry, as do *Gaucher disease* and *Niemann-Pick disease.*

A variety of *achromatopsia* (complete color blindness) with *myopia* is common on the South Pacific island of Pingelap, affecting 5% of the Pingelapese population in the Caroline Islands of Micronesia. *Oguchi disease* is seen primarily, although not exclusively, in Japanese people. Similarly, *sickle cell hemoglobinopathies* are inherited largely among blacks.

The prevalence of *oculocutaneous albinism* is high among the Kuna Indians in Panama. *Hermansky-Pudlak syndrome* occurs with a higher frequency in persons of Puerto Rican ancestry. With this tyrosinase-positive phenotype of autosomal recessively inherited oculocutaneous albinism, findings include a history of easy bruisability and bleeding tendency, associated with a prolonged bleeding time and abnormal platelet aggregation. Some specific human malformations occur with greater frequency in certain races than in others. For example, polydactyly is approximately 10 times more frequent in blacks than in whites, and preauricular sinus may be equally more frequent in blacks.

Patterns of Inheritance

Recessivity Versus Dominance

The terms *dominant* and *recessive* were first used by Gregor Mendel. In classical genetics, a dominant gene is one that is always expressed with similar phenotype, whether the mutant gene is present in a homozygous or heterozygous state. Stated simply, a dominant gene is one that is expressed when present in only a single copy. A gene is called *recessive* when its expression is masked by a normal allele or, more precisely, when it is expressed only in the homozygote (or compound heterozygote) when both alleles at a specific locus are mutant.

A *trait* is the consequence of the gene's action. It is the trait, or phenotypic expression of the gene at a clinical level, rather than the gene itself that is dominant or recessive. A trait is recessive if its expression is suppressed by the presence of a normal gene (as in galactosemia) and dominant if it is apparently unaffected by a single copy of the normal allele (as in Marfan syndrome). If the alleles are different and yet they are both manifested in the phenotype, they are said to be *codominant.* Examples of codominant inheritance include the ABO and MN blood types, leukocyte antigens, and the hemoglobins.

As a result of transcription, a gene may have a greater or lesser effect on the individual or an organ, and therefore the trait may be more or less apparent. Thus, the designation of a trait as either dominant or recessive depends on the testing method used. For example, sickle cell hemoglobinopathy is recessive if the clinical disease is considered, dominant if the sickle preparation test is positive, and codominant if hemoglobin electrophoresis is used to look for the specific product of each allele.

Although, classically, a dominant gene is one that has the same phenotype when the mutant allele is present in either the heterozygous or the homozygous state, most dominant medical diseases stray from this strict definition. For many dominant disorders, individuals who are homozygous for a mutant allele or who harbor 2 mutant alleles (1 on each homologous chromosome) will have more severe expression.

In experiments, the biochemical mechanisms of "dominant" hereditary diseases appear different from those of "recessive" disorders. Recessive traits usually result from enzyme deficiency caused by structural mutations of the gene specifying the affected enzyme. The altered enzyme often can be shown to be structurally abnormal or unstable. Heterozygotes usually have approximately 50% of normal enzyme activity but are clinically unaffected, implying that half of the normal enzyme activity is compatible with near-normal function. If adequate biochemical testing can be performed and the specific enzyme isolated, the reduced enzyme activity can be quantified and the heterozygous genetic state inferred. Thus, clinically unaffected heterozygotes can be detected for such disorders as homocystinuria (decrease in cystathionine β-synthase), galactokinase deficiency (low blood galactokinase activity), classic galactosemia (galactose-1-phosphate uridyl transferase deficiency), gyrate atrophy of the choroid and retina (decreased ornithine-δ-aminotransferase), and Tay-Sachs disease (decreased hexosaminidase A). Table 6-4 outlines several disorders with ocular manifestations for which an enzyme defect is known.

Autosomal Recessive Inheritance

An autosomal recessive disease is expressed fully only in the presence of a mutant gene at the same locus on both homologous chromosomes (ie, homozygosity for a mutant gene) or 2 different mutant alleles at the same locus (compound heterozygosity). A single mutant allele is sufficient to cause a recessive disorder if the normal allele on the homologous chromosome is deleted. A recessive trait can remain latent through several generations until the chance mating of 2 heterozygotes for a mutant allele gives rise to an affected individual. The frequency of heterozygotes for a given disorder will always be considerably greater than that of homozygotes. It is estimated that all human beings inherit about 6 or 7 mutations for different recessive disorders for which they are heterozygotes.

Enzymatic defects

Autosomal recessive diseases often result from defects in enzymatic proteins. Most of the so-called inborn errors of metabolism that result from enzymatic defects are autosomal recessive traits, although a few are X-linked recessive disorders (eg, Lesch-Nyhan syndrome). The defect in *alkaptonuria* involves homogentisic acid oxidase, an enzyme involved in the metabolism of homogentisic acid. Large amounts of homogentisic acid are excreted in the urine, which turns black when mixed with alkali or exposed to light or air. The black urine causes diaper stains, calling attention to the condition. In addition, aggregates of homogentisic acid accumulate in the body, becoming attached to the collagen of cartilage and other connective tissues. The cartilage of the ears and nose and the collagenous sclera are stained black or brownish blue. These manifestations are called

Table 6-4 Known Enzyme Disorders and Corresponding Ocular Signs

Disorder	Defective Enzyme	Ocular Sign
Storage diseases		
Fabry disease	Ceramide trihexosidase (α-galactosidase)	Corneal epithelial verticillate changes; aneurysmal dilation and tortuosity of retinal and conjunctival vessels
Krabbe leukodystrophy	Cerebroside α-galactosidase	Macular cherry-red spot; optic atrophy
Mannosidosis	α-mannosidase	Lenticular opacities
Metachromatic leukodystrophy	Arylsulfatase A	Retinal discoloration, degeneration
Hurler (mucopolysaccharidosis I H)	α-L-iduronidase	Corneal opacity; pigmentary retinal degeneration
Hunter (mucopolysaccharidosis II)	Sulfoiduronate sulfatase	Corneal opacity (mild type); older-age patients
Scheie (mucopolysaccharidosis I S)	α-L-iduronidase	Corneal opacity; pigmentary retinal degeneration
Sanfilippo (mucopolysaccharidosis III)	Heparan sulfate sulfatase	Pigmentary retinal degeneration; optic atrophy
Tay-Sachs disease (GM_2 gangliosidosis, type I)	Hexosaminidase A	Macular cherry-red spot; optic atrophy
Sandhoff disease (GM_2 gangliosidosis, type II)	Hexosidase A and B	Macular cherry-red spot
GM_1 gangliosidosis, type I (generalized gangliosidosis)	β-galactosidase	Macular cherry-red spot; optic atrophy; corneal clouding (mild)
Metabolic disorders		
Alkaptonuria	Homogentisic acid oxidase	Dark sclera
Albinism	Tyrosinase	Foveal hypoplasia; nystagmus; iris transillumination
Intermittent ataxia	Pyruvate dicarboxylase	Nystagmus
Crigler-Najjar syndrome	Glucuronide transferase	Extraocular movement
Ehlers-Danlos syndrome VI	Lysyl hydroxylase	Microcornea; retinal detachment; ectopia lentis; blue scleras
Familial dysautonomia	Dopamine-β-hydroxylase	Alacrima; corneal hypoesthesia; exodeviation; methacholine-induced miosis
Galactokinase deficiency	Galactokinase	Cataracts
Galactosemia	Galactose-1-phosphate uridyl transferase	Cataracts
Gyrate atrophy of the choroid and retina	Ornithine aminotransferase	Degeneration of the choroid and retina; cataracts; myopia
Homocystinuria	Cystathionine synthase	Dislocated lens
Hyperglycinemia	Glycine cell transport	Optic atrophy
Leigh necrotizing encephalopathy	Pyruvate carboxylase	Optic atrophy
Maple syrup urine disease	Branch chain decarboxylase	Ophthalmoplegia; nystagmus
Niemann-Pick disease	Sphingomyelinase	Macular cherry-red spot
Refsum syndrome	Phytanic acid oxidase	Retinal degeneration
Tyrosinosis	Tyrosine aminotransferase	Corneal dystrophy
Sulfite oxidase deficiency	Sulfite oxidase	Ectopia lentis
Tyrosinemia	Tyrosine aminotransferase	Lens opacity

ochronosis. The coloration in the sclera assumes a more or less triangular form, with a limbic base in the region of the palpebral tissue. In the joints, such as those of the spine, the accumulations lead to arthritis. Alkaptonuria is an example of a genetic enzyme block in which the phenotypic features are caused by the accumulation of excess substances just proximal to the block.

In some other disorders with genetic blocks in metabolism, the phenotypic consequences are related to the lack of a normal product distal to the block. An example is *albinism,* in which the metabolic block involves a step between the amino acid tyrosine and the formation of melanin. In still other inborn errors of metabolism, the phenotypic expression results from excessive production of a product through a normally alternative and minor metabolic pathway. *Phenylketonuria,* like alkaptonuria and albinism, is a genetic defect in aromatic amino acid metabolism. The defect is in the enzyme involved in the conversion of phenylalanine to tyrosine. In an affected person, hair and skin pigmentation is reduced. Severe mental retardation is one of the most prominent symptoms. Alternative metabolites of phenylalanine, especially phenylpyruvic acid, are excreted in the urine, providing one basis for diagnosis of the disorder.

The difference in phenotype of these 3 diseases—alkaptonuria, albinism, and phenylketonuria—is noteworthy, although the diseases involve closely related metabolic pathways.

Carrier heterozygotes

The heterozygous carrier of a mutant gene may show minimal evidence of the gene defect, particularly at a biochemical level. Thus, carrier heterozygotes have been detected by a variety of methods:

- identification of abnormal metabolites by electrophoresis (eg, galactokinase deficiency)
- liver biopsy (eg, phenylketonuria)
- hair bulb assay (eg, oculocutaneous albinism and Fabry disease)
- monitoring of enzyme activity in leukocytes (eg, galactose-1-phosphate uridyl transferase in galactosemia), fibroblasts from skin culture (eg, ornithine-δ-aminotransferase deficiency in gyrate atrophy of the retina and choroid), serum, and tears (eg, hexosaminidase A in Tay-Sachs disease)

In contrast to the transmission of dominant traits, most matings resulting in recessive disorders involve phenotypically normal heterozygous parents. Out of 4 offspring produced by carrier parents with the same gene for an autosomal recessive disease, usually 1 will be affected (homozygote), 2 will be carriers (heterozygotes), and 1 will be genetically and phenotypically normal. Thus, clinically normal heterozygous parents will produce offspring with a ratio of 1 clinically affected to 3 clinically normal. There is no predilection for either sex. In 2-child families, the patient with a recessive disease is frequently the only affected family member. For instance, approximately 40%–50% of patients with RP have no family history of the disorder. However, their age of onset, rate of progression, and other phenotypic characteristics are similar to those with defined recessive inheritance patterns.

Once 1 child is born with a recessive disorder, the genetic risk for each subsequent child of the same parents is 25%. This concept has specific implications for genetic counseling. All offspring of an affected individual will be carriers; they are unlikely to be affected with the disorder unless their clinically unaffected parent is also by chance a carrier of the gene. However, because a specific method for identifying a carrier is lacking with most recessive diseases, the normal-appearing sibling of a child with a recessive disorder has a statistical risk of 2 chances in 3 of being a genetic carrier. This liability must be accounted for in any equation to predict the small risk that a normal-appearing sibling will have an affected child.

Consanguinity

The mating of close relatives can increase the probability that their children will inherit a homozygous genotype for recessive traits, particularly for relatively rare ones. For example, the probability that the same allele is present in first cousins is 1 in 8. In the offspring of a first-cousin marriage, 1 of every 16 of the genes is commonly present in a homozygous state. It follows that each offspring from a first-cousin marriage has a 1 in 16 chance of manifesting an autosomal recessive trait within a given family. Approximately 1% of all marriages may be consanguineous. A vigorous search for consanguinity between the parents should be made in any case of a rare recessive disease. Although its occurrence is not rare, incest is a form of consanguinity that is often not acknowledged.

The expression of common recessive genes, by contrast, is less influenced by inbreeding, because most homozygous offspring are the progeny of unrelated parents. This is usually the case with such frequent disorders as sickle cell disease and cystic fibrosis. The characteristics of autosomal recessive inheritance are summarized in Table 6-5.

François J. *Heredity in Ophthalmology.* St Louis: Mosby; 1961:86–92.

Pseudodominance

Occasionally, an affected homozygote mates with a heterozygote. Of their offspring, 50% will be carriers and 50% will be affected homozygotes. Because this segregation pattern mimics that of dominant inheritance, it is called *pseudodominance.* Fortunately, such matings are usually rare and are unlikely to affect more than 2 vertical generations.

Table 6-5 Characteristics of Autosomal Recessive Inheritance

The mutant gene usually does not cause clinical disease (recessive) in the heterozygote.
Individuals inheriting both the genes (homozygote) of the defective type express the disorder.
Typically, the trait appears only in siblings, not in their parents or offspring or in other relatives.
The ratio of normal to affected in a sibship is 3:1. The larger the sibship, the more often will more than one child be affected.
The sexes are affected in equal proportions.
Parents of the affected person may be genetically related (consanguinity); the rarer the trait, the more likely.
Affected individuals have children who, although phenotypically normal, are carriers (heterozygotes) of the gene.

Familial penetrance

Penetrance of recessive disorders within families is rarely if ever incomplete. Expressivity of recessive disorders is characteristically more uniform among affected siblings within families, as each affected individual apparently has a double dose of the same gene. However, age of onset, severity, and rate of progression may vary appreciably among families with the same apparent genetic disease. These variations may reflect intrinsic constitutional differences among families or the modifying effects of unrelated, unknown genes in different families. Alternative (even nonallelic) genes, which cause distantly similar phenotypic diseases, may cause dissimilar expression, as might environmental modifiers.

If the homozygote is defined as a specific base (pair) substitution in a codon, many "autosomal recessive" diseases result from genetically compound heterozygotes—that is, individuals who have 2 different (but both "defective") alleles at a given locus. Whenever detailed biochemical or molecular testing becomes possible, the products of different alleles will show slightly different properties or behaviors. Hemoglobin sickle cell disease and Hurler-Scheie syndrome are well-established compound heterozygote disorders.

Autosomal Dominant Inheritance

When an autosomal allele leads to a regular, clearly definable abnormality in the heterozygote, the trait is termed *dominant*. The first pedigree to be interpreted in terms of mendelian dominant inheritance was a family with brachydactyly (short fingers) reported by Farabee in 1903. Autosomal dominant traits often represent defects in structural nonenzymatic proteins, such as in fibrillin in Marfan syndrome or collagen in Stickler syndrome. In addition, a dominant mode of inheritance has been observed for some malignant neoplastic syndromes, such as retinoblastoma, von Hippel–Lindau disease, tuberous sclerosis, and Gardner syndrome. Although the neoplasias in these diseases are inherited as autosomal dominant traits, the tumors themselves result from loss of function of both alleles of autosomal recessive tumor-suppressor genes.

Almost all bearers of dominant disorders in the human population are heterozygotes. In dominant inheritance, the heterozygote is clinically affected, and a single dose of the mutant gene interferes with normal function. Occasionally, depending on the frequency of the abnormal gene in the population and the phenotype, 2 bearers of the same abnormality marry and produce children. Any offspring of 2 heterozygous parents has a 25% risk of being an affected homozygote. This circumstance has been recorded in achondroplastic dwarfism. The homozygous achondroplastic dwarf has severe cranial and thoracic skeletal disorders and dies at an early age. Because the heterozygote has 1 normal allele and the homozygote has none, it is not surprising that the phenotype of the homozygote is more severely abnormal. Homozygotes (or double heterozygotes) for autosomal dominant RP also appear to have a much more severe form of retinal degeneration.

It has been suggested that dominant diseases are caused by mutations affecting structural proteins, such as cell receptor growth factors (eg, *FGFR2* in Crouzon disease), or by functional deficits generated by abnormal polypeptide subunits (eg, unstable hemoglobins). The dominant disorders aniridia and Waardenburg syndrome result from loss of 1 of the 2 alleles for the developmental transcription factors *PAX6* and *PAX3,* respectively.

However, it is not at all clear exactly how a single gene abnormality can produce the pleiotropic manifestations of such dominant diseases as von Recklinghausen neurofibromatosis or tuberous sclerosis.

In some instances, dominantly inherited traits are not clinically expressed. In other instances—such as with some families with autosomal dominant RP—pedigree analysis infrequently shows a defective gene in individuals who do not manifest any discernible clinical or functional impairment. This situation is called *incomplete penetrance,* or *skipped generation.*

Conclusive evidence of autosomal dominant inheritance requires demonstration of the disease in at least 3 successive generations. Transmission of the disorder from male to male, with both sexes showing the typical disease, must also occur. The characteristics of autosomal dominant inheritance with complete (100%) penetrance are summarized in Table 6-6. In the usual clinical situation, any offspring of an affected heterozygote with a dominant disorder has 1 chance in 2 of inheriting the mutant gene and thereby demonstrating some effect, regardless of sex. The degree of variability in the expression of certain traits is usually more pronounced in autosomal dominantly inherited disorders than in other types of genetic disorders. Moreover, when a clinical disorder is inherited in more than 1 mendelian pattern, the dominantly inherited disorder is, in general, clinically less severe than the recessively inherited one.

Counseling for recurrence risk of autosomal dominant traits must involve thorough examination of not only the affected person (who may have the full syndrome) but also the parents. If 1 parent is even mildly affected, the risk of additional genetically affected siblings rises to 50%. It is unacceptable to miss variable expressivity when parents and other family members can be examined. In some ocular disorders, family members can inherit a gene for a dominant trait and not show clinically apparent manifestations; electrophysiologic testing must be used to detect the impairment. An example is Best vitelliform macular dystrophy, in which clinically normal family members can be diagnosed as having the gene for this disorder only by the presence of an abnormal electro-oculographic light:dark (peak:trough) ratio.

Table 6-6 Characteristics of Autosomal Dominant Inheritance With Complete Penetrance

The trait appears in multiple generations (vertical transmission).

Affected males and females are equally likely to transmit the trait to male and female offspring. Thus, male-to-male transmission occurs.

Each affected individual has an affected parent, unless the condition arose by new mutation in the given individual.

Males and females are affected in equal proportions.

Unaffected persons do not transmit the trait to their children.

The trait is expressed in the heterozygote but is more severe in the homozygote.

The age of fathers of isolated (new mutation) cases is usually advanced.

The more severely the trait interferes with survival and reproduction, the greater the proportion of isolated (new mutation) cases.

Variability in expression of the trait from generation to generation and between individuals in the same generation is expected.

Affected persons transmit the trait to 50% of their offspring on average.

X-Linked Inheritance

A trait determined by genes on either of the sex chromosomes is properly termed *sex-linked*. This genetic pattern became widely known with the occurrence of hemophilia in European and Russian royal families.

The rules governing all modes of sex-linked inheritance can be derived logically by considering the chromosomal basis. Females have 2 X chromosomes, 1 of which will go to each ovum. Males have both an X and a Y chromosome. The male parent contributes his only X chromosome to all his daughters and his only Y chromosome to all his sons. Traits determined by genes carried on the Y chromosome are called *holandric* and are transmitted from a father to 100% of his sons. Among these Y chromosomal genes is the *testis-determining factor* (*TDF*—also called *sex-determining region Y,* or *SRY*). Genes controlling tooth size, stature, and spermatogenesis are also on the Y chromosome. Finally, a gene determining hairy pinnae (ie, hair on the outer rim of the ear) may also be located on the Y chromosome. All other sex-linked traits or diseases are thought to result from genes on the X chromosome and are properly termed *X-linked*. Some X-linked conditions have considerable frequencies in human populations; the various protan and deutan color vision defects were also among the first human traits assigned to a specific chromosome.

The distinctive feature of X-linked inheritance, both dominant and recessive, is the absence of father-to-son transmission. Because the male X chromosome passes only to daughters, all daughters of an affected male will inherit the mutant gene.

X-linked recessive inheritance

A male has only 1 representative of any X-linked gene and therefore is said to be *hemizygous* for the gene, rather than homozygous or heterozygous. Because there is no normal gene to balance a mutant X-linked gene in the male, its resulting phenotype, whether dominant or recessive, will always be expressed. A female may be heterozygous or homozygous for a mutant X-linked gene. X-linked traits are commonly called *recessive* if they are caused by genes located on the X chromosome, as these genes express themselves fully only in the absence of the normal allele. Thus, males (with their single X chromosome) are predominantly affected. All their phenotypically healthy but heterozygous daughters are carriers. By contrast, each son of a heterozygous woman has an equal chance of being normal or hemizygously affected.

A female will be affected with an X-linked recessive trait under a limited number of circumstances:

- She is homozygous for the mutant gene by inheritance (ie, from an affected father and a heterozygous mother).
- Her mother is heterozygous and her father contributes a new mutation.
- She has Turner syndrome, with only 1 X chromosome, and therefore is effectively hemizygous.
- She has a partial deletion of 1 X chromosome, either by rearrangement or by formation of an isochromosome, and is thereby effectively hemizygous.
- She has a highly unusual skewing of inactivation of her normal X chromosome, as explained by the Lyon hypothesis (discussed later in the chapter in Lyonization).
- Her disorder is actually an autosomal genocopy of the X-linked condition.

Table 6-7 summarizes the characteristics of X-linked recessive inheritance, which should be considered if all affected individuals in a family are males, especially if they are related through historically unaffected women (eg, uncle and nephew, or multiple affected half brothers with different fathers).

X-linked dominant inheritance

X-linked dominant traits are caused by mutant genes expressed in a single dose and carried on the X chromosome. Thus, both heterozygous women and hemizygous men are clinically affected. Females are affected nearly twice as frequently as males. All daughters of males with the disease are affected. However, all sons of affected males are free of the trait unless their mothers are also affected. Because only children of affected males provide information in discriminating X-linked dominant from autosomal dominant disease, it may be impossible to distinguish these modes on genetic grounds when the pedigree is small or the available data are scarce. Some X-linked dominant disorders, such as incontinentia pigmenti (Bloch-Sulzberger syndrome), may prove lethal to the hemizygous male. X-linked hypophosphatemic rickets (vitamin D–resistant rickets) is an example of an X-linked dominant disease. The characteristics of X-linked dominant inheritance are summarized in Table 6-8.

Jorde LB, Carey JC, Bamshad MJ, White RL. *Medical Genetics.* Updated ed. for 2006–2007. 3rd ed. Philadelphia: Elsevier Mosby; 2006.

X-linked disorders

Females with X-linked diseases have milder symptoms than males. Occasionally, males may be affected severely enough that they die before the reproductive period, thus preventing transmission of the gene. Such is the case with Duchenne muscular dystrophy, in which most affected males die before their midteens. In other disorders, males are so

---

Table 6-7 Characteristics of X-linked Recessive Inheritance

Usually only males are affected.
An affected male transmits the gene to all of his daughters (obligate carriers) and none of his sons.
All daughters of affected males, even those phenotypically normal, are carriers.
Affected males in a family either are brothers or are related to one another through carrier females (eg, maternal uncles).
If an affected male has children with a carrier female, 50% of their daughters will be homozygous and affected and 50% will be heterozygous and carriers.
Heterozygous females may rarely be affected (manifesting heterozygotes) because of lyonization.
Female carriers transmit the gene on average to 50% of their sons, who are affected, and to 50% of their daughters, who will in turn be carriers.

Table 6-8 Characteristics of X-Linked Dominant Inheritance

Both males and females are affected, but the incidence of the trait is approximately twice as great in females as in males (unless the trait is lethal in the male).
An affected male transmits the trait to all of his daughters and to none of his sons.
Heterozygous affected females transmit the trait to both sexes with equal frequency.
The heterozygous female tends to be less severely affected than the hemizygous male.

---

severely affected that they die before birth, and only females survive. Families with such disorders would include only affected daughters, unaffected daughters, and normal sons at a ratio of 1:1:1. Incontinentia pigmenti is one such lethal genetic disorder. Perinatally, affected females develop an erythematous, vesicular skin eruption, which progresses to marbled, curvilinear pigmentation. The syndrome includes dental abnormalities, congenital or secondary cataracts, proliferative retinopathy and pseudogliomas, and tractional retinal detachment.

Among the most severe X-linked dominant disorders with lethality for the hemizygous males is Aicardi syndrome. No verified birth of males with this entity has ever been reported, although several XXY pseudomales have been reported. Females have profound mental and developmental retardation; muscular hypotonia; blindness associated with a characteristic lacunar juxtapapillary chorioretinal dysplasia and optic disc anomalies; and central nervous system abnormalities, the most common characteristic of which is agenesis of the corpus callosum. No recurrences have been reported among siblings, and parents can be reassured that the risk in subsequent children is minimal. All instances of the disease appear to arise from a new X-dominant lethal mutation, and females do not survive long enough to reproduce. The critical area appears to be on the distal end of the short arm of the X chromosome, because some patients with a deletion in this region have also been shown to have features of Aicardi syndrome.

Maternal Inheritance

When nearly all offspring of an affected woman appear to be at risk for inheriting and expressing a trait, and the daughters are at risk for passing the trait on to the next generation, the pattern of inheritance is called *maternal inheritance*. The disease stops with all-male offspring, whether affected or not. This form of inheritance is highly suggestive of a mitochondrial disorder. The structure and molecular aspects of the mitochondrial genome and a general discussion of mitochondrial disease are covered in Chapter 5, Molecular Genetics.

Lyonization

In classical human genetics, females with a gene for a recessive disease or trait on only 1 X chromosome should have no manifestations of the defect. However, ophthalmic examples of structural and functional abnormalities in females heterozygous for supposedly recessive X-linked traits abound. Such *carrier states,* usually mild but occasionally severe, have been described in carriers of choroideremia, X-linked Nettleship-Falls ocular albinism, X-linked RP, X-linked sutural cataracts, Lowe syndrome, Fabry disease, and color vision defects of the protan and deutan types, among others (Fig 6-4; Table 6-9).

Detection of these carrier states of the X-linked traits has become clinically relevant, especially for sisters and maternal aunts of affected males. In 1961, Mary Lyon (a British geneticist) advanced an explanation for the unanticipated or partial expression of a trait by a heterozygous female. Briefly, lyonization (X-chromosome inactivation) stated that in every somatic cell of a female, only 1 X chromosome is actively functioning. The second

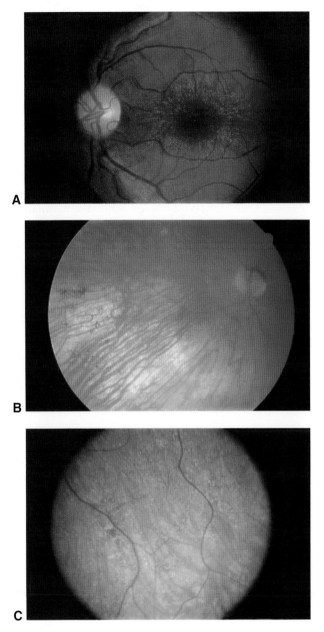

A

Figure 6-4 **A,** Yellow, "gold-dust" tapetal-like reflex in the left retina of a carrier for X-linked retinitis pigmentosa. **B,** Nasal midperipheral retina in the left eye of a carrier for X-linked retinitis pigmentosa, showing patchy bone spicule–like pigment clumping. **C,** Peripheral retina from the left eye of a carrier of choroideremia, showing a "moth-eaten" fundus appearance from areas of hypopigmentation and hyperpigmentation.

(continued)

B

C

X chromosome is inactive and forms a densely staining marginal nuclear structure demonstrated as a Barr body in a buccal smear or in "drumsticks," pedunculated lobules of the nucleus identified in about 5% of the leukocytes of the normal female. Warburg reasoned that X-chromosome inactivation occurs between approximately 6 and 11 days after fertilization, before the process of embryonic lateralization at 11–16 days of embryogenesis. The "decision" to inactivate 1 X chromosome is random, but once it is made, the same X chromosome will be irreversibly inactive in every daughter of each of these "committed"

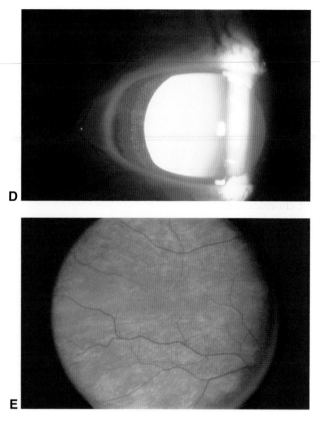

Figure 6-4 D, Characteristic iris transillumination from a carrier of X-linked ocular albinism. **E,** Midperipheral retina from the left eye of a carrier for ocular albinism, showing a chocolate brown pigmentation from areas of apparently enhanced pigmentation and clusters of hypopigmentation.

Table 6-9 Ocular Findings in Carriers of X-Linked Disorders

Disorder	Ocular Findings
X-linked retinitis pigmentosa	Regional fundus pigmentary changes, "gold-dust" tapetal-like reflex; ERG amplitude and implicit time abnormalities
Choroideremia	"Moth-eaten" fundus pigmentary changes, with areas of hypopigmentation, mottling, and pigment clumping in a striated pattern near the equator
Ocular albinism	Chocolate brown clusters of pigment prominent in the midperipheral retina; mottling of macular pigment; iris transillumination
Congenital stationary night blindness with myopia	Reductions in ERG oscillatory potentials
Blue-cone monochromatism	Abnormalities in cone function on ERG, psychophysical thresholds, and color vision testing
Red-green color vision deficiencies (protan and deutan)	Abnormally wide or displaced color match on a Nagel anomaloscope; decrease in sensitivity to red light in protan carriers (Schmidt sign)
Lowe syndrome	Scattered punctate lens opacities on slit-lamp examination
Fabry disease	Fingerprint or whorl-like (verticillate) changes within the corneal epithelium

primordial cells. With only 1 X chromosome "functioning," the active gene is dominant at a cellular level. Thus, a heterozygous female for an X-linked disease will have 2 clonal cell populations (mosaic phenotype), 1 with normal activity for the gene in question and the other with mutant activity.

The proportion of mutant to normal X chromosomes inactivated usually follows a normal distribution, because presumably the inactivations in various cells are random events. Thus, an average of 50% of the paternal X chromosomes and 50% of maternal X chromosomes are inactivated. It is conceivable, however, that in some cases the mutant X is active in almost all cells; in other cases, the mutant X is inactivated in nearly all cells. By this mechanism, a female may express an X-linked disorder, and rare cases are known of women who have a classic color deficiency or X-linked ocular albinism, X-linked RP, or choroideremia.

Some possible clinical implications of X inactivation are the following:

- The abnormalities in carrier females from different families and even within the same family may vary greatly in degree because of random inactivation and the resultant tissue derivatives containing differing proportions of the active X cells.
- A large population sample should have as many severely affected as mildly affected heterozygous carriers.
- In some tissues, both normal and abnormal areas could be found if a known biochemical defect could be mapped in a carrier, especially if the gene product is nondiffusible. For example, each hair bulb is ultimately derived from a single primordial cell. Therefore, biochemical analysis of hair roots may demonstrate the mutant phenotype directly: In Fabry disease, X-linked Nettleship-Falls ocular albinism, and Lesch-Nyhan syndrome, the scalp is a mosaic of hairs that have either normal or defective enzyme activity but not an intermediate activity.
- In certain diseases, interactions between cells with the normal X active alter the ability of cells with the mutant X active to survive. The enzyme hypoxanthine phosphoribosyltransferase travels from "normal" skin fibroblasts through gap junctions to mutant cells, allowing them to survive. In other situations, normal cells survive by favorable growth characteristics. In bone marrow and white blood cells, there is progressive elimination of the abnormal X-active cells in the heterozygote and protective survival of normal X-active cells.

Carriers of the X-linked variety of Nettleship-Falls ocular albinism may have a mottled mosaic fundus: in the pigmented retinal epithelial cells, the normal X chromosome is active; in the nonpigmented cells, the mutant X is active. However, these distinguishing features of the carrier state are not always present. The possibility that the patient is a carrier cannot be entirely eliminated if a given sign is not present, because a female might have undergone chance inactivation of the mutant X chromosome in most of her primordial cells, which evolved into the specific tissue observed and may appear phenotypically normal. This subtlety is even more important in evaluating family members with X-linked disease if the phenotypic carrier state is age-dependent; thus, even in obligate carrier females for Lowe syndrome, lenticular cortical opacities are not necessarily seen before the third decade of life.

Krill AE. X-chromosomal-linked diseases affecting the eye: status of the heterozygote female. *Trans Am Ophthalmol Soc.* 1969;67:535–608.

Warburg M. Random inactivities of the X chromosome in intermediate X-linked retinitis pigmentosa. Two hypotheses. *Trans Ophthalmol Soc U K.* 1971;91:553–560.

Polygenic and Multifactorial Inheritance

In chromosomal and mendelian (single-gene) disorders, genetic analysis of phenotypic, biochemical, or molecular parameters is imperative. However, a simple mode of inheritance cannot be assigned and a recurrence risk cannot be predicted for many common normal characteristics or disorders for which genetic variability clearly exists. Such traits as stature, facial features, refractive error, IOP, iris color, and intelligence are usually distributed as a continuous variation over a wide range without sharp distinction between normal and abnormal phenotypes. This distribution contrasts with the bimodal curve noted in conditions transmitted by a single gene. Common diseases are often superimposed on this substrate of normal variation, perhaps with a threshold level beyond which individuals may be regarded as abnormal. Consequently, the level of blood sugar in diabetes mellitus, the level of IOP for glaucoma, or the intermedial canthal distance for telecanthus is somewhat arbitrary. Such conditions are often termed *polygenic,* implying that they result from the operation of multiple collaborating genes, each with rather minor additive but individually indeterminate effects.

The term *multifactorial* denotes a combination of genetic and environmental factors in the etiology of disease without specifying the nature of the genetic influence. Examples of these factors in humans include intelligence, stature, blood pressure, atherosclerosis, and refractive index of the eye. The distinction between polygenic and multifactorial inheritance is one not of exclusion but rather of emphasis: most diseases can be thought of as constituting a spectrum of varying degrees of relative importance of the genetic and nongenetic factors in their causation.

Counseling for recurrence may be difficult in this type of inheritance. Ideally, empirical data are summarized from exhaustive analyses of similarly affected families in the population. Regrettably, such empirical data are rarely available for ophthalmic disorders. However, several general guidelines can be offered. If 1 offspring has the defect (such as cleft lip/palate) and the parents are normal, the chance that a subsequent child will inherit a similar set of genes and thus manifest the same type of malformation is considerably higher than the frequency of the defect in the general population but much lower than the risk of a mendelian defect. The usual estimate for such recurrence is 5% or less for common polygenic diseases. In addition, the more severe the abnormality in the index case, the higher the risk of recurrence of the trait in relatives, presumably because either a greater number of deleterious genes are at work or a fixed population of more harmful genes exists. The risk that an affected individual will have an affected offspring is also approximately 5%, similar to the recurrence risk in siblings. The risk of recurrence in future children is increased when more than 1 member of a family is affected, which is not true for mendelian disorders. Such observations have been offered for various forms of strabismus, glaucoma, and significant refractive errors.

Polygenic traits with a threshold (either present or absent) may be much more frequent in 1 sex if the threshold is sex-influenced. For example, isolated cleft lip is more common in males and isolated cleft palate is more common in females. The risk of recurrence should be higher among relatives of index cases of the less susceptible sex, who are genetically more highly predisposed or who carry more deleterious genes. For example, perinatal pyloric stenosis is much more common in males than females. Thus, if a female infant is affected, she presumably has either more deleterious genes or a higher personal liability to manifest the trait and, accordingly, a greater likelihood of having an affected sibling or relative.

Finally, if the malformation or disorder has occurred in both paternal and maternal relatives, the recurrence risk is distinctly higher because of the consanguineous sharing of multiple unspecifiable but potentially harmful genes in their offspring. Such empirical risks clearly increase the likelihood of diabetes mellitus in the offspring of 2 affected parents, even if neither parent has an antecedent family history of the disease.

Jorde LB, Carey JC, Bamshad MJ, White RL. *Medical Genetics.* Updated ed. for 2006–2007. 3rd ed. Philadelphia: Elsevier Mosby; 2006.

Pedigree Analysis

Recording a family history for general medical and eye disease is an essential part of an ophthalmologic consultation. Family data can be summarized in a pedigree chart, a shorthand method for recording data for visual reference. The word *pedigree* is derived from the French expression *pied de grue,* or "crane's foot," from the branching pattern of the diagram.

The affected individual who brings a family to the attention of the physician is the *proband* (propositus or proposita). The person seeking counseling is most frequently identified as the *consultand.* The most commonly used symbols for drawing a pedigree are shown in Figure 6-5. In human pedigree charts, the usual practice is to place the male symbol first on the left; breeding records of other species generally list the female symbol first.

Accurate completion of the pedigree drawing is essential to its interpretation. The health history of family members may be as important as the ocular history. The interviewer should inquire specifically about abortions, stillbirths, and deceased family members. Often, information on these individuals is erroneously omitted, and prenatal or postnatal lethal disorders or relevant medical and genetic causes of death are overlooked. Ages at death may be useful in specific situations and can be recorded directly near the appropriate symbols. For example, a clinician evaluating a child with ectopia lentis and no family history of similar ocular disease can find the identification of a relative deceased from a dissecting thoracic aortic aneurysm in his fourth decade of life very informative, leading to a tentative consideration of Marfan syndrome in the differential diagnosis. The casual observation in a young adult of multiple patches of congenital hypertrophy of the RPE in each eye may stimulate the recognition of a parent deceased at age 50 from metastatic adenocarcinoma of the colon, and a sibling deceased from a brain tumor at 10 years

PEDIGREE SYMBOLS

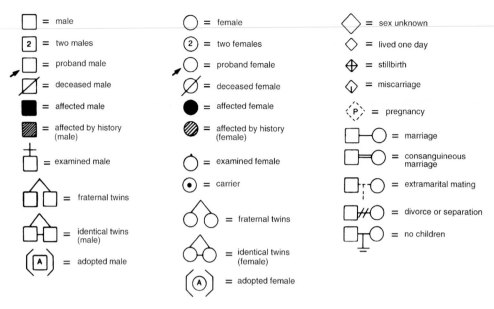

Figure 6-5 Symbols commonly used for pedigree analysis.

of age, thus leading to a diagnosis of Gardner syndrome and referral to a gastroenterologist for further diagnostic evaluation.

The interviewer should always clarify whether brothers and sisters are half siblings or full siblings. This procedure may not only limit the possible patterns of inheritance but also identify other individuals at risk for the disorders under consideration. Occasionally, information about parentage must be pursued aggressively (but always privately and confidentially). In the United States in 1990, 28% of babies—3 of every 11—were born to parents who were not legally married. The frequency of offspring born to teenage mothers outside of conventional marriages ranges from 30% to 80%. Both incest and nonpaternity are sensitive issues, but clearly neither is rare in our society. The national nonpaternity rate is estimated at 5%, but in some urban settings it may be as high as 15%. In considering rare autosomal recessive diseases, the interviewer must ask specifically about consanguinity in the following ways:

- searching for common last names in the families of both parents
- finding identical birthplaces for the parents
- identifying similar parental backgrounds from known ethnic or religious isolates

Genetic Counseling

The ophthalmologist who understands the principles of human genetics has a foundation for counseling patients about their diseases. Genetic counseling imparts knowledge of human disease, including a genetic diagnosis and its ocular and systemic implications, and information about the risk of occurrence or recurrence of the disorder within the family. It also encourages an open discussion of the options for reproduction. All genetic counseling is predicated on certain essential requirements.

- *Accurate diagnosis:* The physician must be sufficiently aware of the range of human ocular pathology to derive an accurate and specific diagnosis. It is impossible to counsel or refer patients on the basis of "congenital nystagmus" or "color blindness" or "macular degeneration"; these are signs, not diagnoses.
- *Complete family history:* A family history will narrow the choices of possible inheritance patterns, but it may not necessarily exclude new mutational events, isolated occurrences of recessive diseases, and chromosomal rearrangements in individual circumstances. The ophthalmologist must examine (or arrange to have examined) the parents, siblings, and other family members for mild manifestations of dominant diseases or characteristic carrier states in X-linked disorders. Identification of 1 young adult with the findings of Usher syndrome—prelingual deafness; night blindness; visual field constriction; and, ultimately, deterioration of central vision—obligates the ophthalmologist to evaluate a younger sibling who is congenitally deaf but "historically" has no eye problems. The probability is overwhelming that the sibling has the same disease. Only an ophthalmologist will be cognizant of and attentive to the atypical findings of hereditary ocular disorders.
- *Understanding the genetic and clinical aspects of the disorder:* The ophthalmologist should appreciate, perhaps more intimately than any other physician, how some clinically similar diseases inherited in the same pattern may be the result of different and even nonallelic defects. For example, the visual implications of and prognosis for tyrosinase-positive and tyrosinase-negative oculocutaneous albinism are considerably different. Some entities that are clinically similar may be inherited differently and thus have a different impact on other family members. In both its autosomal dominant and recessive modes, pseudoxanthoma elasticum is often a late-onset disease that has serious implications for cardiovascular disease, stroke, and gastrointestinal bleeding. Informed counseling falls short if the ophthalmologist advises only about visual disability associated with angioid streaks without attention to the complete disease and risks to other family members.

Issues in Genetic Counseling

The ophthalmologist must remember that an individual affected by a heritable condition may represent a homozygous recessive trait; thus, the ophthalmologist should search for parental consanguinity or ambiguous parentage (nonpaternity, incest, and even occult adoption) or for a new mutation and should inquire about advanced paternal (or maternal grandparental) age. Heterogeneity may confuse the diagnosis. Somatic mutations also occur, as with segmental neurofibromatosis or unilateral unifocal retinoblastoma. Nonpenetrance or mild expressivity in other family members should be excluded by diligent examination. Chromosomal abnormalities and phenocopies caused by infections or drugs may account for the isolated affected person. Nonetheless, the ophthalmologist's obligation to explain the disorder begins with accurate diagnosis and establishment of the mode of heritability.

Counseling can be considered successful if the patient or family, having acquired the facts, makes a reproductive decision that is reasonable and appropriate. The counselor is an informer, not an adviser. Properly done, genetic counseling is nondirective. It is inappropriate, perhaps even unethical, to tell the patient what to do (for instance, not to have any children).

In any circumstance, the counseling ophthalmologist should outline the options for family planning when it is necessary. The ophthalmologic practitioner's responsibilities are to

- suspect and establish the diagnosis of inherited disease
- inform the patient of the findings and their implications for health
- provide accurate answers to direct and implied questions about risks of recurrence and burden of disease

Some people may accept a high statistical risk and have children. This decision must be based on how they perceive the social and psychologic burdens of the disorder. Attitude toward reproduction may be considerably different for a female carrier of protanopia than for a female carrier of X-linked RP or choroideremia, even though the statistical risk for an affected son is the same for each carrier.

Some people may elect to delay childbearing in hopes of medical advances in prenatal diagnosis or postnatal treatment of a disorder. Others may choose, for a variety of personal and ethical considerations, not to have natural offspring and may proceed with contraception, termination of pregnancy, sterilization, or adoption.

Artificial insemination by donor is a useful option in family planning if the father has a dominant disease or if both parents are carriers of a biochemically detectable recessive disorder. However, it is clearly not applicable if the mother is the carrier of an X-linked disorder or is the individual affected by an autosomal dominant mutation. Finally, although its acceptance and legal implications may lag behind, embryo adoption (transplantation) and surrogate motherhood may soon become useful alternatives for some families.

Prenatal Diagnosis

Prenatal diagnosis with amniocentesis or chorionic villus sampling for biochemically identifiable disorders (eg, Tay-Sachs disease, many mucopolysaccharidoses, and about 100 other diseases) is also useful in the proper genetic settings. However, because most genes are expressed in a tissue-specific manner, biochemical diagnostic techniques are limited to diseases for which the gene products are expressed in amniocytes.

Other possible indications for amniocentesis include advanced maternal age, with its increased risk of chromosomal abnormalities; elevated maternal serum α-fetoprotein, suggesting a neural tube defect; and the presence of a familial disease detectable by DNA analysis.

Amniocentesis is usually performed at 15–16 weeks of gestation, when enough fluid and cells can be obtained for culture and the maternal risk of abortion is relatively low. The risk of spontaneous abortion or fetal morbidity from the procedure is about 0.5%. Earlier prenatal diagnosis of chromosomal abnormalities, at about 10 weeks of gestation, is available through the use of chorionic villus sampling. In this procedure, tissue from the placenta is obtained under ultrasound visualization. It is then cultured and karyotyped in a manner similar to that used for amniocentesis. As a first-trimester procedure, chorionic villus sampling allows for an earlier diagnosis and a safer means of pregnancy termination. The rate of spontaneous abortion associated with this procedure is estimated at 1%–2%. Because the yield of DNA is greater than that from the 20 mL of amniotic fluid withdrawn in amniocentesis, direct DNA analysis of cells can often be done without prior cell culture. Thus, information can be obtained considerably sooner than with amniocentesis.

Pharmacogenetics

The study of heritable factors that determine how drugs are chemically metabolized in the body is called *pharmacogenetics.* This field addresses genetic differences among population segments that are responsible for variations in both the therapeutic and adverse effects of drugs. Investigations in pharmacogenetics are important not only because they may lead to more rational approaches to therapy but also because they facilitate a deeper understanding of drug pharmacology. Part V of this section, Ocular Pharmacology, offers more detail.

The drug isoniazid provides an example of how pharmacogenetics works. This antituberculosis drug is normally inactivated by the liver enzyme acetyltransferase. A large segment of the population, which varies by geographic distribution, has a reduced amount of this enzyme; these individuals are termed *slow inactivators.* When they take isoniazid, the drug reaches higher-than-normal concentrations, causing a greater incidence of adverse effects. Family studies have shown that a reduced level of acetyltransferase is inherited as an autosomal recessive trait.

Several other well-documented examples demonstrate how pharmacogenetics works. One example involves 10% of the male African-American population, a high percentage of male Sephardic Jews, and males from a number of other ethnic groups. These individuals have an X-linked recessive trait that causes affected males to have glucose-6-phosphate dehydrogenase enzyme deficiency in their erythrocytes. As a consequence, a number of drugs (including sulfacetamide, vitamin K, acetylsalicylic acid, quinine, chloroquine, and probenecid) may produce acute hemolytic anemia in these individuals. Pharmacogenetic causes have also been ascribed to variations in response to ophthalmic drugs, such as the increased IOP seen in a segment of the population after prolonged use of topical corticosteroids.

Several drugs have been shown to cause greater reaction in children with Down syndrome than in children without the syndrome. As a result of supersensitivity, some children with Down syndrome have died after systemic administration of atropine. This supersensitivity is also seen with the topical use of atropine. In these patients, atropine exerts a greater-than-normal effect on pupillary dilation. In several children with Down syndrome being treated for strabismus, hyperactivity has occurred several hours after local instillation of 0.125% echothiophate iodide.

One of the earliest examples of an inherited deficit in drug metabolism involved succinylcholine, a strong muscle relaxant that interferes with acetylcholinesterase, the enzyme that catabolizes acetylcholine at neuromuscular junctions. Normally, succinylcholine is rapidly destroyed by plasma cholinesterase (sometimes called *pseudocholinesterase*) so that its effect is short-lived—usually no more than a few minutes. Some people are homozygous for a recessive gene that codes for a form of cholinesterase with a considerably lower substrate affinity. Consequently, at therapeutic doses of succinylcholine, almost no destruction occurs, and the drug continues to exert its inhibitory effect on acetylcholinesterase, resulting in prolonged periods of apnea.

Jorde LB, Carey JC, Bamshad MJ, White RL. *Medical Genetics.* Updated ed. for 2006–2007. 3rd ed. Philadelphia: Elsevier Mosby; 2006.

Clinical Management of Genetic Disease

Genetic disease may not be curable, but in most cases the patient benefits considerably from the physician's appropriate medical management. Such care should include all of the following steps.

Accurate Diagnosis

Unfortunately, because health care providers may not be as knowledgeable about genetic diagnoses as they are about other areas of medicine, many cases are not precisely diagnosed or, worse yet, are diagnosed incorrectly. A case of deafness and pigmentary retinopathy may be called rubella syndrome when the patient really has Usher syndrome. Such a syndrome associated with RP may not be recognized in patients with RP. For example, patients with RP and congenital polydactyly (surgically corrected in infancy) may not be recognized as having Bardet-Biedl syndrome. Besides the obvious reasons, the correct diagnosis in such cases is important to ensure that the patient's educational and lifetime support needs are truly met.

Complete Explanation of the Disease

Patients are often very disturbed when they do not understand the nature of their disease. A careful explanation of the disorder, as currently understood, will often dispel myths that patients may have about their disease and their symptoms.

Virtually all genetic disorders confer burdens that may interfere with certain activities later in life. The appropriate time to discuss these burdens with patients and family members is often when they first ask about the consequences of a disease. Such explanations need to be tempered with compassion and with an understanding of the possible emotional and psychological effects of this information.

Treatment of the Disease Process

Although definitive cures—that is, reversing or correcting of underlying genetic defects—are yet to emerge for various heritable disorders, some conditions in which metabolic defects have been identified can often be managed through 5 fundamental approaches:

1. dietary control
2. chelation of excessive metabolites

3. enzyme or gene product replacements
4. vitamin and cofactor therapy
5. drug therapy to reduce accumulation of harmful products

Some genetic disorders affecting the eye that arise from an inborn error of metabolism can effectively be managed by dietary therapy. These include familial hyperlipoprotein-emia, tyrosinosis, homocystinuria, Refsum disease, phenylketonuria, fructose or lactose intolerance, galactokinase deficiency, and galactosemia. Implementing a galactose-free diet can reverse some of the main clinical signs of galactosemia, such as hepatospleno-megaly, jaundice, and weight loss. Progression of cortical cataracts can be avoided, and less extensive lens opacities may even regress with a galactose-free diet. With time, galac-tosemic patients are able to metabolize galactose through alternative pathways, obviating the need for lifelong dietary restriction. In phenylketonuria, mental retardation can be prevented by early phenylalanine restriction.

Disorders that result from enzyme or transport protein deficiencies may lead to the accumulation of a metabolite or metal that harms various tissues. For example, in Wilson disease, decreased levels of serum ceruloplasmin result in poor transport of free copper (Cu^{2+}) ions and in storage of copper in tissues such as the brain, liver, and cornea. Resultant clinical signs can be reversed, at least partially, after the administration of D-penicillamine, a chelator of Cu^{2+} ions. Other copper chelators such as British antilewisite (BAL) can be used, along with copper-deficient diets, to reverse the clinical signs of Wilson disease (he-patolenticular degeneration).

Although no cure yet exists for most of the metabolic diseases, enzyme replacement therapy for types I and VI have been useful in reducing nonneurologic symptoms and pain in some of the affected indivduals. Also, plasma infusions in patients with Fabry dis-ease have succeeded in temporarily decreasing plasma levels of the accumulated substrate ceramide trihexoside, although clinical improvement was not detected. Further in-depth investigations are necessary before intervention with this type of therapy becomes mean-ingful, because circulating enzymes from infusions are rapidly degraded or excreted by the kidneys. Nevertheless, a slow-release depot preparation administered intramuscularly is at least feasible in providing short-term improvement in some metabolic disorders.

Organ transplantation can be considered as a form of regionalized enzyme replace-ment. In patients with cystinosis, cystine crystals accumulate in the kidney. If a normal kidney, with its rich source of enzymes, is transplanted into a patient with cystinosis, cys-tine does not accumulate in the cells of the renal tubules, and renal function tends to remain normal. In a complementary approach, stem cell transplantation is being investi-gated to treat various diseases, including those of the eye.

In addition to enzyme replacement, synthetic or recombinant gene product replace-ment can effectively manage a gene defect. Hemophilia, for example, can be treated through the administration of a missing clotting factor (VIII). The value of gene product replacement is demonstrated in the use of thyroid hormone for hypothyroidism, insu-lin for diabetes, erythropoietin for anemia, and growth hormone for pituitary dwarfism. However, caution is needed in light of the possible spread of AIDS caused by HIV if the gene product is extracted from pooled human tissues.

Vitamin therapy appears to be of benefit in 2 autosomal recessive disorders. In at least some patients with homocystinuria, vitamin B_6 (pyridoxine) administration has been shown to decrease homocystine accumulation in plasma and to reduce the severity of the disorder. Vitamin A and vitamin E therapy have been noted to benefit some patients with abetalipoproteinemia with regard to neurologic impairment; such therapy is also likely to slow or lessen the development and progression of retinal degeneration. More long-term therapeutic trials are necessary to better define the efficacy of vitamin therapy for these and perhaps other metabolic disorders.

Various genetically determined disorders can be managed by use of an appropriate drug. For example, excess accumulation of uric acid in primary gout can be prevented or reduced by (1) blocking the activity of the enzyme xanthine oxidase with the drug allopurinol or (2) increasing excretion of uric acid by the kidneys with the use of probenecid. In addition, a reduction in serum cholesterol found with familial hypercholesterolemia can often be achieved with the use of various cholesterol-lowering drugs or substances that bind bile acids in the gastrointestinal tract.

Appropriate management of sequelae and complications

Some of the sequelae of genetic diseases, such as glaucoma in Rieger syndrome or cataracts in patients with RP, can be successfully managed to preserve or partially restore vision. However, patients need to understand how treatment of the sequelae or complications may differ in their situation, especially if treatment affects the expected outcome.

Genetic Counseling

As discussed earlier in the chapter, the physician has an important obligation to either provide genetic counseling or arrange for the service by referral to a geneticist.

Referral to Providers of Support for Disabilities

Individuals and families often receive considerable benefit from referral to local, regional, or national agencies, support groups, or foundations that provide services for those with a particular disease. These organizations include local and state agencies for the blind or visually impaired, special school education programs, and appropriate consumer groups. Particularly when a disability is chronic and progressive, these agencies or support groups can greatly aid the individual or family in adjusting to changing visual disabilities.

Internet: *http://ncbi.nlm.nih.gov/Omim* through the *Online Mendelian Inheritance in Man* home page website (under OMIM Allied Resources).

PART IV

Biochemistry and
Metabolism

Introduction

Considerable progress has been made in the biochemistry of vision over the past 15 to 20 years, as witnessed by the numerous reviews, research articles, and books that have been published during this time. Part IV, Biochemistry and Metabolism, was written for both practitioners and residents in ophthalmology, as well as for students and researchers seeking a concise picture of the current state of knowledge in the biochemistry of the eye. With the recent growth in new information about vision biochemistry has come increasing specialization among ophthalmic researchers. These chapters cover most areas of research in ocular biochemistry, including tear film, cornea, iris and ciliary body, aqueous humor, lens, vitreous, retina, retinal pigment epithelium, and free radicals and antioxidants. The text attempts to relate basic science to clinical problems that may be faced during residency training and in subsequent practice.

CHAPTER 7

Tear Film

The primary functions of the tear film are to provide a smooth optical surface at the air–eye interface; to serve as a medium for removal of debris; to protect the ocular surface; and to supply oxygen, growth factors, and other compounds to the corneal epithelium. The tear film carries tear constituents and debris to the puncta. In addition, it contains a vast number of antimicrobial agents, lubricates the cornea–eyelid interface, and prevents desiccation of the ocular surface. Human tears are distributed among

- the marginal tear strip (or *tear meniscus*)
- the preocular film covering the exposed bulbar conjunctiva and cornea (precorneal tear film)
- the conjunctival sac (between the lids and bulbar conjunctiva)

The *precorneal tear film* is a trilaminar structure consisting of an anterior lipid layer, a middle aqueous layer, and a posterior mucin layer. Measurements of tear-film thickness have differed widely. Original measurements of the precorneal tear film gave an average thickness of approximately 8–9 µm, with the aqueous layer constituting nearly all the thickness (Fig 7-1). More recent, and presumably more accurate, studies using optical coherence tomography (OCT) and reflectometry have found the tear film to be only about 3.4 µm thick. The separation between the mucin and aqueous layers may not be distinct because mucins absorb electrolytes and water. The steady-state volume of tears is 7.4 µL for the unanesthetized eye and 2.6 µL for the anesthetized eye; this volume decreases with age. Some properties of the normal human tear film are given in Table 7-1.

Lipid Layer

The anterior layer of the tear film (approximately 100 molecules thick) contains polar and nonpolar lipids secreted primarily by the *meibomian (tarsal) glands* (Fig 7-2). These glands are located in the tarsal plate of the upper and lower eyelids and are supplied by parasympathetic nerves that are cholinesterase-positive and contain vasoactive intestinal polypeptide (VIP). Sympathetic and sensory nerves are present but sparsely distributed. Neuropeptide Y (NPY)-positive nerves are also abundant. There are approximately 30–40 meibomian glands in the upper eyelid and 20–30 smaller glands in the lower eyelid. Each gland orifice opens onto the skin of the eyelid margin, between the tarsal *gray line* and the mucocutaneous junction. The sebaceous glands of Zeis, located at the eyelid margin close to the eyelash roots, also secrete lipid, which is incorporated into the tear film.

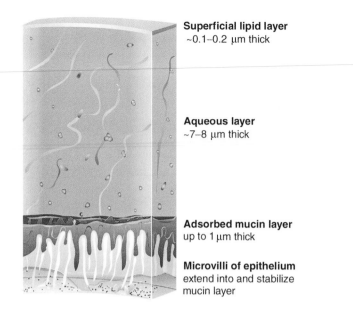

Superficial lipid layer
~0.1–0.2 µm thick

Aqueous layer
~7–8 µm thick

Adsorbed mucin layer
up to 1 µm thick

Microvilli of epithelium
extend into and stabilize
mucin layer

Figure 7-1 Schematic drawing of the structure of the tear film showing the outer lipid layer, middle aqueous layer, inner mucus layer, and microvilli on the apical cells of the ocular surface epithelium. *(From Marshall D. Tear layer mechanics. In: Bennett ES, Weissman BA, eds.* Clinical Contact Lens Practice. *Philadelphia: JB Lippincott; 1991:2.)*

Table 7-1 **Properties of Human Tear Film**

Composition	Water	98.2%
	Solid	1.8%
Thickness	Total	3.4 µm
	Lipid layer	0.1–0.2 µm
Volume	Unanesthetized	7.4 µL
	Anesthetized	2.6 µL
Secretory rate	Unanesthetized	
	Schirmer	3.8 µL/min
	Fluorophotometry	0.9 µL/min
	Anesthetized	
	Schirmer	1.8 µL/min
	Fluorophotometry	0.3 µL/min
Turnover rate	Normal	12%–16%/min
	Stimulated	300%/min
Evaporation rate		0.06 µL/cm^2/min
Osmolarity		296–308 mOsm/L
pH		6.5–7.6
Electrolytes (mmol/L)	Na$^+$	134–170
	K$^+$	26–42
	Ca^{2+}	0.5
	Mg^{2+}	0.3–0.6
	Cl$^-$	120–135
	HCO$_3^-$	26

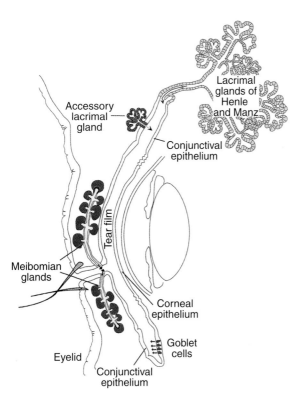

Figure 7-2 Schematic drawing of the major tear glands and ocular surface epithelia that contribute to the tear film. Shown are the meibomian glands (secrete oily layer), main lacrimal gland, accessory lacrimal gland, conjunctival epithelium, corneal epithelium (secretes aqueous layer), and conjunctival goblet cells (secrete mucus layer). *(From Dartt DA, Sullivan DA. Wetting of the ocular surface. In: Albert DM, Jakobiec FA, eds.* Principles and Practice of Ophthalmology. *Philadelphia: Saunders; 1994:967.)*

The lipid layer has the following functions:

- retard evaporation
- contribute to the optical properties of the tear film because of its position at the air–tear film interface
- maintain a hydrophobic barrier *(lipid strip)* that prevents tear overflow by increasing surface tension
- prevent damage to lid margin skin by tears

Because the polar lipids are charged compounds *(phospholipids)*, they are located at the aqueous–lipid interface. The fatty acids of the phospholipids interact with the other hydrophobic lipids (cholesterol and wax esters, which make up the bulk of the lipid layer) through noncovalent, noncharged bonds. Tear lipids are not susceptible to lipid peroxidation because they contain extremely low levels of polyunsaturated fatty acids.

Aqueous Layer

The middle aqueous layer is secreted by the main and accessory lacrimal glands (see Fig 7-2). It consists of electrolytes, water, and proteins. The main lacrimal gland is divided into 2 anatomical parts, the *orbital* and the *palpebral* portions, by the *levator aponeurosis.* The *glands of Krause,* which constitute two thirds of the accessory lacrimal glands, are located in the lateral part of the upper fornix. A number of Krause glands are also present in the lower fornix. The *glands of Wolfring* are variably located along the proximal margin of each tarsus. The accessory lacrimal glands are structurally like the main lacrimal gland.

The main lacrimal gland is richly innervated by parasympathetic nerves containing the neurotransmitters acetylcholine and VIP. The sympathetic innervation is less dense than the parasympathetic and contains norepinephrine and NPY as neurotransmitters. The sensory nerves are sparsely supplied with the neurotransmitters substance P and calcitonin gene–related peptide (CGRP). The accessory lacrimal glands are densely innervated, but the majority of nerves are unidentified. Some of this innervation consists of nerves containing VIP, substance P, and CGRP. Corneal innervation is predominantly sensory, but there is also sympathetic and (to a lesser extent) parasympathetic innervation. The conjunctival epithelium is innervated by parasympathetic, sympathetic, and sensory nerves.

The aqueous layer of tears consists of electrolytes, water, protein, and a variety of other solutes secreted by the main and accessory lacrimal glands, as well as by the corneal and conjunctival epithelia. In addition, with conjunctival inflammation and in response to drugs such as histamine, the blood vessels of the conjunctiva can leak a plasmalike fluid into the aqueous layer of tears.

Electrolytes and small molecules regulate the osmotic flow of fluids between the corneal epithelial cells and the tear film, buffer tear pH, and serve as enzyme cofactors in controlling membrane permeability. The Na^+ concentration of tears parallels that of serum; the concentration of K^+ is 5–7 times greater than that in serum. Na^+, K^+, and Cl^- regulate the osmotic flow of fluids from the cornea to the tear film. Bicarbonate regulates tear pH. Other tear electrolytes (Fe^{2+}, Cu^{2+}, Mg^{2+}, Ca^{2+}, PO_4^{3-}) are enzyme cofactors.

Tear-film solutes include urea, glucose, lactate, citrate, ascorbate, and amino acids. All enter the tear film via the systemic circulation, and their concentrations parallel those of serum levels. Fasting tear glucose levels are 3.6–4.1 mg/cc in those with and without diabetes. However, after a 100-mg oral glucose load, tear glucose levels exceed 11 mg/cc in 96% of diabetic persons tested.

Proteins in the tear film include immunoglobulin A (IgA) and secretory IgA (sIgA). IgA is formed by plasma cells in interstitial tissues of the main and accessory lacrimal glands and by the substantia propria of the conjunctiva. The secretory component is produced within lacrimal gland acini, and sIgA is secreted into the lumen of the main and accessory lacrimal glands. IgA plays a role in local host-defense mechanisms of the external eye, as shown by increased levels of IgA and IgG in human tears associated with ocular inflammation. Other immunoglobulins in tears are IgM, IgD, and IgE. Vernal conjunctivitis causes elevated tear and serum levels of IgE, increased IgE-producing plasma cells in the giant papillae of the superior tarsal conjunctiva, and elevated histamine. Increased levels of tear histamine support the concept of conjunctival mast-cell degranulation triggered by IgE–antigen interaction.

Lysozyme, lactoferrin, group II phospholipase A_2, lipocalins, and defensins are important tear antimicrobial constituents. Also present in tears is interferon, which inhibits viral replication and may be efficacious in limiting the severity of ulcerative herpetic keratitis.

Tears also contain a wide array of cytokines and growth factors, including transforming growth factor βs, epidermal growth factor, β fibroblast growth factor, interleukin 1α and 1β, and tumor necrosis factor α. These may play a role in the proliferation, migration, and differentiation of corneal and conjunctival epithelial cells. They may also regulate wound healing of the ocular surface.

The aqueous layer has the following functions:

- supply oxygen to the avascular corneal epithelium
- maintain a constant electrolyte composition over the ocular surface epithelium
- provide an antibacterial and antiviral defense
- smooth minute irregularities of the anterior corneal surface
- wash away debris
- modulate corneal and conjunctival epithelial cell function

Mucin Layer

The mucin layer of the tear film coats the microplicae of the superficial corneal epithelial cells and forms a fine network over the conjunctival surface. It contains mucins, proteins, electrolytes, and water. Functions of the mucin layer include the following:

- convert the corneal epithelium from a hydrophobic to a hydrophilic layer, which is essential for the even and spontaneous distribution of the tear film
- interact with the tear lipid layer to lower surface tension, thereby stabilizing the tear film
- trap exfoliated surface cells, foreign particles, and bacteria (by the loose mucin network covering the bulbar conjunctiva)
- lubricate the eyelids as they pass over the globe

Tear mucins are secreted principally by the conjunctival goblet cells and the stratified squamous cells of the conjunctival and corneal epithelia and minimally by lacrimal glands of Henle and Manz (see Fig 7-2). Goblet-cell mucin production is 2–3 μL/day, which contrasts with the 2–3 mL/day of aqueous tear production. Both conjunctival and tear mucins are negatively charged, high-molecular-weight glycoproteins. Tear dysfunction may result when tear mucins are deficient in number (avitaminosis A, conjunctival destruction), excessive in number (hyperthyroidism; foreign-body stimulation; allergic, vernal, and giant papillary conjunctivitis), or biochemically altered (keratoconjunctivitis).

Tear Secretion

The lacrimal secretory system was once thought to have 2 components: *basic secretors* and *reflex secretors*. Basic secretion was ascribed to the accessory lacrimal glands of Krause and Wolfring; and reflex secretion, to the main lacrimal gland. However, it is now thought that all lacrimal glands respond as a unit. In addition, the cornea and conjunctiva can also respond by secreting electrolytes, water, and mucins. Although the meibomian glands are innervated, it is not known whether nerves mediate lipid secretion from these glands.

Reflex tear secretion is neurally mediated and induced in response to physical irritation (superficial corneal and conjunctival sensory stimulation by mechanical, thermal, or chemical means), psychogenic factors, and bright light via the optic nerve. Induction of sensory nerves by a local neural reflex activates the parasympathetic and sympathetic nerves that innervate the tear glands and epithelia, causing secretion.

Parasympathetic and sympathetic nerves release their neurotransmitters, which interact with specific G-protein–linked receptors in the lacrimal glands, cornea, and conjunctiva; these receptors then activate their respective signaling pathways. There are 2 main signaling pathways: Ca^{2+}/protein kinase C–dependent and cyclic adenosine monophosphate (cAMP)–dependent (Figs 7-3, 7-4). In most tissues, the Ca^{2+}/protein kinase C–dependent pathway is activated by acetylcholine and, except in the main lacrimal gland, by norepinephrine. Acetylcholine, released from parasympathetic nerves, activates muscarinic receptors; norepinephrine, released from sympathetic nerves, activates α_1-adrenergic receptors. Stimulation of muscarinic and α_1-adrenergic receptors activates a guanine nucleotide–binding protein (G protein) of the $G\alpha_{q/11}$ subtype, which then

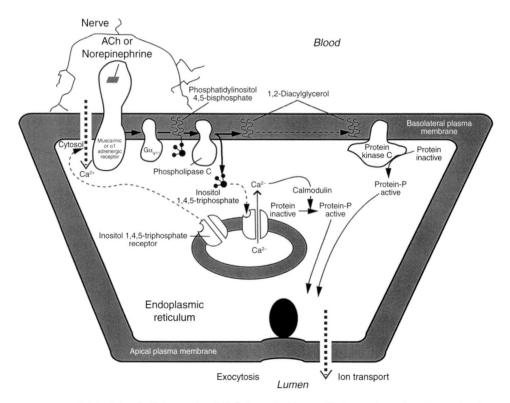

Figure 7-3 Epithelial cell. Schematic of Ca^{2+}/protein kinase C–dependent signal transduction pathway activated by cholinergic and α_1-adrenergic agonists in epithelial cells to stimulate mucin, protein, or electrolyte and water secretion. *ACh* = acetylcholine, $G\alpha_{q/11}$ = q/11 subtype of guanine nucleotide–binding protein, *Protein-P* = phosphorylated (activated) protein. *(From Dartt DA. Regulation of tear secretion.* Adv Exp Med Biol. *1994;350:4.)*

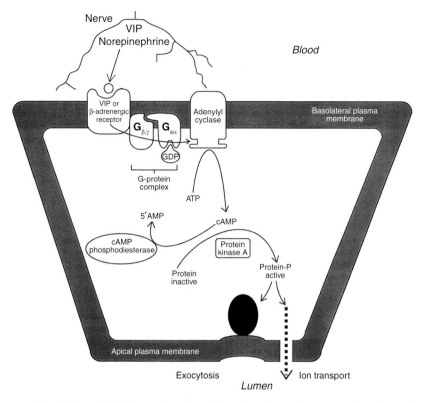

Figure 7-4 Epithelial cell. Schematic of 3′,5′-cyclic adenosine monophosphate *(cAMP)*-dependent signaling pathway activated by vasoactive intestinal polypeptide *(VIP)* or norepinephrine to stimulate mucin, protein, or electrolyte and water secretion in epithelial cells. *5′ AMP* = adenosine 5′-monophosphate, *ATP* = adenosine 5′-triphosphate, $G_{\beta,\gamma}$ = β- and γ-subunits of guanine nucleotide-binding protein, $G_{s\alpha}$ = stimulatory α-subunit of guanine nucleotide-binding protein, *GDP* = guanosine 5′-diphosphate, *Protein-P* = phosphorylated (activated) protein. *(Modified from Dartt DA. Regulation of tear secretion.* Adv Exp Med Biol. *1994;350:5.)*

turns on phospholipase C. Phospholipase C breaks down a membrane lipid—phosphatidylinositol 4,5,-bisphosphate—into inositol 1,4,5-trisphosphate (IP_3) and diacylglycerol. IP_3 releases intracellular Ca^{2+}. The depletion of Ca^{2+} from intracellular stores causes the influx of extracellular Ca^{2+} to refill these stores. Ca^{2+} (either by itself or by activating Ca^{2+}-calmodulin–dependent protein kinases) stimulates protein and/or electrolyte and water secretion. The increase in diacylglycerol activates protein kinase C, a family of 11 isozymes that stimulate protein and/or electrolyte and water secretion.

The cAMP-dependent pathway is activated by VIP and norepinephrine. VIP, released from parasympathetic nerves, interacts with VIP receptors; norepinephrine, released from sympathetic nerves, activates β-adrenergic receptors. Stimulation of VIP or β-adrenergic receptors activates G protein $G_{s\alpha}$ subtypes, which in turn stimulate adenylyl cyclase. Activation of adenylyl cyclase produces cAMP from ATP. cAMP activates cAMP-dependent protein kinases to stimulate protein and/or electrolyte and water secretion. The action of cAMP is terminated when it is broken down by cAMP-dependent phosphodiesterases.

Another mechanism for stimulating tear secretion (in addition to nerves) is peptide and steroid hormones. Peptide hormones, including α-melanocyte-stimulating hormone and adrenocorticotropic hormone (ACTH), stimulate protein secretion from the main lacrimal gland. These hormones activate the cAMP-dependent pathway described for VIP and β-adrenergic receptors. The steroid hormones, specifically the androgens, stimulate secretion of sIgA from the main lacrimal gland and lipid secretion from the meibomian glands. Androgens diffuse into the nucleus and bind to receptors, which are members of the steroid/thyroid hormone/retinoic acid family of transcription factors. The monomeric-activated androgen-receptor complex then associates with the response elements in the regulating region of the target gene (eg, for sIgA secretion, the target would be the secretory component gene). This association promotes dimerization of 2 androgen-receptor complexes, a process that then activates gene transcription and eventually protein synthesis.

Eyelid movement is important in tear-film renewal, distribution, turnover, and drainage. As the eyelids close in a complete blink, the superior and inferior fornices are compressed by the force of the preseptal muscles, and the eyelids move toward each other, with the upper eyelid moving over the longer distance and exerting force on the globe. This force clears the anterior surface of debris and any insoluble mucin and expresses secretions from meibomian glands. The lower eyelid moves horizontally in a nasal direction and pushes tear fluid and debris toward the superior and inferior puncta. When the eyelids are opened, the tear film is redistributed. The upper eyelid pulls the aqueous phase of the tear film by capillary action. The lipid layer spreads as fast as the eyelids move, so that no area of the tear film is left uncovered by lipid. The lipid layer increases tear-film thickness and stabilizes the tear film. Polar lipids, present in the meibomian secretions, concentrate at the lipid–water interface and enhance the stability of the lipid layer.

Tear Dysfunction

A qualitative or quantitative abnormality of the tear film may occur as a result of

- change in the amount of tear-film constituents
- change in the composition of tear film
- uneven dispersion of the tear film because of corneal surface irregularities
- ineffective distribution of the tear film caused by eyelid–globe incongruity

The amount or composition of the tear film can change because of aqueous deficiency, mucin deficiency or excess (with or without associated aqueous deficiency), and/or lipid abnormality (meibomian gland dysfunction). For example, increases in tear-film osmolarity have been observed in patients with keratoconjunctivitis sicca (KCS, or dry eyes) or blepharitis and in those who use contact lenses. The preocular tear film is dispersed unevenly with an irregular corneal or limbal surface (inflammation, scarring, dystrophic changes) or poor contact lens fit. Eyelid–globe incongruity results from congenital, traumatic, or neurogenic eyelid dysfunction or absent or dysfunctional blink mechanism.

Diagnostic tests for tear dysfunction include the tear breakup time, lissamine green staining, rose bengal staining, osmolarity tests, and Schirmer tests.

The tear-constituent imbalance can be corrected by decreasing the evaporation of tears (through reduced room temperature or increased humidity) and changing contact lenses for glasses. Tear-film instability (secondary to aqueous and/or mucin deficiency) can be reduced by the use of topical tear substitutes. Reduction of tear drainage by punctal occlusion prolongs the effect of artificial tears and preserves the natural tears. Thus, tear dysfunction is managed by creating a more regular corneal or conjunctival contour or by facilitating eyelid–globe congruity. Unfortunately, all these treatments are palliative (and not curative) in nature.

There is increasing evidence that KCS is associated with ocular surface inflammation. In various studies, adhesion molecule expression by conjunctiva epithelial cells, T-cell infiltration of the conjunctiva, and increases in soluble mediators (cytokines and proteases) in the tear film have been found in patients with KCS (Fig 7-5). Preliminary clinical studies have shown that using hypotonic tear substitutes to treat patients with KCS may reduce tear osmolarity and improve ocular symptoms. Moreover, therapy with a multitude of anti-inflammatory agents (including corticosteroids, cyclosporine, matrix metalloproteinases, and doxycycline) has been observed to improve the clinical symptoms of patients with KCS (Fig 7-6). Recently, topical cyclosporine A emulsion (Restasis) was approved by the FDA for treating the inflammatory component of dry eye. This fungal-derived peptide emulsion has been shown effective in stimulating aqueous tear production and reducing symptoms of blurred vision in patients with KCS. No significant adverse systemic or ocular events (except for burning symptoms) were observed.

BCSC Section 7, *Orbit, Eyelids, and Lacrimal System,* discusses the lacrimal system in depth, with numerous illustrations.

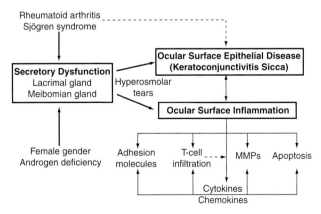

Figure 7-5 Inflammatory mediators in keratoconjunctivitis sicca. *MMPs* = matrix metalloproteinases. *(Reproduced with permission from Pflugfelder SC. Antiinflammatory therapy for dry eye. Am J Ophthalmol. 2004;137(2):338.)*

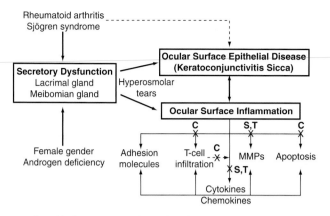

Figure 7-6 Targets of anti-inflammatory therapies for keratoconjunctivitis sicca. *C* = CsA (cyclosporin A), *MMPs* = matrix metalloproteinases, *S* = corticosteroids, *T* = tetracycline. *(Reproduced with permission from Pflugfelder SC. Antiinflammatory therapy for dry eye. Am J Ophthalmol. 2004;137(2):340.)*

Iester M, Orsoni GJ, Gamba G, et al. Improvement of the ocular surface using hypotonic 0.4% hyaluronic acid drops in keratoconjunctivitis sicca. *Eye.* 2000;14(Pt 6):892–898.

Pflugfelder SC. Antiinflammatory therapy for dry eye. *Am J Ophthalmol.* 2004;137(2):337–342.

Tiffany JM. Tears and conjunctiva. In: Harding JJ, ed. *Biochemistry of the Eye.* London: Chapman & Hall Medical; 1997:1–15.

Tsubota K. Tear dynamics and dry eye. *Prog Retin Eye Res.* 1998;17(4):565–596.

CHAPTER 8

Cornea

The cornea is a remarkable structure, with a high degree of transparency and excellent self-protective and reparative properties. The cornea is made up of the following histologic layers (Fig 8-1):

- epithelium with basement membrane
- Bowman's layer
- stroma (or *substantia propria*)
- Descemet's membrane
- endothelium

The human cornea has a rich afferent innervation. The long posterior ciliary nerves (branches of V_1, the ophthalmic division of CN V) penetrate the cornea in 3 planes: scleral, episcleral, and conjunctival. Peripherally, approximately 70–80 branches of the long posterior ciliary nerves enter the cornea and lose their myelin sheath 1–2 mm from the limbus. A plexus posterior to Bowman's layer sends branches anteriorly into the epithelium.

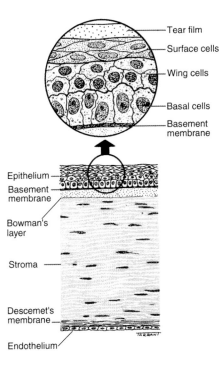

Epithelium

Basement membrane

Bowman's layer

Stroma

Descemet's membrane

Endothelium

Tear film
Surface cells
Wing cells
Basal cells
Basement membrane

Figure 8-1 Diagram of different layers of the cornea. *(Reproduced with permission from Kanski JJ. Clinical Ophthalmology: A Systematic Approach. 3rd ed. Oxford: Butterworth-Heinemann; 1994:100.)*

Oxygen to the cornea is provided by the preocular tear film, lid vasculature, and aqueous humor. The primary metabolic substrate for the epithelial cells, stromal keratocytes, and endothelium is glucose. The stroma receives glucose primarily from the aqueous humor by carrier-mediated transport through the endothelium; the epithelium receives glucose by passive diffusion through the stroma. The preocular tear film and limbal vessels supply approximately 10% of the glucose used by the cornea. Glucose is metabolized in the cornea by all 3 metabolic pathways:

1. tricarboxylic acid (TCA) cycle
2. anaerobic glycolysis
3. hexose monophosphate (HMP) shunt

In the epithelium and endothelium, the HMP pathway breaks down 35%–65% of the glucose, but the keratocytes of the stroma metabolize very little glucose via this pathway. The keratocytes appear to lack 6-phosphogluconate dehydrogenase, an important enzyme in the HMP pathway. The TCA cycle is much more active in the endothelium than in the epithelium. Pyruvic acid, the end product of glycolysis, is converted either to CO_2 and H_2O (via the TCA cycle under aerobic conditions) or to lactic acid (under anaerobic conditions). Production of lactic acid increases in conditions of oxygen deprivation, as in the case of tight-fitting contact lenses of low oxygen permeability. Accumulation of lactic acid in the cornea has detrimental visual consequences, such as edema (due to an increase in an osmotic solute load) or stromal acidosis, which can change endothelial morphology and function.

Human corneas possess a remarkably high level of aldehyde dehydrogenase and transketolase. Together, these 2 proteins constitute 40%–50% of the soluble proteins in corneal stroma. Like enzyme crystallins of the lens, both aldehyde dehydrogenase and transketolase are thought to contribute to the optical properties of the cornea. Both proteins are also thought to protect corneal cells against free radicals and oxidative damage by absorbing UVB irradiation.

Epithelium

The *epithelium* is typically about 65 μm thick and constitutes 5%–10% of total corneal thickness. It is composed of 5–6 layers, which include 1–2 layers of superficial squamous cells, 2–3 layers of broad wing cells, and the innermost layer of the columnar basal cells. Surface projections (microvilli and microplicae) are present on the apical surface of the most superficial cell layer of epithelium. These projections are coated with filamentous material known as *glycocalyx*. Mucin glycoproteins, the major constituents of glycocalyx, are thought to promote both stability of the tear film and wettability of the corneal surface. Plasma membrane proteins and the lipids of corneal epithelial cells, like those of other cell types, are heavily glycosylated and play an important role in cell–cell adhesion as well as in the adhesion of the basal cells of corneal epithelium to the underlying basement membrane. The sugar residues of the plasma membrane glycoproteins and the glycolipids of corneal epithelium also play a role in wound-healing mechanisms, by mediating corneal epithelial sheet migration over the wound surface following ocular injury; and in pathogenesis of corneal infection, by serving as attachment sites for microbes.

Hydrophilic molecules penetrate the epithelium poorly, but they may pass through intercellular tight junctions if the polar molecule is less than 500 daltons (D) in apparent molecular mass. Knowing the ionic dissociation constant of a molecule is important for determining its permeability across the cornea. To diffuse across the epithelium, organic molecules should exist in an uncharged state. However, a charged molecule more readily penetrates the stroma. Therefore, to penetrate the cornea and enter the anterior chamber, an organic molecule should be able to dissociate at physiologic pH and temperature (ie, within the stroma).

Bowman's Layer

Bowman's layer is immediately posterior to the epithelial basal lamina. This layer is 8–12 μm thick and is composed of randomly packed type I and type V collagen fibers that are 30 nm in diameter. The fibers are enmeshed in a matrix consisting of proteoglycans and glycoproteins. Bowman's layer is secreted during embryogenesis by the anterior stromal keratocytes and epithelium. It is acellular, and it does not regenerate when damaged. It is thought that this layer, by virtue of its acellularity and packing distribution, serves to prevent exposure of stromal corneal keratocytes to growth factors secreted by epithelial cells, such as transforming growth factor βs (TGF-βs). This is notable because, during excimer laser photorefractive keratectomy (PRK) for correction of myopia, Bowman's layer (along with anterior corneal stromal tissue) is removed from the center of the cornea and thus the anterior dome of the cornea becomes flatter. Similarly, Bowman's layer is lost during laser subepithelial keratomileusis (LASEK) for myopia correction. In this procedure, corneal haze is a common and significant postoperative complication (especially if steroids are not used for months), presumably because stromal keratocytes are exposed to regenerating epithelial growth factors and metaplase into fibroblasts. However, during laser in situ keratomileusis (LASIK), Bowman's layer is transected but still retained, with ablation occurring intrastromally on the stromal bed surface; and thus central corneal haze is extremely rare in uncomplicated LASIK.

Stroma

The *stroma* makes up 90% of the corneal thickness. Stromal cells are known as *keratocytes.* Depending on a person's age, keratocytes constitute 10%–40% of corneal volume. Usually, these cells reside between the collagen lamellae. The stroma is made up of roughly 200 layers of lamellae, which are 1.5–2.5 μm in thickness and are composed of collagen fibrils enmeshed in a matrix consisting of proteoglycans, proteins, and glycoproteins. The stromal fibrils within each lamella are narrow and uniform in diameter. In humans, the average fibril diameter is 30 nm.

Collagen fibrils within each lamella run parallel to each other from limbus to limbus. Adjacent lamellae are positioned at roughly right angles to each other: less than 90° in the anterior stroma but almost 90° in the posterior stroma. That is, alternate arrays of fibrils are nearly perpendicular, and they are observed tangentially in electron micrographs of cross sections of corneal stroma. Also, collagen fibrils in each lamella are regularly spaced, with a center-to-center distance of 55–60 nm. The narrow and uniform diameter of collagen fibrils and their regular arrangement are characteristic of collagen of the corneal stroma and are necessary for the transparency of this tissue. Type I is the major collagen component of the corneal stroma, constituting approximately 70% of the total stromal dry weight. Immunohistochemical and biochemical studies have demonstrated that normal adult corneal stroma also contains collagen types V, VI, VII, XII, and XIV. Type III collagen production is associated uniquely with stromal wound healing.

After collagen, proteoglycans are the second most abundant biological constituents of the cornea, constituting approximately 10% of the dry weight of the cornea. It is the proteoglycans that confer hydrophilic properties to the stroma. Proteoglycans are glycosylated proteins with at least 1 glycosaminoglycan (GAG) chain covalently bound to the protein core. GAGs are composed of repeating disaccharides. The GAGs found in corneal stroma include

- keratan sulfate
- chondroitin sulfate
- dermatan sulfate

Two major proteoglycan populations have been identified in corneal stroma, 1 containing keratan sulfate chains, the other containing both dermatan sulfate and chondroitin sulfate chains. Regulation of spacing between the stromal collagen fibrils is thought to result from highly specific interactions between the proteoglycans and the collagen fibrils; when these interactions are disturbed, the ability of the cornea to remain transparent is profoundly affected.

Matrix metalloproteinases (MMPs) are a family of Zn^{2+}-dependent enzymes responsible for degradation of the components of the extracellular matrix (including proteoglycans and various types of collagens) during normal development as well as in disease processes. Of more than a dozen known metalloproteinases, only MMP-2 proenzyme has been found in the normal healthy cornea. However, after corneal injury, additional MMPs (including MMP-1, MMP-3, and MMP-9) are synthesized. The proteinase inhibitors of the cornea play a key role in corneal protection by restricting damage during corneal inflammation, ulceration, and wound healing. The following proteinase inhibitors have thus far been identified in the cornea:

- α_1-proteinase inhibitor
- α_1-antichymotrypsin
- α_2-macroglobulin
- plasminogen activator inhibitors 1 and 2
- tissue inhibitors of metalloproteinases

Many of these inhibitors are synthesized by resident cells of the cornea; some are derived from tears, aqueous humor, and limbal blood vessels.

Descemet's Membrane and Endothelium

Descemet's membrane is a 10-μm-thick specialized basement membrane present between the endothelium and the posterior stroma. It is secreted by endothelium and comprises an anterior banded portion and a posterior nonbanded portion. Type IV is the most abundant collagen in Descemet's membrane. The corneal endothelium is a single layer posterior to Descemet's membrane and is composed of polygonal cells 20 μm in diameter. In young adults, the normal endothelial cell count is approximately 3000/mm². The number of endothelial cells decreases with aging, with a concomitant spreading and thinning of the remaining cells. A group of tight junctions forms the apical junctional complex between cells that occludes the lateral extracellular spaces from the aqueous humor. Approximately 20–30 short microvilli per cell extend from the apical plasma membrane into the aqueous humor. The endothelium functions as a permeability barrier between the aqueous humor and the corneal stroma and as a pump to maintain the cornea in a dehydrated state by generating the negative hydrostatic pressure that also serves to hold free corneal flaps (eg, LASIK flaps) in place. In vivo, the endothelium derives sufficient oxygen from the aqueous humor to maintain normal pump function.

If the endothelium is injured, healing occurs mainly via cell migration, rearrangement, and enlargement of the residual cells. Substantial cell loss or damage results in irreversible edema because human corneal endothelial cells have a limited ability to divide after birth. Infiltration of polymorphonuclear leukocytes in response to severe corneal injury induces endothelial cells to become fibroblastic and to synthesize *retrocorneal fibrous membrane* (RCFM). This RCFM forms between Descemet's membrane and the corneal endothelium and causes a significant loss of visual acuity. Unlike normal corneal endothelial cells, which accumulate little type I collagen protein, the fibroblastic cells isolated from the RCFM predominantly express type I collagen.

Panjwani N. Cornea and sclera. In: Harding JJ, ed. *Biochemistry of the Eye*. London: Chapman & Hall Medical; 1997:16–51.

CHAPTER 9

Iris and Ciliary Body

Introduction

The iris and ciliary body are the anterior parts of the *uveal tract*, which is continuous with the choroid posteriorly.

The iris is a highly pigmented tissue that functions as a movable diaphragm between the anterior and posterior chambers of the eye, regulating the amount of light that reaches the retina. It is a delicate, dynamic structure, capable of precise and rapid changes in pupillary diameter in response to both light and specific pharmacologic stimuli.

The ciliary body produces and regulates the composition of aqueous humor and thus directly influences the ionic environment and metabolism of the lens, cornea, and trabecular meshwork.

Protein Types Expressed in Human Ciliary Body

Using *expressed sequence tags (ESTs)* to identify active molecules from a human ciliary body library, researchers found that the largest group (37%) contains unidentified sequences with unknown functions. Of the known compounds, the functions of major groups of expressed genes include

- protein synthesis, folding, secretion, and degradation (20%)
- energy supply and biosynthesis (12%)
- contractility and cytoskeleton structure (6%)
- cellular signaling and cell cycle regulation (7%)
- nerve cell–related tasks (2%), including neuropeptide processing and putative nonvisual phototransduction and circadian rhythm control

Escribano J, Coca-Prados M. Bioinformatics and reanalysis of subtracted expressed sequence tags from the human ciliary body: identification of novel biological functions. Review. *Mol Vis.* 2002;8:315–332.

Iris–Ciliary Body Smooth Muscle

Unlike smooth muscle elsewhere in the body, which is derived from mesoderm, the smooth muscle in the iris and ciliary body is derived from neuroectoderm. The biochemistry of the smooth muscles of the iris includes the following:

- contraction–relaxation
- receptor characterization

253

- second-messenger formation and regulation
- protein phosphorylation
- phospholipid metabolism
- arachidonic acid (AA) release and eicosanoid biosynthesis

The ciliary body is the main pharmacologic target in the treatment of glaucoma. Many treatments employed to lower intraocular pressure (IOP) in glaucoma, such as adrenergic and cholinergic drugs and prostaglandins (PGs), work through receptors and their respective signal transduction pathways. The iris–ciliary body is rich in many types of receptors that bind to various agonists and antagonists, including adrenergic, muscarinic cholinergic, and peptidergic; PG; serotonin; platelet-activating factor; and growth factor receptors.

The following discussion concerns biochemical aspects of the iris–ciliary body such as aqueous humor formation, eicosanoids, and membrane signal transduction and second-messenger systems. Chapter 2 of this volume discusses and illustrates all of the various structures mentioned in this chapter.

Aqueous Humor Dynamics

Aqueous humor, the transparent fluid that fills the anterior and posterior chambers, is secreted by the nonpigmented ciliary epithelium from a substrate of blood plasma. Aqueous is the major nutrient source for the avascular lens and cornea and provides a route for the removal of waste products. Aqueous humor is essentially protein-free, which allows for optical clarity. The total protein level in human aqueous humor, about half of which is albumin, is very low—only about 1/500 of that in plasma. Other components include growth factors; several enzymes, such as carbonic anhydrase, lysozyme, diamine oxidase, plasminogen activator, dopamine β-hydroxylase, phospholipase A_2 and PGs, cyclic adenosine monophosphate (cAMP), catecholamines, steroid hormones, and hyaluronic acid.

Ocular fluids are separated from blood by barriers formed by tight junctions between epithelial and endothelial cells. These barriers are called either blood–aqueous or blood–retina, depending on their location in the eye. Because of these barriers, the composition and amounts of all materials entering and leaving the eye can be carefully controlled, except for materials that exit through the Schlemm canal. Perturbations of these blood–ocular barriers result in the mixing of blood constituents with ocular fluids, which may be the cause of plasmoid aqueous, retinal exudates, or retinal edema.

Aqueous humor enters the posterior chamber from the ciliary processes by means of active and passive physiologic mechanisms:

- *passive:* diffusion and ultrafiltration
- *active:* energy-dependent secretion, including carbonic anhydrase II (CA II) activity

Diffusion involves the movement of ions like sodium across a membrane toward the side with the most negative potential. Ultrafiltration is the nonenzymatic component of aqueous formation that depends on IOP, blood pressure, and the blood osmotic pressure in the ciliary body. CA II in humans is present in pigmented and nonpigmented epithelium. Its inhibitors cause a reduction in the rate of entry of sodium and bicarbonate into the aqueous, leading to a reduction in aqueous flow. The formation of aqueous humor is largely a product of *active secretion* by the inner, nonpigmented ciliary epithelium and involves membrane-associated Na^+,K^+-ATPase.

The following observations support the involvement of active-transport mechanisms in secretion:

- Aqueous concentrations of Na^+, K^+, Cl^-, *myo*-inositol, certain amino acids, and glucose are maintained by specific active-transport systems located in the ciliary epithelium.
- The high level of ascorbic acid in the aqueous humor suggests that an active pump mechanism secretes it into the aqueous.
- Both the iris and the ciliary body accumulate ρ-aminohippuric acid from the aqueous against a concentration gradient (the accumulation shows saturation kinetics; ρ-aminohippuric acid is inhibited at 0°C and depressed by cyanide, dinitrophenol, ouabain, iodopyracet, and probenecid).
- The low protein concentration of aqueous humor relative to serum results from the exclusion of large molecules by the blood–aqueous barrier. The presence of such a barrier requires active-transport systems either for moving substances across the cellular layer into the eye or for removing those substances from the aqueous humor.
- The rate of aqueous humor formation differs among species, being approximately 2 μL/min in humans. IOP is maintained by continuous aqueous formation and drainage, which allows the surrounding tissues to remove the waste products of metabolism. Inhibitors of enzymatic processes decrease aqueous humor inflow by different amounts and thus provide additional evidence for active secretory processes. Carbonic anhydrase inhibitors and β-blockers (discussed later in this chapter) are used systemically and topically in the treatment of glaucoma to reduce the rate of aqueous humor formation. See Chapter 17 of this volume and BCSC Section 10, *Glaucoma,* for more detail.

Eicosanoids

Types and Actions

Eicosanoids, which include PGs, prostacyclin (PGI_2), thromboxanes (TXA_2), and leukotrienes, are an important family of compounds with hormonal activity. They are synthesized as a result of phospholipase A_2 (PLA_2) stimulation, which causes the release of arachidonic acid (AA) from membrane glycerolipids (Fig 9-1). These agents affect both the male and the female reproductive systems, the gastrointestinal system, the cardiovascular and renal systems, the nervous system, and the eye. PGI_2 and TXA_2 are natural biological antagonists. PGI_2, which is synthesized mainly in the endothelial cells of vascular

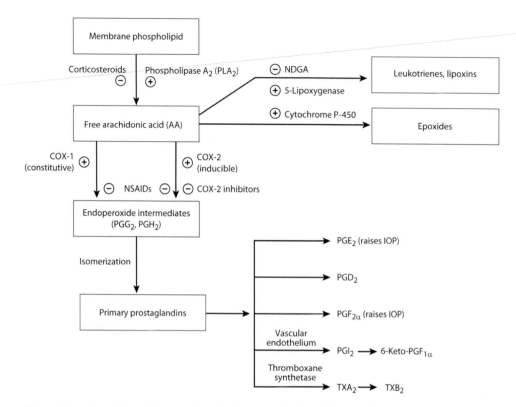

Figure 9-1 An outline of the synthesis of prostaglandins (PGs) and leukotrienes from arachidonic acid. In response to stimulation of a target cell with a relevant stimulus (eg, a cytokine, neurotransmitter, various pharmacologic agents), phospholipase A_2 is activated, and arachidonic acid is released from the sn-2 position of membrane phospholipids. Arachidonic acid is then converted by cyclooxygenase 1 *(COX-1)* or cyclooxygenase 2 *(COX-2)* to PGH_2, and then PGH_2 is isomerized to biologically active prostanoid products. Arachidonic acid can also be metabolized through the 5-lipoxygenase and cytochrome P-450 pathways to generate leukotrienes and epoxides, respectively. Phospholipase A_2 can be inhibited by corticosteroids such as dexamethasone; COX-1, by nonsteroidal anti-inflammatory drugs *(NSAIDs)* such as indomethacin and aspirin; COX-2, by DUP697, SC58125, L-745-337, and NS398; and the 5-lipoxygenase pathway, by nordihydroguaiaretic acid *(NDGA)*. TXA_2 = thromboxane A_2, TXB_2 = thromboxane B_2. *(Courtesy of Ata Abdel-Latif, PhD.)*

tissues, is a potent vasodilator, a potent platelet-antiaggregating agent, and a stimulator of adenylate cyclase. In contrast, TXA_2, which is synthesized mainly by platelets, is a potent vasoconstrictor and a platelet-aggregating agent.

Prostaglandins have profound effects on inflammation in the eye, aqueous humor dynamics, and blood–ocular barrier functions. PGs of the E and F subtypes and AA, when administered intracamerally or topically at high concentrations, cause miosis, an elevation of IOP, an increase in aqueous protein content, and the entry of white cells into the aqueous and tear fluid. Evidence indicates that some antiglaucoma drugs, such as epinephrine, may affect IOP by influencing the production of PGs. More recently, PGs and their derivatives have been found to be useful as antiglaucoma agents. For example, several PGF_2 receptor agonists (latanoprost, bimatoprost, travoprost) have been shown to decrease IOP by 27%–35%. Unlike β-blockers, CA inhibitors, and $α_2$-agonists, PG analogues act on enhancement of outflow rather than formation of aqueous humor.

Synthesis

Arachidonic acid can be released from plasma membrane phospholipids through a wide variety of stimuli: inflammatory, immunologic, neural, chemical, or simple mechanical agitation. Free AA reacts either with cyclooxygenase (also known as *PG synthetase*), the first enzyme of the PG biosynthetic sequence, or with lipoxygenase to generate hydroperoxy fatty acids (see Fig 9-1). Note that these are 2 isoforms of cyclooxygenase (COX-1 and COX-2). In the cyclooxygenase reaction, the released arachidonate is converted into endoperoxides (PGG_2 and PGH_2) by the membrane-bound cyclooxygenase. The endoperoxides are then converted to TXA_2 by thromboxane synthetase or to various PGs by isomerase or reductase enzymes.

Most nonsteroidal anti-inflammatory drugs (NSAIDs), such as indomethacin and aspirin, can block PG biosynthesis from AA via the COX-1 reaction. The NSAIDs bind irreversibly to the cyclooxygenase enzyme. Topical NSAIDs have been used in the treatment of anterior segment inflammation, aphakic and pseudophakic cystoid macular edema, allergic conjunctivitis, and other pain after refractive surgery. Flurbiprofen 0.03% (Ocufen) and suprofen 1% (Profenal) drops are used preoperatively for the prevention of PG-mediated pupillary miosis during ocular surgery. Diclofenac 0.1% (Voltaren Ophthalmic) has been approved for the treatment of postoperative inflammation following cataract extraction. Ketorolac tromethamine 0.5% (Acular) is indicated for the relief of itching from allergic conjunctivitis. Several studies support the use of either diclofenac 0.1% or ketorolac 0.5% to reduce the severity and duration of pseudophakic macular edema thought to be due to ciliary body–derived cytokines and in relieving corneal pain after radial keratotomy.

Prostaglandin biosynthesis, via the COX-2 reaction, can also be blocked by recently developed COX-2 inhibitors. Previously developed NSAIDs (eg, ibuprofen, naproxen) inhibit both COX-1 and COX-2 and compete with arachidonate in binding to the cyclooxygenase-active site. These compounds are effective anti-inflammatory agents, but they are also all quite ulcerogenic when given systemically. In response, pharmaceutical firms have developed new cyclooxygenase inhibitors that selectively inhibit COX-2 (while sparing inhibition of COX-1). These efforts were initially driven by 2 notions, which subsequently proved to be correct:

1. COX-2 is the relevant enzyme in inflammation (it is expressed at low levels under normal physiologic conditions and regulated only in response to pro-inflammatory signals).
2. Constitutively expressed COX-1 (but not COX-2) is present in a variety of tissues (including the inner lining of the stomach).

Indeed, COX-2 inhibitors have been reported to be anti-inflammatory and analgesic and to lack gastrointestinal toxicity. Moreover, they provide time-dependent, reversible inhibition of the COX-2 enzyme. However, oral COX-2 inhibitors, including rofecoxib

(Vioxx), celecoxib (Celebrex), and valdecoxib (Bextra), have been reported to increase the risks of cardiovascular toxicity and complications (eg, myocardial infarction). Because each of these different COX-2 inhibitors has been found to be associated with cardiovascular events, the complication appears to be a class effect.

Leukotrienes

Leukotrienes are also formed from AA through the lipoxygenase pathway. Their actions in intraocular tissues and fluids has not yet been thoroughly investigated. Leukotrienes C_4 and D_4 have been identified as the major active constituents of the slow-reacting substance of anaphylaxis (SRS-A) and are powerful smooth-muscle contractors that alter muscle permeability. They are much more active than histamine. NSAIDs do not inhibit lipoxygenase, but nordihydroguaiaretic acid (NDGA) does.

Prostaglandin Receptors

There is a large family of G-protein–coupled, 7-transmembrane PG receptors. Complex specificity and regulatory functions arise because individual receptors have differing and overlapping specificities for individual PGs, they are specifically distributed among different cells and tissues, and there are different coupling mechanisms in different cells. The variety of PGs and the variability in receptors, which was described earlier, leads to very complicated and incompletely understood pathophysiologic functions for most PGs.

In general, PGs play key roles in regulation of smooth-muscle contractility; in mediation of pain and fever; in regulation of blood pressure and platelet aggregation; and in other physiologic defense mechanisms, including immune and inflammatory responses. Inhibition of cyclooxygenases, and therefore prostaglandins, is the mechanism for much of the analgesic, anti-inflammatory, antipyretic, and antithrombotic effects of NSAIDs.

Abdel-Latif AA. Release and effects of prostaglandins in ocular tissues. *Prostaglandins Leukot Essent Fatty Acids.* 1991;44(2):71–82.

Colin J. The role of NSAIDs in the management of postoperative ophthalmic inflammation. *Drugs.* 2007;67(9):1291–1308.

Drazen JM. COX-2 inhibitors—a lesson in unexpected problems. *N Engl J Med.* 2005;352(11): 1131–1132.

Rho DS. Treatment of acute pseudophakic cystoid macular edema: diclofenac versus ketorolac. *J Cataract Refract Surg.* 2003;29(12):2378–2384.

Neurotransmitters, Receptors, and Signal Transduction Pathways

In the iris–ciliary body, the sphincter and ciliary muscles have parasympathetic innervation by the third cranial (oculomotor) nerve, and cholinergic impulses are transmitted to the muscle by acetylcholine (ACh). In the ciliary processes, nonmedullated nerve fibers, many of them adrenergic, surround the blood vessels. The dilator muscle fibers of the iris are innervated by the sympathetic nerves from the superior cervical ganglion, and the adrenergic nerve impulses are transmitted to the muscle cells by norepinephrine (NE).

The neurons that synthesize, store, and release ACh are called *cholinergic neurons*; those that synthesize, store, and release NE are called *adrenergic neurons*.

There are also 2 major types of autonomic receptors: cholinergic receptors receive input from cholinergic neurons; adrenergic receptors, from adrenergic neurons. These receptors are further divided as shown in Table 9-1. The receptors of both the iris sphincter and the ciliary muscle are of the cholinergic muscarinic type, and the iris dilator is mainly of the α-adrenergic receptor type. In addition, the iris muscles contain sensory nerves. The sensory neurotransmitters include substance P and calcitonin gene–related peptide (CGRP), which may be involved in trophic effects, inflammatory reactions, and direct or indirect regulation of iris muscle tone in many species, including humans.

Miotics

Miotic agents, which constrict the pupil, act either by stimulating the sphincter (cholinergic agonists) or by blocking the dilator (adrenergic blockers).

Cholinergic agonist miotics

Sphincter stimulators produce responses similar to ACh. They contract the sphincter (resulting in an increase in pupillary contraction) and the ciliary muscles (resulting in accommodation). Sphincter activity can be affected by 2 mechanisms:

1. direct action on the muscles through ACh, carbachol, and pilocarpine
2. inhibition of acetylcholinesterase (AChE), either reversibly with physostigmine (Eserine) or neostigmine (Prostigmin), or irreversibly with diisopropyl fluorophosphate (DFP) or echothiophate iodide (Phospholine Iodide). The AChE inhibitors allow ACh to accumulate at the parasympathetic third nerve endings and produce accommodative spasm.

Table 9-1 Cholinergic and Adrenergic Receptors

Receptors	Agonists	Blocking Agents
Cholinergic (sphincter)	Acetylcholine	
Muscarinic	Muscarine	Atropine
Nicotinic	Nicotine	d-Tubocurarine
Adrenergic (dilator)	Norepinephrine	
Alpha*	Phenylephrine	Phentolamine and phenoxybenzamine
α_1	Phenylephrine	Prazosin, thymoxamine, dapiprazole
α_2	Apraclonidine	Yohimbine
Beta	Isoproterenol	Propranolol and timolol
β_1	Tazolol	Betaxolol
β_2	Albuterol	Butoxamine

The cholinergic agonists and the adrenergic blockers listed cause miosis; the adrenergic agonists and the cholinergic blockers listed cause dilation.

* The prefixes α_1 and α_2 have been proposed for post- and presynaptic α-adrenoceptors, respectively. According to the present view, the classification into α_1 and α_2 subtypes is based exclusively on the relative potencies and affinities of agonists and antagonists, regardless of their function and localization.

Adrenergic antagonist miotics

Two mechanisms for the action of dilator blockers are available:

1. inhibition of the release of NE at the myoneural junction by guanethidine (Ismelin), which acts by depleting NE stores at the nerve terminals (once these stores are depleted, miosis follows)
2. blockage of the α-adrenergic receptors of the dilator muscle by thymoxamine, dapiprazole, phenoxybenzamine, dibenamine, or phentolamine, which prevent contraction and produce miosis (miosis is due to the unopposed action of the iris sphincter, which is tonically innervated)

The pupillary dilator muscle has predominantly α-adrenergic receptors, whereas the ciliary muscle is under parasympathetic control. Thymoxamine and dapiprazole, which are selective α_1-adrenergic blocking agents, can cause miosis through dilator-muscle paralysis without affecting the ciliary muscle–controlled facility of outflow, IOP, or amplitude of accommodation. Thymoxamine has been advocated for many uses but is not commercially available in the United States. Until recently, dapiprazole was commercially available for reversal of pupillary dilation after pharmacologic mydriasis. With thymoxamine or dapiprazole, the pupil returns to its predilated state in 30 minutes (versus 3–4 hours without these agents). These agents will not prevent angle-closure glaucoma, but they are able to move the pupil through the more dangerous mid-dilated state more quickly than when they are not used.

Mydriatics

Mydriatic agents, which dilate the pupil, act by stimulating the dilator (adrenergic agonists) or by blocking the sphincter (cholinergic blockers).

Adrenergic agonist mydriatics

Dilator stimulators increase dilator activity in 3 ways:

1. by increasing NE release, as with hydroxyamphetamine, which causes NE to be released rapidly, thus resulting in mydriasis
2. by interfering with NE reuptake, as with cocaine, which, in addition to acting as a local anesthetic, prevents NE reuptake (inactivation) and thus prolongs or potentiates the action of released NE
3. by directly stimulating the α_1-receptors of the dilator, as with phenylephrine (Neo-Synephrine)

Cholinergic antagonist mydriatics

An adrenergic agent is only mydriatic, but an anticholinergic is mydriatic and cycloplegic. An effective anticholinergic (sphincter-blocking) agent that produces both mydriasis and cycloplegia is atropine, which blocks the action of ACh and pilocarpine at the muscle. Its effects are long lasting (a single drop may last for days). A drug that produces rapid cycloplegia but has a relatively short action is tropicamide. Cyclopentolate is a blocker of intermediate action and duration. Other agents include homatropine and scopolamine (see Chapter 17, Table 17-2).

Calcium Channels and Channel Blockers

Calcium channels are membrane-bound protein receptors that contain multiple subunits, one of which is the active site for binding of calcium channel blockers. Calcium plays a major role in influencing cellular function, and the most common pathway for entry into cells is through the calcium channels. Six subclasses of calcium channel blockers have been identified: L, T, N, P, Q, and R. The L-type blocker is predominant in skeletal, cardiac, and vascular smooth muscle. Calcium channel blockers bind to membrane-bound calcium channels and inhibit the influx of extracellular calcium in vascular smooth muscle, thereby causing direct arteriolar vasodilation and depression of myocardial contractility. They are widely used for the treatment of hypertension and, in therapeutic doses, do not affect glucose tolerance, lipoproteins, uric acid, or serum electrolytes. Topically applied calcium channel blockers lower IOP. Because normal-tension glaucoma may be associated with vasospastic disease, calcium channel blockers may play a role in the treatment of this poorly understood condition. See also BCSC Section 10, *Glaucoma*.

Netland PA, Erickson KA. Calcium channel blockers in glaucoma management. *Ophthalmol Clin North Am.* 1995;8:327–334.

Membrane Receptors and Intracellular Communications

Signal Transduction

Receptors for neurotransmitters and peptide hormones are located on the surface of the cell, whereas receptors for steroid hormones are intracellular, so steroid hormones must be able to enter the cell to have an effect. Both the iris and the ciliary body contain adrenergic, muscarinic cholinergic, peptidergic, PG, serotonin, and purinergic receptors.

Membrane receptors have several characteristics:

- They recognize and bind to first messengers, or *ligands*—molecules such as hormones, peptides, drugs, and neurotransmitters.
- They are ligand-specific, but many can cause positive or negative responses depending on their location (ie, different cell types may have different responses to the same messenger).
- The number of receptors occupied by ligands determines the magnitude of the cell response.

Receptor–Effector Coupling

The response of the cell to the ligand depends on signal transduction across the plasma membrane to the cell interior, which occurs by several basic mechanisms, including

- A ligand (eg, neurotransmitters such as glycine, glutamate, γ-aminobutyric acid) binds to a receptor that functions as an ion channel (a ligand-gated ion channel) and causes it to open, allowing cations to pass into the cells.
- Receptors that have integral enzyme (eg, tyrosine kinase) activity are activated by ligand binding.

- G-protein–coupled receptors activate effector proteins, which include ion channels and enzymes.

The G-protein–coupled receptor mechanism involves a cascade of 3 steps: A ligand excites a receptor protein to activate a G protein, which in turn activates an effector protein (E). The effector proteins are usually enzymes such as adenylate cyclase, phospholipase C (PLC), phospholipase A_2, or phosphodiesterase (PDE). These produce second messengers such as cyclic nucleotides (eg, cAMP, cGMP) and lipid-derived molecules (eg, PGs, discussed earlier in this chapter, and IP_3, discussed next). Rhodopsin, one of the most studied G-protein–coupled receptors, is discussed in detail in Chapter 13.

Cyclic AMP and Polyphosphoinositide Turnover

Activated β-adrenergic and CGRP receptors *stimulate* the adenylate cyclase system via the stimulatory G proteins ($G_{s\alpha}$); others, such as M_2-muscarinic and α_2-adrenergic receptors, *inhibit* this effector enzyme via an inhibitory G protein ($G_{i\alpha}$) (Fig 9-2).

The primary control for many intracellular events is the concentration of free Ca^{2+} in the cytosol. Many Ca^{2+}-mobilizing hormones and neurotransmitters, such as ACh, NE, and $PGF_2\alpha$, act by changing the intracellular Ca^{2+} concentration. Activation of Ca^{2+}-mobilizing receptors, such as M_3-muscarinic and α_1-adrenergic receptors, causes the

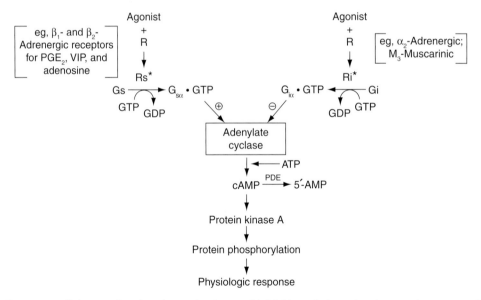

Figure 9-2 Scheme showing the activation and inhibition of the adenylate cyclase second-messenger system. Adenosine diphosphate *(ADP)* ribosylation of $G_{s\alpha}$ by cholera toxin maintains $G_{s\alpha}$ in the active state, whereas ADP ribosylation of $G_{i\alpha}$ by pertussis toxin results in inactivation of $G_{i\alpha}$. *5′-AMP* = adenosine 5′-monophosphate; *ATP* = adenosine triphosphate; *cAMP* = 3′,5′-cyclic adenosine monophosphate; *GDP* = guanosine diphosphate; *Gs and Gi* = stimulatory and inhibitory G proteins, respectively; *GTP* = guanosine triphosphate; *PDE* = phosphodiesterase; *PGE_2* = prostaglandin E_2; *Rs* and Ri** = activated receptor complexes; *VIP* = vasoactive intestinal polypeptide. *(Courtesy of Ata Abdel-Latif, PhD.)*

release of Ca^{2+} from the sarcoplasmic reticulum (SR) via the polyphosphoinositide second messenger IP_3. Phosphatidylinositol 4,5-bisphosphate (PIP_2) turnover also has a role in the regulation of $[Ca^{2+}]_1$ (Fig 9-3).

In the iris sphincter, as well as in other types of smooth muscle, activation of muscarinic receptors leads to IP_3 production, Ca^{2+} mobilization, and muscle contraction. In contrast, activation of β-adrenergic receptors leads to cAMP formation, reduction in intracellular Ca^{2+} concentration, and muscle relaxation. Contraction–relaxation responses are regulated by increases in the level of cAMP. In the iris sphincter, PGs can trigger either IP_3 production and muscle contraction or cAMP formation and muscle relaxation, depending on the type of PG, species, cell type, and tissue. Such interactions between the 2 signaling systems could constitute the biochemical basis for the multiple functions observed for PGs in a wide variety of systems. The sympathetic nervous system, via alterations in cAMP concentrations, can modulate the cholinergic stimulation of IP_3 production and muscle contraction.

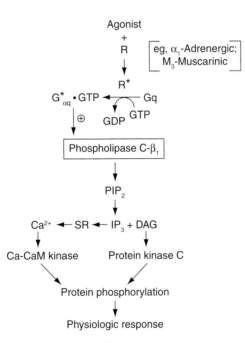

Figure 9-3 Scheme showing agonist-stimulated breakdown of phosphatidylinositol 4,5-bisphosphate *(PIP₂)* into inositol 1,4,5-triphosphate *(IP₃)* and diacylglycerol *(DAG)*. The agonists bind to the Ca^{2+}-mobilizing receptor to activate the G protein G_q to $G^*_{\alpha q}$ and stimulate phospholipase C-β₁ to hydrolyze PIP_2 into IP_3 and DAG. IP_3 diffuses through the cytosol and binds to the IP_3 receptor on the sarcoplasmic reticulum *(SR)* to release Ca^{2+} from a specific Ca^{2+} pool. Ca^{2+} binds to calmodulin *(CaM)*; Ca^{2+}-calmodulin then activates a protein kinase to phosphorylate a protein substrate and provoke a cellular response. IP_3 is then rapidly metabolized by a series of dephosphorylation and phosphorylation pathways. DAG acts by binding to protein kinase C. Once activated, protein kinase C translocates to the plasma membrane and there phosphorylates a number of proteins on serine and threonine residues. Phorbol esters mimic the action of DAG on protein kinase C; in fact, the enzyme is presumed to be the receptor for phorbol esters. *GDP* = guanosine diphosphate, *GTP* = guanosine triphosphate, *R** = activated receptor complex. *(Courtesy of Ata Abdel-Latif, PhD.)*

Receptors

Examples of ocular receptors, their subtypes, and their signal transduction mechanisms are given in Table 9-2. In recent years, a number of reports have appeared on the biochemical and pharmacologic characterization of these receptors. Understanding ocular receptors and their transduction mechanisms will help us design better therapeutic agents for the treatment of glaucoma. This can be appreciated from the summary on the mode of action of the various antiglaucoma agents provided in Table 9-3. The therapeutic actions of these drugs are mediated through specific receptors.

> Abdel-Latif AA. Iris–ciliary body, aqueous humor and trabecular meshwork. In: Harding JJ, ed. *Biochemistry of the Eye.* London: Chapman and Hall Medical; 1997:52–93.

Table 9-2 Ocular Receptor Subtypes and Their Signal Transduction Mechanisms

Receptor	Receptor Subtypes and Their Signal Transduction Mechanisms			
β-Adrenoceptor	β_1 cAMP ↑	β_2 cAMP ↑	β_3 cAMP ↑	
α_1-Adrenoceptor	α_1A $IP_3/Ca^{2+}/DAG$	α_1B $IP_3/Ca^{2+}/DAG$	α_1D $IP_3/Ca^{2+}/DAG$	
α_2-Adrenoceptor	α_2A cAMP ↓	α_2B cAMP ↓	α_2C cAMP ↓	α_2D cAMP ↓
Muscarinic cholinergic	M_1 $IP_3/Ca^{2+}/DAG$	M_2 cAMP ↓	M_3 $IP_3/Ca^{2+}/DAG$	M_4 cAMP ↓
Calcitonin gene-related peptide	$CGRP_1$ cAMP ↑	$CGRP_2$ cAMP ↑		
Endothelin	ET_A $IP_3/Ca^{2+}/DAG$ cAMP ↓	ET_B $IP_3/Ca^{2+}/DAG$		
Prostaglandin	DP, EP (EP_1, EP_2, EP_3, EP_4), FP, IP, TP Increase in cAMP or IP_3 depending on the receptor subtype			

Table 9-3 Mode of Action of Antiglaucoma Agents That Act Through Receptors

Primary Mechanism of Action	Drug Class	Examples
1. Decrease aqueous humor production	a. β-Adrenergic antagonists	Timolol, betaxolol, carteolol, levobunolol
	b. α_2-Adrenergic agonists	Apraclonidine, brimonidine
2. Increase trabecular outflow	a. Miotics	Pilocarpine
	b. Adrenergic agonists	Epinephrine, dipivalyl epinephrine
3. Increase uveoscleral outflow	a. Prostaglandins	Latanoprost, bimatoprost, travoprost
	b. α-Adrenergic agonists	Apraclonidine, brimonidine

CHAPTER 10

Aqueous Humor

The aqueous humor is important in the physiology of the mammalian eye. It provides nutrients (eg, glucose and amino acids) to support the function of tissues of the anterior segment, such as the avascular lens, cornea, and trabecular meshwork; it also removes the metabolic wastes from these tissues (eg, lactic acid, pyruvic acid). Aqueous humor also helps to maintain appropriate IOP. These functional properties are essential to the eye's structural integrity. In addition, because the aqueous humor is devoid of blood cells and of more than 99% of the plasma proteins, it provides an optically clear medium for the transmission of light along the visual path.

Aqueous Dynamics

The aqueous humor is secreted by the ciliary epithelium at a flow rate of 2–3 µL/min. The ciliary epithelium is a bilayer of polarized epithelial cells lining the surface of the ciliary body; the 2 cell layers are *nonpigmented ciliary epithelium (NPE)*, which faces the aqueous humor through the cells' basal plasma membrane; and *pigmented ciliary epithelium (PE)*, which faces the stroma, also through the cells' basal plasma membrane. Therefore, the apical plasma membranes of both NPE and PE cells appose each other, establishing cell-to-cell communication through numerous gap junctions. Of the 2 cell layers that constitute the ciliary epithelium, the NPE cells establish a blood–aqueous barrier by the presence of tight junctions proximal to the apical plasma membrane, thus preventing the free passage of plasma proteins and other macromolecules from the stroma to the posterior chamber. In contrast, the PE cell layer is considered a leaky epithelium, as it allows the movement of solutes through the intercellular space between the PE cells.

Composition of the Aqueous Humor

Table 10-1 summarizes the composition of aqueous humor. It is clear from the values given in the table that the fluid and electrolyte composition is similar to that of plasma. However, the aqueous secretion is not an ultrafiltrate of plasma (as was once speculated), because it is produced by energy-dependent processes in the epithelial layer of the ciliary body; this mode of production allows precise control to be maintained over the composition of fluid bathing structures essential for normal vision.

Macknight AD, McLaughlin CW, Peart D, Purves RD, Carré DA, Civan MM. Formation of the aqueous humor. *Clin Exp Pharmacol Physiol.* 2000;27(1–2):100–106.

Table 10-1 Composition of Aqueous Humor

Components (mmol/kg H$_2$O)	Plasma	Aqueous Posterior	Anterior	Vitreous
Rabbit				
Na	143	159	138	134
K	4.6	4.7	4.3	4.6
Cl	108	97	101	105
HCO$_3$	25	34	30	26
Ascorbate	0.04	1.4	1.1	0.46
Lactate	10.3	9.9	9.3	12
Glucose	6	6	6	4.6
Human				
Na	146	163		144
Cl	109	134		114
HCO$_3$	28	20		20–30
Ascorbate	0.04	1.06		2.21
Glucose	6	3		3.4

From Macknight AD, MacLaughlin CW, Peart D, Purves RD, Carré DA, Civan MM. Formation of the aqueous humor. *Clin Exp Pharmacol Physiol.* 2000;27(1–2):100–106.

The ionic composition of aqueous humor is determined by selective active-transport systems (eg, Na$^+$,K$^+$-2Cl$^-$ symport, Cl$^-$-HCO$_3^-$ and Na$^+$,H$^+$ antiports, cation channels, water channels, Na$^+$,K$^+$-ATPase, K$^+$ channels, Cl$^-$ channels, H$^+$-ATPase) that participate in secretion of aqueous humor by the ciliary epithelium. The systems' activity and cellular distribution along the cell membranes of PE and NPE cells determine unidirectional net secretion from the stroma to the posterior chamber, a process that involves 3 steps:

1. uptake of solute and water at the stromal surface by PE cells
2. transfer from PE to NPE cells through gap junctions
3. transfer of solute and water by NPE cells into the posterior chamber

Likewise, it is thought that there is a mechanism for transporting solute and water from the posterior chamber back into the stroma. In this unidirectional reabsorption, another set of transporters may be involved in extruding Na$^+$,K$^+$ and Cl$^-$ back into the stroma.

Krupin T, Civan MM. Physiologic basis of aqueous humor formation. In: Ritch R, Shields MB, Krupin T, eds. *The Glaucomas.* 2nd ed. Vol 1. St Louis: Mosby; 1996:251–280.

Molecular studies have shown that the secretory properties of the ciliary epithelium are not limited to ions and electrolytes but extend to a wide range of molecules of different molecular mass. A common feature for many of these molecules is their synthesis locally in the ciliary epithelium and then their secretion by the NPE cells through the regulatory pathway into the aqueous humor. Among the proteins identified whose mRNA expression has been demonstrated are

- plasma proteins (eg, complement component C4, α_2-macroglobulin, selenoprotein P, apolipoprotein D, plasma glutathione peroxidases, angiotensinogen)

- proteinases (eg, cathepsin D, cathepsin O)
- a component of the visual cycle (eg, cellular retinaldehyde–binding protein, or *CRALBP*)
- a neurotrophic factor (eg, pigment epithelium–derived factor)
- neuropeptide-processing enzymes (eg, carboxypeptidase E, peptidyl-glycine-α-amidating monoxygenase)
- neuroendocrine peptides (eg, secretogranin II, neurotensin, galanin)
- bioactive peptides and hormones (eg, atrial natriuretic peptide, brain natriuretic peptide)

These findings support the view that the ciliary epithelium exhibits neuroendocrine properties that are directly related to the makeup of the aqueous humor and its regulation. The aqueous humor composition is in dynamic equilibrium, determined both by its rate of production and outflow and by continuous exchanges with the tissues of the anterior segment. It contains the following:

- inorganic ions and organic anions
- carbohydrates
- glutathione and urea
- proteins
- growth-modulatory factors
- oxygen and carbon dioxide

Inorganic Ions

The concentrations of sodium, potassium, and magnesium in the aqueous are similar to those in plasma, but the level of calcium is only half that of plasma. The 2 major anions are chloride and bicarbonate. Phosphate is also present in the aqueous (aqueous:plasma ratio: $\approx$0.5 or less), but its concentration is too low to have any significant buffering capacity. Iron, copper, and zinc are all found in the aqueous humor at essentially the same levels as in plasma, approximately 1 mg/mL.

Organic Anions

Lactate is the most abundant of organic anions in the aqueous, and its concentration is always higher than that in plasma. Plasma and aqueous levels of lactate are directly related, and the contribution resulting from the glycolytic metabolism of intraocular tissues is significant.

Ascorbic acid (vitamin C) is perhaps the most unique constituent of the aqueous humor. In most mammalian species, its concentration ranges from 0.6 to 1.5 mmol/L, levels that are some 10–50 times higher than that in plasma. Furthermore, levels of ascorbic acid in the aqueous humor of diurnal mammals may be 20 times higher than ascorbic acid levels in nocturnal mammals. Ascorbic acid is an important antioxidant, both in the aqueous humor and in tissues of the anterior segment. Ascorbic acid is actively transported by the ciliary epithelial cells from the stroma side into the posterior chamber by a Na$^+$-dependent L-ascorbic acid transporter.

Carbohydrates

Glucose concentration in the aqueous is roughly 70% of that in plasma. The rate of entry of glucose into the posterior chamber is much more rapid than would be expected from its molecular size and lipid solubility, suggesting that its passage across the ciliary epithelium occurs by facilitated diffusion. Saturation studies have demonstrated that a specific carrier is involved, but no evidence of active transport has been detected, nor has insulin been found to affect the entry of glucose into the aqueous. Aqueous glucose levels are increased in people with diabetes, leading to higher concentrations in the lens, with short-term refractive and longer-term cataract implications. Inositol, important for phospholipid synthesis in the anterior segment, occurs at a concentration approximately 10 times that in plasma.

Glutathione and Urea

Glutathione, an important tripeptide with a reactive sulfhydryl group, is found in the aqueous humor. Its concentration in primates ranges from 1 to 10 μmol/L. Blood contains a high concentration of glutathione, but virtually all glutathione resides within the erythrocytes, and plasma has only a low concentration of 5 μmol/L or less. Although aqueous glutathione may be derived by diffusion from the blood or by an active-transport system in the ciliary epithelium analogous to that of the lens, it probably also arises by loss from the lens and cornea. Glutathione acts as a stabilizer of the redox state of the aqueous by reconverting ascorbate to its functional form after oxidation, as well as by removing excess hydrogen peroxide. Glutathione also serves as a substrate in the enzymatic conjugation by a group of cytosolic enzymes involved in the cellular detoxification of electrophilic compounds. These enzymes (glutathione S-transferases) are important in protecting tissues from oxidative damage and oxidative stress and are highly expressed in the ocular ciliary epithelium.

The concentration of urea in the aqueous is between 80% and 90% of that in plasma. This compound is distributed passively across nearly all biological membrane systems, and its high aqueous:plasma ratio indicates that this small molecule (molecular weight of 60 kD) crosses the epithelial barrier quite readily. Urea is effective in the hyperosmotic infusion treatment for glaucoma. However, mannitol (with a molecular weight of 182 kD) is preferred to urea because it crosses the barrier more easily.

Proteins

The nonpigmented ciliary epithelial cell layer establishes a blood–aqueous barrier that prevents the diffusion of plasma proteins from the stroma into the posterior chamber; nevertheless, plasma proteins do enter the aqueous humor, and one possible route for this is through the root and anterior surface of the iris.

Normal aqueous contains approximately 0.02 g of protein per 100 mL, as compared with the typical plasma level of 7 g/100 mL. The most abundant plasma proteins identified in aqueous humor are albumin and transferrin, which together may account for 50% of all the protein content.

However, there is compelling evidence that proteins that make up the aqueous humor might actually have been synthesized within the ciliary body and secreted directly into the aqueous humor. Molecular techniques (such as the screening of cDNA libraries constructed from the intact human and bovine ciliary bodies) have resulted in the isolation and identification of numerous protein-encoding genes. These studies, therefore, challenge the long-held view that plasma proteins in the aqueous humor are transported into the aqueous from outside the eye. Among cDNAs isolated from the ciliary body–encoding plasma proteins are

- complement component C4, which participates in immune-mediated inflammation responses
- α_2-macroglobulin, which serves as a carrier protein and is involved in proteinase inhibition, clearance, and targeting; and processing of foreign peptides
- apolipoprotein D, which binds and transports hydrophobic substances, including cholesterol, cholesteryl esters, and arachidonic acid
- selenoprotein P, which has antioxidant properties

Proteinases and inhibitors

A number of proteinases and proteinase inhibitors have also been identified in the aqueous humor. These proteinases include cathepsin D and cathepsin O, which are synthesized and secreted by the ciliary epithelial cells. Cathepsin D is involved in the degradation of neuropeptides and peptide hormones and has been found in high levels in the cerebrospinal fluid of patients with Alzheimer disease. Less is known about cathepsin O; it may be involved in normal cellular protein degradation and turnover. Of the proteinase inhibitors, α_2-macroglobulin and α_1-antitrypsin are perhaps the most extensively studied. An imbalance in equilibrium between proteinases and proteinase inhibitors could lead to an alteration in aqueous humor composition, which may result in disease (eg, glaucoma).

Enzymes

Activators, proenzymes, and fibrinolytic enzymes are present in the aqueous, and these enzymes could play a role in the regulation of outflow resistance. Both plasminogen and plasminogen activator are found in human and monkey aqueous, but only traces of plasmin have been reported. In addition to the proteins already mentioned, other enzymes have been reported in the aqueous humor. Several of these are of interest chiefly because of their increased levels in certain pathologic conditions, such as retinoblastoma, wherein tissue damage results in the release of intracellular enzymes. The frequent absence of coenzymes or the substrates of such enzymes from the aqueous (as in the case of nicotinamide adenine dinucleotide for lactic dehydrogenase or of oxaloacetate for glutamic-oxaloacetic transaminase) leads to the conclusion that these enzymes have no significant catalytic role in the normal aqueous. However, 3 enzymes in the aqueous appear to be exceptions to this nonreactive role:

1. *Hyaluronidase* may be important in the normal regulation of the resistance to outflow through the trabecular meshwork because its injection into the anterior chamber has been shown to increase outflow facility in some species.
2. *Carbonic anhydrase* is present in trace amounts. Because it is an enzyme with an extremely high turnover, even a low concentration may be significant in the catalysis of the equilibrium between bicarbonate and CO_2 plus water.

3. *Lysozyme* provides significant antibacterial protection. Most likely, lysozyme originates only in part from the blood; in cases of ocular inflammation, the intraocular
level may be raised tenfold or more, reaching concentrations well above those in
plasma.

Neurotrophic and neuroendocrine proteins

The ciliary epithelia, which are derived from neuroectoderm, are functionally similar to
neuroendocrine glands elsewhere in the body. Bioactive neuroendocrine markers identified from human ciliary body cDNA subtraction studies, such as neurotensin, angio-
tensin, endothelins, and natriuretic peptides, have systemic vascular hemodynamic effects
and, by implication, may have similar roles in IOP regulation or aqueous secretion. Some
authors have linked circadian IOP rhythms to these markers, but this has not been clearly
established because corneal biomechanical properties also fluctuate.

The neuroendocrine properties of the ciliary epithelium could also determine the
composition of the aqueous humor. Neuropeptide-processing enzymes include prohor-
mone convertases, carboxypeptidase E, and peptidylglycine α-amidating monooxygenase;
among neuropeptides and peptide hormones are secretogranin II, galanin, neurotensin,
and natriuretic peptides. These compounds, synthesized as large precursors, are cleaved
to bioactive peptides and secreted by the ciliary epithelial cells into the aqueous in a regulated, calcium-dependent manner. The function of these bioactive peptides in the aqueous
humor secretion is not clearly understood.

Coca-Prados M, Escribano J, Ortego J. Differential gene expression in the human ciliary epithelium. *Prog Retin Eye Res.* 1999;18(3):403–429.
Cowdrey G, Firth M, Moss R, Karim A, Thompson G, Firth G. The analysis of aqueous humor
constituents using capillary zone electrophoresis. *Exp Eye Res.* 1998;67(4):449–455.

Growth-Modulatory Factors

The physical and chemical properties of the aqueous humor play a substantial role in
modulating the proliferation, differentiation, functional viability, and wound healing of
ocular tissues. These properties are largely influenced by a number of growth-promoting
and differentiation factors that have been identified or quantified in aqueous humor. They
include

- transforming growth factor βs 1 and 2 (TGF-β_1 and -β_2)
- acidic and basic fibroblast growth factor (aFGF and bFGF)
- insulin-like growth factor I (IGF-I)
- insulin-like growth factor binding proteins (IGFBPs)
- vascular endothelial growth factor (VEGF)
- transferrin

The growth factors in the aqueous humor perform diverse, synergistic, and sometimes opposite biological activities. Normally, the lack of significant mitosis of the corneal
endothelium and trabecular meshwork in vivo is probably controlled by the complex coordination of effects and interactions among the different growth-modulatory substances
present in the aqueous humor (see Part V, Ocular Pharmacology). Disruption in the balance among various growth factors that occurs with the production of plasmoid aqueous

humor may explain the abnormal hyperplastic response of the lens epithelium and corneal endothelium observed in chronic inflammatory conditions and traumatic insults to the eye. Ultimately, however, the effect of a given growth factor in the aqueous humor is determined primarily by the growth factor's bioavailability. Bioavailability depends on many factors, including the expression of receptors on target tissues, interactive effects with components of the extracellular matrix, and the levels of circulating and matrix-bound proteases.

The role of several growth factors has been studied in patients with diabetes mellitus. IGFBPs are elevated fivefold in human patients with diabetes (without retinopathy), and IGF-I levels are elevated in patients with diabetic retinopathy. These elevations suggest that the increase in vitreal IGFBPs is not the result of a preexisting end-stage retinopathy but is rather an early ocular event in the diabetic process.

Vascular Endothelial Growth Factors

The VEGF family of glycoproteins includes VEGF-A, -B, -C, -D and placental growth factor (PlGF). VEGF-A, which has 9 isoforms, is currently the most studied; it is the only one induced by hypoxia and is a critical regulator of angiogenesis and a potent inducer of vascular permeability. Three VEGF receptors have been identified:

1. VEGFR1 has both positive and negative angiogenic effects.
2. VEGFR2 is the primary mediator of the mitogenic, angiogenic, and vascular permeability effects of VEGF-A.
3. VEGFR3 mediates the angiogenic effects on lymphatic vessels.

VEGF-A and its receptors are also present in tissues and organ systems in normal adults, underlining its physiologic role. VEGF may also have roles in retinal leukostasis and neuroprotection.

VEGF-A levels are increased not only in patients with active ocular neovascularization from proliferative diabetic retinopathy but also after occlusion of the central retinal vein and with iris neovascularization. The expression of VEGF-A is increased by hypoxia in retinal endothelial cells, retinal pericytes, Müller cells, and RPE cells. In addition, a soluble VEGF-dependent mechanism has been shown to mediate RPE barrier dysfunction in cocultures of RPE with endothelial cells (ECs). This EC–RPE contact-induced disruption of barrier properties takes place with ocular conditions such as choroidal neovascularization, wherein ECs pass through Bruch's membrane and contact the RPE. Also, aqueous VEGF-A levels increase in response to anterior segment ischemia in animal models, in addition to the well-described response to retinal hypoxia.

Bhisitkul RB. Vascular endothelial growth factor biology: clinical implications for ocular treatments. *Br J Ophthalmol.* 2006;90(12):1542–1547.

Oxygen and Carbon Dioxide

Oxygen is present in the aqueous humor at a partial pressure of about 55 mm Hg, roughly one third of its concentration in the atmosphere. It is derived from the blood supply to the ciliary body and iris, for there is no net flux of oxygen from the atmosphere across the cornea. Indeed, the corneal endothelium is critically dependent on the aqueous oxygen supply for the active fluid-transport mechanism that maintains corneal transparency. The lens and the endothelial lining of the trabecular meshwork also derive their oxygen supply from the aqueous humor.

The carbon dioxide content of the aqueous humor is in the range of 40–60 mm Hg, which contributes approximately 3% of the total bicarbonate. The relative proportions of CO_2 and HCO_3^- determine the pH of the aqueous, which in most species has been found to be in the range of 7.5–7.6. CO_2 is continuously lost from the aqueous by diffusion across the cornea into the tear film and atmosphere. The Na^+,K^+-Cl^- cotransporter is also important both in the trabecular meshwork and for control of aqueous outflow.

Gong H, Tripathi RC, Tripathi BJ. Morphology of the aqueous outflow pathway. *Microsc Res Tech.* 1996;33(4):336–367.

Spector A, Ma W, Wang RR. The aqueous humor is capable of generating and degrading H_2O_2. *Invest Ophthalmol Vis Sci.* 1998;39(7):1188–1197.

Clinical Implications of Breakdown of the Blood–Aqueous Barrier

With compromise of the blood–aqueous barrier in conditions such as ocular insult (trauma or intraocular surgery), as well as uveitis and other inflammatory disorders, the protein content of aqueous humor may increase 10–100 times, especially in the high-molecular-weight polypeptides. The levels of inflammatory mediators, immunoglobulins, fibrin, and proteases rise, and the balance among the various growth factors is disrupted (see Chapter 17). The clinical sequelae include fibrinous exudate and clot (with or without a macrophage reaction and formation of cyclitic membranes) and synechiae formation (peripheral and posterior), as well as an abnormal neovascular response, which further exacerbates breakdown of the barrier. Chronic disruption of the blood–aqueous barrier is implicated in the abnormal hyperplastic response of the lens epithelium, corneal endothelium, trabecular meshwork, and iris, and in the formation of complicated cataracts. Degenerative and proliferative changes may occur in various ocular structures as well. The use of anti-inflammatory steroidal and nonsteroidal drugs, cycloplegics, protease activators or inhibitors, growth and antigrowth factor agents, and even surgical intervention may be necessary to combat these events.

CHAPTER 11

Lens

The lens is a transparent, avascular body that, in concert with the cornea, focuses incident light onto the sensory elements of the retina. To perform this function, the lens must be transparent and must have an index of refraction higher than that of the surrounding fluids. Maintenance of transparency depends on precise organization of the cellular structure of the lens and a high degree of short-range order of the protein matrix of the lens-fiber cytoplasm. Transparency must be maintained as the lens changes shape during accommodation. The high refractive index is due to the presence of a very high concentration of protein in the lens cells, especially of the soluble proteins called *crystallins*. Further, because there is little if any turnover of protein in the central region of the lens (where the oldest, denucleated cells are found), the proteins of the human lens must be extremely stable to remain functionally viable for a lifetime. When we consider the lens's mode of growth and the stresses to which the lens is chronically exposed, it is remarkable that in most people, lenses retain good transparency. Nearly all humans develop opacities by the seventh or eighth decade of life.

This chapter discusses the structure and composition of the lens as well as aspects of membrane function, metabolism, and regulatory processes within the lens. Additional information on the lens and on cataractogenesis is provided in BCSC Section 11, *Lens and Cataract*.

Structure of the Lens

Capsule

The lens is enclosed in an elastic basement membrane called the *lens capsule* (Fig 11-1). The capsule is noncellular and is composed primarily of type IV collagen, with smaller amounts of other collagens and extracellular matrix components (including glycosaminoglycans, laminin, fibronectin, and heparan sulfate proteoglycan). The capsule is a very thick basement membrane, particularly on the anterior side of the lens, where the epithelial cells continue to secrete capsular material throughout life. On the posterior side of the lens, where there is no epithelium, the posterior fiber cells have limited capacity to secrete such material. The zonular fibers, from which the lens is suspended, insert into the capsule near the equator on both the anterior and posterior sides. The capsule is not a barrier to diffusion of water, ions, other small molecules, or proteins up to the size of serum albumin (molecular weight of 68,000 kD).

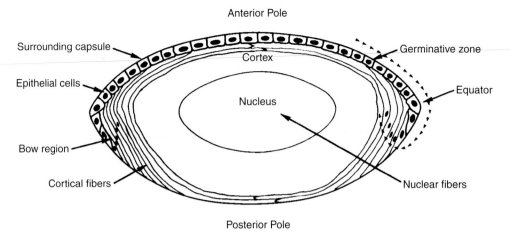

Figure 11-1 Schematic representation of the mammalian lens in cross section. *Small arrowheads* indicate direction of cell migration from the epithelium to the cortex. *(Reproduced with permission from Anderson RE, ed.* Biochemistry of the Eye. *San Francisco: American Academy of Ophthalmology; 1983:112.)*

Epithelium

A single layer of epithelial cells covers the anterior surface of the lens. These cells have full metabolic capacity and play the primary role in regulating the water and ion balance of the entire lens. Although the cells of the central epithelium are not mitotically active, a germinative zone exists as a ring anterior to the equator, where the epithelial cells divide. The new cells migrate toward the equator and begin to differentiate into lens fibers.

Cortex and Nucleus

Aside from the single layer of epithelial cells on its anterior surface, the lens is composed of lens fibers, very long ribbonlike cells. All fibers are formed from epithelial cells at the lens equator; hence, younger fibers are always exterior to older ones. The lens structure can be equated with the growth rings of a tree in that the oldest cells are in the center, with progressively younger layers, or shells, of fiber cells toward the periphery. Unlike the case with many tissues, no cells are sloughed from the lens, and cells produced before birth remain at the center of the lens throughout life.

As new fiber cells are elongating and differentiating into mature fibers, their cell nuclei form the *bow zone*, or *bow region*, at the lens equator. Elongating fibers greatly increase their volume and their surface area and express large amounts of both lens crystallins and a lens-fiber–specific membrane protein called the *major intrinsic protein (MIP)*. As the fibers become fully elongated and make sutures at each end with fibers that have elongated from the opposite side of the lens, they become mature, terminally differentiated fiber cells. The cell nuclei disintegrate, as do mitochondria and other organelles. This process happens quite abruptly by mechanisms that remain obscure. What is understood is that the elimination of cellular organelles is necessary in the central portion of the lens because such bodies are sufficiently large to scatter light and thereby degrade visual acuity. It should also be noted that with the loss of cell nuclei, the mature fibers lose the machinery required for the synthesis of proteins. The fiber mass of the adult lens can be divided into the *cortex* (ie, the outer fibers, laid down after the age of about 20 years) and the *internal nucleus* (ie, the cells produced from embryogenesis through adolescence).

Chemical Composition of the Lens

Membranes

The chemical composition of lens-fiber plasma membranes suggests that they are both very stable and very rigid. A high content of saturated fatty acids, a high cholesterol:phospholipid ratio, and a high concentration of sphingomyelin all contribute to the tight packing and low fluidity of the membrane. Although lipids make up only about 1% of the total lens mass, they constitute about 55% of the plasma membrane's dry weight, with cholesterol being the major neutral lipid. As the lens ages, the protein:lipid and cholesterol:phospholipid ratios increase as a result of phospholipid loss, especially in the nucleus.

Lens Proteins

The lens probably has the highest protein content of any tissue. In some species, more than 50% of lens wet weight is protein. Lens crystallins, a diverse group of proteins expressed in high abundance in the lens-fiber cells and thought to play critical roles in providing the transparency and refractile properties essential to lens function, constitute 90%–95% of total lens protein. In addition to the crystallins, the lens also has a full complement of enzymes and regulatory proteins that are present primarily in the epithelium and in immature fiber cells, where most metabolic activity occurs.

Crystallins

Crystallins are water-soluble proteins so-named for their high abundance in the "crystalline lens." Until the 1980s, crystallins were considered lens-specific proteins, lacking biological activity, which were highly evolved structural elements forming the transparent protein matrix of the lens. It is now clear that most (if not all) crystallins are expressed in other tissues as well and have specific biological functions distinct from their roles in the lens as refractile elements.

All crystallins now appear to be "borrowed" proteins, recruited by the lens for a function completely distinct from their biological functions in other tissues. Although the specific criteria that make a protein suitable to function as a crystallin are not well understood, crystallins must have 2 obvious attributes: (1) Crystallins must be very stable structures because the proteins of the lens are probably the longest-lived proteins in the body. (2) Crystallins must remain soluble under conditions of high protein concentration without forming large aggregates, which would be light-scattering centers within the lens.

Crystallins can be divided into 2 groups. One group includes α-crystallin and the β,γ,-crystallin family, both of which appear to be present in all vertebrate lenses. The second group is the taxon-specific crystallins, which are each present at crystallin levels only in phylogenetically restricted groups of species.

Andley UP. Crystallins in the eye: function and pathology. *Prog Retin Eye Res.* 2007;26(1): 78–98.

α-Crystallin α-Crystallin is the largest of the crystallins, having a native molecular mass in the 600–800 kD range. It is composed of 2 subunits, αA and αB, which are approximately 20 kD in mass and which are nearly 55% identical in sequence. Native α-crystallin has a wide range of molecular masses, apparently because it is a dynamic structure wherein the number of subunits varies somewhat and subunit exchange occurs among the native multimers. Probably because of this molecular mass variability, α-crystallin has thus far resisted attempts at crystallization, so a definitive 3-dimensional structure for the molecule has not been determined.

α-Crystallin is a member of the small "heat-shock protein" family; as a result, the expression of αB is inducible by heat and other stresses. Both αA and αB have a chaperone-like activity whereby they bind proteins that are beginning to denature and prevent further denaturation and aggregation. Zinc ions enhance the chaperone function and stability of α-crystallin. Because protein aggregates in the lens will scatter light and cause loss of transparency, the antiaggregative function of α-crystallin is crucial to the long-term maintenance of transparency in the fibers of the lens nucleus, where synthesis of new protein is impossible and where protein molecules must exist for decades.

β,γ-Crystallins Until the primary sequences of the various β- and γ-crystallins were determined, they were thought to be 2 unrelated families of proteins. However, it is now known that the 2 groups are related members of the same protein superfamily. The β-crystallins, a complex group of oligomers composed of polypeptides, have molecular masses ranging from 23 to 32 kD.

The γ-crystallins are monomeric proteins with molecular masses near 20 kD. Most expression of γ-crystallins occurs early in development; thus, they tend to be most concentrated in the nuclear region of the lens. Given its compact and symmetric structure (which can pack very densely), γ-crystallin tends to be highly concentrated in aged, hard lenses, which have little to no accommodative ability.

Although no specific biological functions have been identified for the β- and γ-crystallins, at least some of them are expressed outside the lens, suggesting that such functions do exist. Members of the superfamily have also been identified in microorganisms, where they are expressed during spore or cyst formation (suggesting a possible role in stress response).

Taxon-specific crystallins In addition to the α- and β,γ-crystallins found in all vertebrate lenses, other proteins are expressed in large quantities in various phylogenetic groups. Most taxon-specific crystallins are oxidoreductases, which bind pyridine nucleotides, and their presence in the lens tremendously increases the concentration of the bound nucleotide. Reduced nucleotides absorb UV light and could serve to protect the retina from UV-induced oxidation; or, these strongly reducing compounds could be part of the antioxidant defenses of the lens. It is noteworthy that taxon-specific crystallins generally occur only in strongly diurnal species that are chronically exposed to increased oxidative stress. Taxon-specific proteins actually function as enzymes and are expressed at increased levels in the lens. For example, ε-crystallin was found to be actually lactate dehydrogenase and to be catalytically active.

Cytoskeletal and membrane proteins

Although the great majority of proteins in the normal lens are water-soluble, a number of important structural proteins can be solubilized only in the presence of chaotropic agents or detergents. These water-soluble proteins include the cytoskeletal elements *actin* (actin filaments), *vimentin* (intermediated filaments), and *tubulin* (microtubules), as well as 2 additional proteins called *filensin* and *phakinin*, which have been found only in lens-fiber cells and which compose a cytoskeletal structure unique to the lens called the *beaded filament*. The filamentous structures of the cytoskeleton provide structural support to the cells and also play critical roles in such processes as differentiation, motility and shape change, and organization of the cytoplasm.

Lens-fiber membranes have one quantitatively dominant protein, which has received a great deal of attention, called MIP (as discussed earlier in the chapter). MIP is expressed only in lens-fiber cells and was once thought to be a gap junction protein; in fact, it is not a connexin but rather an aquaporin, a member of a large, diverse family of proteins involved in regulating water transport. Current data suggest that MIP functions as a water channel.

Posttranslational modifications to lens proteins

The proteins of the lens are probably the longest-lived in the body, with the oldest ones (in the center of the lens nucleus) having been synthesized before birth. As would be expected, these proteins become structurally modified in a variety of ways: oxidation of sulfur and aromatic residue side chains, inter- and intrapolypeptide cross-links, glycation, racemization, phosphorylation, deamidation, and carbamylation. Many of these modifications occur quite early in life and are probably part of a programmed modification of the crystallins that is required for their long-term stability and functionality. There is evidence that certain of these processes (phosphorylation, thiol oxidation) are reversible and may serve a regulatory function, although this remains to be proven.

What is known is that with increasing age (particularly in some cataracts), certain oxidative modifications do accumulate, contributing to the cross-linking of crystallin polypeptides, alterations in fluorescent properties, and an increase in protein-associated pigmentation. In particular, the formation of disulfide cross-links in the proteins of the lens nuclear region is associated with formation of protein aggregates, light scattering, and cataract.

Physiologic Aspects

Because of its avascularity and its mode of growth, the lens faces some unusual problems. All nutrients must be obtained from the surrounding fluids; likewise, all waste products must be released into those fluids. Most of the cells of the adult lens have reduced metabolic activity and lack the membrane machinery to independently regulate ionic homeostasis. Elucidating how the lens maintains ionic balance and how solutes move from cell to cell throughout the lens is critical to understanding the normal biology of the organ as well as the process of cataractogenesis.

In the normal lens, sodium is low ($\approx$10 mmol/L) and potassium is high ($\approx$120 mmol/L); in the aqueous humor, sodium is about 150 mmol/L and potassium, about 5 mmol/L. When normal regulatory mechanisms are abrogated, potassium leaks out of the lens and sodium floods in, followed by chloride. Water then enters in response to the osmotic gradient, causing loss of transparency by disrupting the normally smooth gradient of refractive index. The ionic balance in the lens is maintained primarily by the Na^+,K^+-ATPase pump, an intrinsic membrane protein that hydrolyzes adenosine triphosphate (ATP) to transport sodium out of and potassium into the lens. Functional Na^+,K^+-ATPase pumps are found primarily at the anterior surface of the lens, in the epithelium and the outer, immature fibers. Studies using ouabain, a specific inhibitor of the pump, have established the pump's role as the primary determinant of the normal ionic state of the lens. Lens cells also contain membrane channels that pass ions; in particular, K^+-selective channels have been studied by patch-clamp techniques and found to be present primarily in the epithelial cells.

Communication between lens cells is provided by gap junctions, which are thought to account for most ion and small-molecule movement between cells. True gap junctions occur in the lens and are composed of members of the connexin family. Junctions between epithelial cells are composed of connexin 43; fiber–fiber gap junctions contain connexins 46 and 50. MIP also forms junctionlike structures, although these apparently do not provide direct communication from cell to cell.

Within the fiber mass, gap-junctional coupling is greatest in the outer layers of the lens, where the junctions can be uncoupled by lowering the pH. In the lens nuclear region, such uncoupling does not occur. This supports the idea that the lens nucleus may be a syncytium, resulting from membrane fusion between adjacent fibers.

Some years ago, the vibrating probe technique was used to demonstrate that currents of ions flow around and through the normal lens. As depicted in Figure 11-2, the currents flow in at the anterior and posterior poles and out at the equatorial region of the lens. The source of these currents is not completely understood, but it is apparent that the various ion pumps and channels near the lens surface and the communicating pathways between cells play important roles in establishing and maintaining the currents. It has been suggested that fluid flow would follow the flow of ions and that this would, in effect, provide the lens with a circulatory system able to do the work done by blood vessels in other tissues. That is, nutrients could be carried deep into the lens and waste products moved toward the surface. This model implies that the homeostasis of the cells throughout the lens depends on these ionic currents; if that is true, the maintenance and regulation of the currents would be crucial to the functional integrity of the lens.

Lens Metabolism and Formation of Sugar Cataracts

Energy Production

Energy, in the form of ATP, is produced in the lens primarily through anaerobic glycolysis in metabolically active cells in the anterior lens. This is necessitated by the fact that

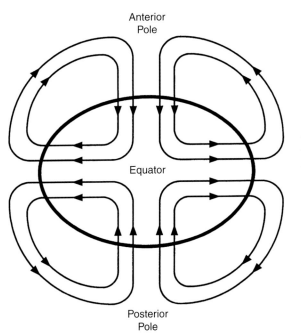

Anterior
Pole

Equator

Posterior
Pole

Figure 11-2 Schematic representation of ionic current flow around and through the lens. The flow is inward at the anterior and posterior poles and outward at the equatorial area. *(From Mathias RT, Rae JL, Baldo GJ. Physiological properties of the normal lens. Physiol Rev. 1997;77(1):21–50.)*

the oxygen tension in the lens is much lower than that in other tissues, because oxygen reaches the avascular lens only via diffusion from the aqueous humor.

Most of the glucose entering the lens is phosphorylated to glucose-6-phosphate by hexokinase, the rate-limiting enzyme of the glycolytic pathway. Under normal conditions, most glucose-6-phosphate passes through glycolysis, wherein 2 molecules of ATP are formed per original molecule of glucose. A small proportion of glucose-6-phosphate is metabolized through the pentose phosphate pathway (hexose monophosphate shunt). This pathway is activated under conditions of oxidative stress because it is responsible for replenishing the supply of nicotinamide adenine dinucleotide phosphate (NADPH) that becomes oxidized through the increased activity of glutathione reductase under such conditions.

Carbohydrate Cataracts

Much of the research activity on lens carbohydrate metabolism has been stimulated by interest in "sugar cataracts," which are associated with diabetes and galactosemia. True diabetic cataract is a rapidly developing bilateral "snowflake" cataract (see BCSC Section 11, *Lens and Cataract*, Chapter 5, Fig 5-16) occurring in the lens cortex of patients with poorly controlled type 1 diabetes mellitus. People with adult-onset diabetes do not develop this type of cataract but do have a higher prevalence of age-related cataract with a slightly earlier onset. It is likely that for such persons, diabetes is simply an additional factor contributing to the development of age-related cataracts.

Defects in galactose metabolism also cause sugar cataracts. Classic galactosemia is caused by a deficiency of galactose-1-phosphate uridyltransferase. Infants with this inborn error of metabolism develop bilateral cataracts within a few weeks of birth unless milk (lactose) is removed from the diet. Cataracts are also associated with a deficiency of galactokinase. Under certain conditions wherein sugar levels are elevated significantly, some glucose (or galactose) is metabolized through the polyol pathway (Fig 11-3). Aldose reductase is the key enzyme for the pathway, and it converts the sugars into the corresponding sugar alcohols. Because aldose reductase has a very high K_m (apparent affinity constant) for glucose (or galactose), under normal conditions little or no activity occurs through this pathway; however, under conditions of hyperglycemia, aldose reductase competes with hexokinase for glucose (or galactose).

Studies using animal models have established the importance of the polyol pathway in experimental sugar cataracts. Animals with diabetes mellitus (either natural or induced) develop cataracts that are associated with the presence of sorbitol in the lens and with influx of water. The osmotic hypothesis was proposed to account for these facts. It invokes the activity of aldose reductase as central to the pathology by markedly increasing the sorbitol content of the lens. Sorbitol is largely unable to penetrate cell membranes and is thus trapped inside the cells. Because its further conversion to fructose by polyol dehydrogenase is slow, sorbitol builds up in lens cells under conditions of hyperglycemia such that it creates an osmotic pressure that draws water into the lens, swelling the cells, damaging membranes, and causing cataract.

Confirmation of the theory has come from a variety of sources. First, ease of induction of cataract by hyperglycemia varies from species to species, depending on the level of aldose reductase activity in the lens. Rats, the most commonly used animal in studies,

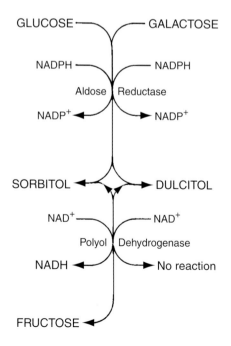

Figure 11-3 Sorbitol pathway for glucose and galactose metabolism. The reduction of glucose and galactose to sorbitol and dulcitol, respectively, is catalyzed by aldose reductase using the reduced form of nicotinamide adenine dinucleotide phosphate (NADPH) as cofactor. The second step is the oxidation of sorbitol (dulcitol is not a substrate) to fructose, catalyzed by polyol dehydrogenase using NAD+ as cofactor. This step is reversible in the human lens, as indicated by the *arrows*.

have a high level of aldose reductase activity and develop cataracts readily; mice, with almost no aldose reductase activity in the lens, do not form sugar cataracts. Second, rats fed diets high in galactose develop cataract more rapidly and severely than do diabetic rats. This correlates with the fact that dulcitol levels in their lenses reach higher levels than does sorbitol in diabetic rats because galactose is a better substrate than glucose for aldose reductase. In addition, dulcitol is not further metabolized because it is not a substrate for polyol dehydrogenase. Most convincingly, a number of potent inhibitors of aldose reductase have been developed that can completely prevent cataract in diabetic or galactose-fed animals.

Unfortunately, although it is certain that aldose reductase activity is the critical factor in the cascade leading to sugar cataract in these animal models, the situation is not at all clear with respect to human diabetic cataracts. The levels of aldose reductase are much lower in the human lens than in the lenses of the animals used in sugar cataract models, but the levels of polyol dehydrogenase are much higher. There is controversy as to whether sorbitol can accumulate in the lenses of people with diabetes mellitus to levels capable of causing a significant osmotic influx of water. Oxidative stress and/or glycation of proteins in the lens may also be involved in human cataracts associated with diabetes.

Garland DL, Duglas-Tabor Y, Jimenez-Asensio J, Datiles MB, Magno B. The nucleus of the human lens: demonstration of a highly characteristic pattern by two-dimensional electrophoresis and introduction of a new method of lens dissection. *Exp Eye Res.* 1996;62(3):285–291.

Mathias RT, Rae JL, Baldo GJ. Physiological properties of the normal lens. *Physiol Rev.* 1997;77(1):21–50.

Piatigorsky J. Gene sharing in lens and cornea: facts and implications. *Prog Retin Eye Res.* 1998;17(2):145–174.

Piatigorsky J, Hejtmancik JF. In: Albert DM, Miller JW, Azar DT, Blodi BA, eds. *Albert & Jakobiec's Principles and Practice of Ophthalmology.* 3rd ed. Philadelphia: Elsevier Saunders; 2008;chap 105.

Quinlan RA, Sandilands A, Procter JE, et al. The eye lens cytoskeleton. *Eye.* 1999;13(Pt 3b): 409–416.

Slingsby C, Clout NJ. Structure of the crystallins. *Eye.* 1999;13(Pt 3b):395–402.

Wistow G. *Molecular Biology and Evolution of Crystallins: Gene Recruitment and Multifunctional Proteins in the Eye Lens.* Austin, TX: RG Landes; 1995.

CHAPTER 12

Vitreous

The vitreous body is a specialized connective tissue whose functions include

- serving as a transparent gel occupying the major volume of the globe
- acting as a conduit for nutrients and other solutes to and from the lens

The basic physical structure of the vitreous is a gel composed of a collagen framework interspersed with hydrated hyaluronan, also known as hyaluronic acid, molecules. The hyaluronan contributes to the viscosity of the vitreous humor and is thought to help stabilize the collagen network, although most of the hyaluronan can be removed enzymatically without collapse of the gel.

The relative amounts of collagen apparently determine whether the vitreous is a liquid or gel, with the rigidity of the gel being greatest in regions of highest collagen concentration. The collagen fibrils supply a resistance to tensile forces and give plasticity to the vitreous; the hyaluronan resists compression and confers viscoelastic properties. Regeneration of the vitreous after a vitrectomy occurs very slowly, if at all.

Composition

The vitreous contains approximately 98% water and 0.15% macromolecules, including collagen, hyaluronan, and soluble proteins. The remainder of the solid matter consists of ions and low-molecular-weight solutes. The 2 major structural components are collagen and hyaluronan; however, several noncollagenous structural proteins and glycoproteins have been identified in the vitreous, including versican, link protein, fibulin-1, nidogen-1, fibronectin, and 2 novel glycoproteins—opticin and VIT1. These last 2 proteins were initially identified after extraction of a pellet of collagen fibrils obtained from the bovine vitreous after centrifugation. In addition, the human vitreous contains hyaluronidase and at least 1 matrix metalloproteinase (*MMP-2*, or *gelatinase*), suggesting that turnover of vitreous structural macromolecules can occur.

Collagen

Vitreous collagen fibrils are composed of 3 different collagen types:

1. *Type II,* which forms the major component of the fibrils
2. *Type IX,* which is located on the surface of the fibril
3. *Type V/XI,* which may be located such that its amino terminus projects from the surface of the fibril (Fig 12-1)

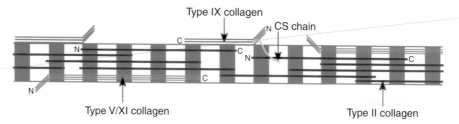

Figure 12-1 Model for the structure of a collagen fibril from the vitreous. Note that 3 different collagen types (II, IX, and XI) are assembled to form the fibril. Type II collagen forms the major structure of the vitreous with stagger to form overlap and gap regions. Type IX is located on the surface of the fibril such that part of the molecule projects from the surface. It is in an antiparallel direction compared with the type II collagen molecules. Type IX also has a single chondroitin sulfate chain *(CS)* that may project from the surface of the fibril. Type V/XI collagen is also located close to the surface of the fibril with a part of the molecule projecting from the gap region. However, the location of this molecule is controversial; other models suggest it is located in the center of the fibril, where it may form a microfibril. *C* = carboxyl terminus, *N* = amino terminus. *(Adapted from Olsen BR. New insights into the function of collagens from genetic analysis.* Curr Opin Cell Biol. *1995;7(5):720–727.)*

At present, 19 types of collagen are known, and the genes for several more have been identified. Type V/XI collagen is unique to the vitreous in that native triple-helical molecules can be isolated that contain the α_1 (XI) and α_2 (V) chains. The vitreous collagens are closely related to the collagens of hyaline cartilage. They differ from the types I, III, XII, and XIV collagens commonly found in scar tissue and in tissues such as dermis, cornea, and sclera.

The precise mechanism by which the diameter of the vitreous collagen fibrils is controlled remains poorly understood, although type V/XI collagen is thought to play a critical role. In most connective tissues, the collagen fibrils (as observed in the electron microscope) show an axial periodicity of 67 nm, but vitreous collagen fibrils rarely show this periodicity with direct staining, although the periodicity can be observed with negative staining. The collagen fibrils of the vitreous are only loosely attached to the internal limiting membrane (ILM) of the retina; however, at the vitreous base, the fibrils are firmly anchored to the peripheral retina and pars plana, as well as to the margins of the optic disc.

The origin of vitreous collagen in mammals is not well established. In vitro, human retinal Müller cell lines synthesize collagens of the vitreous and vitreoretinal interface. It has been shown in the chicken that during early development, the cells of the neural retina synthesize and probably secrete type II collagen. However, other cells (hyalocytes?) present within the vitreous cavity may also contribute. In the developing chicken eye, in situ hybridization of the retina initially yields positive results for type II collagen, whereas transcripts for type IX collagen are present only at the region of the ciliary body. Later in development, type II collagen mRNA also becomes localized only to the presumptive ciliary region. The origin of type V/XI collagen within the vitreous is unknown.

Hyaluronan

Hyaluronan is a polysaccharide (glycosaminoglycan) that has a repeating unit of glucuronic acid and N-acetylglucosamine linked with a β-1,3 glycosidic bond. The repeating units are further linked with β-1,4 glycosidic bonds to form a long, linear, unbranched molecular chain. At physiologic pH, hyaluronan is a weak polyanion because of the ionization of the carboxyl groups present in each glucuronic acid residue. In free solution, hyaluronan occupies an extremely large volume relative to its weight and probably occupies all of the space in the vitreous except for the space occupied by the collagen fibrils. Hyaluronan molecules of the vitreous may undergo lateral interactions with each other, and such interactions may be stabilized by noncollagenous proteins. Link protein, which binds to hyaluronan in cartilage, is known to be present in the vitreous in small amounts. Hyaluronan is present in nearly all vertebrate connective tissues and is nontoxic, noninflammatory, and nonimmunogenic.

Both the concentration and the molecular weight of hyaluronan in the vitreous vary, depending on the species, location in the vitreous body, and type of analysis. Hyaluronan in human vitreous can achieve a molecular weight of greater than 1×10^6.

The source of hyaluronan is also poorly understood. In primate eyes, hyaluronan synthesis has been identified in the posterior pars plana, the neural retina, and the hyalocytes (macrophage-like cells) of the vitreous. Three forms of hyaluronan synthetase are known, but which isoform is responsible for synthesizing the hyaluronan of the vitreous has not been determined. In all animal species that have been analyzed, the hyaluronan concentration is highest in the posterior cortical layer near the retina and lowest in the anterior portion behind the lens.

Laurent TC, ed. *The Chemistry, Biology and Medical Applications of Hyaluronan and Its Derivatives.* Miami: Portland Press; 1998.

Soluble and Fibril-Associated Proteins

Many proteins remain in solution after the collagen fibrils and other insoluble elements present in the vitreous gel are removed by filtration or centrifugation. Serum albumin is the major soluble vitreous protein, followed by transferrin. Poorly defined glycoproteins make up 20% of the total vitreous protein and are thought to originate from surrounding tissues and not from blood. Other proteins include neutrophil elastase inhibitor (which may play a role in resisting neovascularization) and tissue plasminogen activator (which may have a fibrinolytic role in the event of vitreous hemorrhage). Serum albumin is thought to originate from the plasma, whereas transferrin at least partially originates from the region of the ciliary body. The concentration of soluble proteins estimated from a number of species is approximately 1.0 mg/mL. However, the concentration of serum proteins in the vitreous gel depends on the integrity of the retinal vasculature and the degree of any intraocular inflammation that may be present. Consequently, the concentration of soluble proteins within the vitreous cavity can rise dramatically if the blood–retina barrier is compromised.

Some structural proteins are specifically associated with the collagen fibrils and are isolated by extraction of collagen fibrils after centrifugation of the vitreous. These include a novel leucine-rich-repeat glycoprotein called *opticin,* produced in the posterior nonpigmented ciliary epithelium, and another novel glycoprotein called *VIT1.* The latter contains 2 von Willebrand A domains and is closely related to a protein of the cochlear gene,

COCH, called *cochlin.* Both opticin and VIT1 are thought to play key roles in the structure of the collagen fibril, and VIT1 may also interact with hyaluronan.

Zonular Fibers, Lipids, and Low-Molecular-Weight Solutes

Some zonular fibers are present in the anterior vitreous and can be observed by electron microscopy. However, most of these fibers form the zonular apparatus, which is the structural connection between the lens and the ciliary body. The major structural protein of these fibers is a large linear protein called *fibrillin,* which possesses an unusually high cysteine content.

Lipids account for about 7% wet weight of the pellet obtained after centrifugation of the vitreous. The major fatty acids in human vitreous include palmitate (25%), stearate (18%), oleate (23%), and arachidonate (17%). Little variation occurs with age.

Ions and organic solutes originate from adjacent ocular tissues and blood plasma. The barriers that control entry into the vitreous include the vascular endothelium of retinal vessels, the RPE, and the inner layer of the ciliary epithelium. The concentrations of Na^+ and Cl^- are similar to those in plasma, but the concentration of K^+ is somewhat higher than that in plasma.

Bishop PN. Structural macromolecules and supramolecular organisation of the vitreous gel. *Prog Retin Eye Res.* 2000;19(3):323–344.

Mayne R, Brewton RG, Ren Z-X. Vitreous body and zonular apparatus. In: Harding JJ, ed. *Biochemistry of the Eye.* London: Chapman & Hall Medical; 1997:135–143.

Biochemical Changes With Aging and Disease

Vitreous Liquefaction and Posterior Vitreous Detachment

The human vitreous gel undergoes progressive liquefaction with age, so that typically by the age of 80–90 years, more than half of the vitreous is liquid. Myopia is associated with faster vitreous liquefaction, which leads to early posterior vitreous detachment (PVD). The process of vitreous liquefaction has, as a crucial component, the breakdown of the thin (12–15 nm) collagen fibrils into smaller fragments; implicated in this process is less "shielding" of type II collagen due to the age-related exponential loss of type IX collagen. Some proteolytic enzymes, such as plasminogen, may have elevated vitreous concentrations with increasing age, but others, such as MMP-2, do not. The fragments aggregate into thick fibers, or *fibrillar opacities,* which are visible by low-powered slit-lamp microscopy. As liquefaction proceeds, the collagen fibrils become condensed into the residual gel phase and are absent from (or in low concentration in) the liquid phase. In terms of hyaluronan concentration or molecular weight, there are no differences between the gel and liquid phases. With increasing age, there is a weakening of adhesion at the vitreoretinal interface between the cortical vitreous gel and the inner limiting lamina. These combined processes eventually result in PVD in approximately 50% of the population.

PVD is a separation of the cortical vitreous gel from the ILM as far anteriorly as the posterior border of the vitreous base; the separation does not extend into the vitreous base owing to the unbreakable adhesion between the vitreous and retina in that zone. PVD is often a sudden event, during which liquefied vitreous from the center of the vitreous body passes through a hole in the posterior vitreous cortex and then dissects the residual cortical gel away from the inner limiting lamina. As the residual vitreous gel collapses anteriorly within the vitreous cavity, retinal tears sometimes occur at areas where the retina is more strongly attached to the vitreous than the surrounding retina can withstand, which subsequently can result in rhegmatogenous retinal detachment. A PVD can protect against proliferative diabetic retinopathy by denying a scaffold for fibrovascular proliferation emanating from the disc and the retina.

A PVD can be achieved surgically during macular hole surgery. However, it is now clinically recognized that in many eyes thought to have a PVD, collagen fibrils are still extensively attached to the ILM; and even after production of an acute PVD during vitreous surgery, some collagen fibrils typically remain adherent to the ILM. Removal of the ILM itself is now more frequently the goal in limiting the extent of traction maculopathy.

Myopia

When the axial length of the globe is greater than 26 mm, both collagen and hyaluronan concentrations are approximately 20%–30% lower than their concentrations in emmetropic eyes. In a model of negative power lens–induced myopic response in the tree shrew, hyaluronan was found to rapidly decrease when the lens was applied and equally rapidly recover when the myopia-inducing lens was removed. Associated with these changes were biomechanical alterations in the sclera and increased axial length.

Vitreous as an Inhibitor of Angiogenesis

Numerous studies have shown that the normal vitreous is an inhibitor of angiogenesis. This inhibitory activity is decreased during diabetic vitreoretinopathy. However, the molecular basis of the phenomenon remains poorly understood. Known inhibitors of angiogenesis, such as thrombospondin I and pigment epithelium–derived factor, are present within the mammalian vitreous and may inhibit angiogenesis in normal eyes. In contrast, VEGF, a promoter of angiogenesis, is markedly elevated in the vitreous of patients suffering from proliferative diabetic vitreoretinopathy.

Physiologic Changes After Vitrectomy

Both the normal vitreous and the vitreous cavity after vitrectomy are 99% water. Most of the changes in ocular physiology after vitrectomy result from altered viscosity in the vitreous cavity, which decreases between 300- and 2000-fold when the vitreous is removed. Not only do growth factors and other compounds such as antibiotics transfer between the posterior and anterior segments more easily, but they are also cleared more quickly from the eye. This effect is proportional to the change in diffusion coefficient, which is of the same magnitude as the viscosity change. In addition, fluid currents may be present that may move solutes even more rapidly.

In particular, oxygen movement is more rapid, and the normal oxygen gradient between the well-oxygenated anterior segment and the posterior segment flattens significantly, with greatly increased oxygen tension at the retina. This process has been proposed as a mechanism by which vitrectomy may improve the outcome of retinal ischemic diseases such as diabetic macular edema. It has also been proposed that increased oxygen tension at the posterior pole of the lens may be part of postvitrectomy cataractogenesis.

Injury With Hemorrhage and Inflammation

If blood penetrates the vitreous cortex, platelets come in contact with vitreous collagen, aggregate, and initiate clot formation. The clot in turn stimulates a phagocytic inflammatory reaction, and the vitreous becomes liquefied in the area of a hemorrhage. In severe cases, hemoglobin-laden macrophages may cause secondary glaucoma by blocking the trabecular outflow channels. Rigid, degenerated blood cells, called *ghost cells,* can also cause secondary glaucoma (see BCSC Section 10, *Glaucoma*).

If the vitreous is largely liquefied (as in myopic, aphakic, or senile eyes), the clot that is formed is loosely aggregated, and early resolution is more likely. Hemorrhage into vitreous gel is less freely dispersed, and a more compact clot is formed. The subsequent inflammatory reaction varies in degree for unknown reasons and may result in proliferative vitreoretinopathy.

Streeten BAW, Wilson DJ. Disorders of the vitreous. In: Garner A, Klintworth GK, eds. *Pathobiology of Ocular Disease.* 2nd ed. 2 vols. New York: M. Dekker; 1994:701–742.

Involvement of Vitreous in Macular Hole Formation

With the development of optical coherence tomography (OCT) and, more recently, ultra-high resolution OCT (UHR OCT), it is possible to directly visualize the vitreous cortex and the retina in the region of the macula. The results of studies using OCT suggest that macular holes sometimes originate from traction generated by attachment of the vitreous specifically to the fovea, with the subsequent generation of additional tangential tractional force along the ILM, causing hole enlargement. Lamellar macular holes may have a similar pathogenesis.

Madreperla SA, McCuen BW. *Macular Hole: Pathogenesis, Diagnosis, and Treatment.* Boston: Butterworth-Heinemann; 1998.

Witkin AJ, Ko TH, Fujimoto JG, et al. Redefining lamellar holes and the vitreomacular interface: an ultrahigh-resolution optical coherence tomography study. *Ophthalmology.* 2006;113(3): 388–397.

Genetic Disease Involving the Vitreous

In Stickler syndrome or Marshall syndrome, the vitreous collapse is premature, which may induce retinal detachment (see BCSC Section 12, *Retina and Vitreous*). Mutations in both the α_1 (II) and α_1 (XI) collagen chains have been shown to be responsible for this condition. However, other families with these ocular conditions have also been identified in which the genetic basis is still not understood.

Snead MP, Yates JR. Clinical and molecular genetics of Stickler syndrome. *J Med Genet.* 1999; 36(5):353–359.

Enzymatic Vitreolysis

Considerable interest exists in enzyme preparations that may aid in the clearing of blood from the vitreous and in potentially performing noninvasive vitrectomy or producing a PVD in young eyes (see BCSC Section 12, *Retina and Vitreous*). Enzymes that have been proposed for injection into the vitreous cavity include hyaluronidase, plasmin, dispase, and chondroitinase.

Sebag J. Pharmacologic vitreolysis. *Retina.* 1998;18(1):1–3.

CHAPTER 13

Retina

The retina is composed of 2 laminar structures, an outer RPE and an inner neural retina. (This chapter discusses the neurosensory retina; the RPE is discussed in Chapter 14.) These laminar structures arise from an invagination of the embryonic optic cup that folds an ectodermal layer into apex-to-apex contact with itself. The 2 layers form a hemispheric shell on which the visual image is focused by the anterior segment of the eye. The neural retinal cell types are as follows:

- photoreceptors—rods and 3 types of cones
- bipolar cells—rod on-bipolars and cone on- and off-bipolars
- interneurons—horizontal and amacrine cells
- ganglion cells and their axons, forming the optic nerve
- astroglia, oligodendroglia, Schwann cells, microglia, and vascular endothelium and pericytes

Neural Retina—The Photoreceptors

Rod Phototransduction

Catching light and converting its minute amount of energy into a neural response distinguishes the retina from all other neural structures, which it otherwise resembles. This combined process occurs within a specialized organelle of the photoreceptor cell, the *outer segment*. Most of our knowledge of phototransduction comes from information known about rods, which are sensitive nocturnal light detectors. Much more biochemical material can be obtained from rods than from cones because rods are much more numerous in most retinas. In addition, they contain much more membrane than do cones, which contributes to the rods' higher sensitivity.

The outer segment of a rod is composed primarily of plasma-membrane material organized in an unusual way. Most of the membrane is in the form of membrane sacs flattened along the long axis of the outer segment. There are about 1000 sacs within a rod outer segment and about a million rhodopsin molecules in each sac. The sacs float within the cytoplasm of the outer segment like a stack of coins disconnected from the plasma membrane. The sacs contain the protein machinery to capture and amplify light energy. This abundance of outer-segment membrane increases the number of rhodopsin molecules, which can absorb light. Some deep-sea fish, which need great sensitivity to detect the small amount of light available, have much longer rods than do humans.

Light is absorbed by rhodopsin concentrated in the outer-segment membrane of rods. Rhodopsin is a freely diffusible membrane protein similar to α- and β-adrenergic receptors. It has 7 helical loops embedded in the lipid membrane (Fig 13-1). Phosphorylation sites exist on the cytoplasmic side of the protein, where rhodopsin is inactivated and sugar is attached on the intradiscal side. At amino acid 296 on the seventh membrane loop, the 11-*cis*-retinal chromophore is bound to a lysine by a protonated Schiff base linkage. Each molecule responds to a single quantum of light. Rhodopsin absorbs green light best at wavelengths of approximately 510 nm. It absorbs blue and yellow lights less well and is insensitive to longer wavelengths (red light). The tuning of rhodopsin to this part of the electromagnetic spectrum is due to the amino-acid sequence of the protein and the binding of the 11-*cis* isomer of retinaldehyde, which creates a molecular antenna.

Once rhodopsin absorbs a quantum of light, the 11-*cis* double bond of retinal is broken and the opsin molecule undergoes a series of rapid configurational changes that lead to an activated state, *metarhodopsin II*. Activated rhodopsin starts a reaction that controls the inflow of cations into the rod outer segment. The target of this reaction is a cyclic guanosine monophosphate (cGMP)–gated cationic channel located on the outer membrane of the outer segment. This channel controls the flow of Na^+ and Ca^{2+} ions into the rod. In the dark, Na^+ and Ca^{2+} ions flow in through this channel, which is kept open by cGMP. Ionic balance is maintained by a Na^+,K^+-ATPase pump in the inner segment and a Na^+,K^+-Ca exchanger in the outer-segment membrane, both of which require metabolic energy. Depolarization of the rod causes the transmitter glutamate to be released from its synaptic terminal, starting the neural signals for vision.

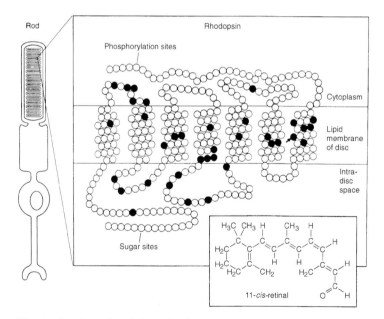

Figure 13-1 The rhodopsin molecule is embedded in the lipid membrane of the outer segment with 7 helical loops. Each circle is an amino acid, with the highly conserved ones in *black*. An *arrow* shows the lysine to which the vitamin A chromophore is linked. Phosphorylation sites occur on the cytoplasmic and sugar attachment sites on the intradiscal (extracellular) ends of the rhodopsin molecule. *(Courtesy of Peter Gouras, MD.)*

Light-activated rhodopsin drives a second molecule, transducin, by causing an exchange of guanosine diphosphate (GDP) for guanosine triphosphate (GTP). One rhodopsin molecule can activate a hundred transducin molecules, amplifying the reaction. Activated transducins excite a third protein, rod phosphodiesterase (rod PDE), which hydrolyzes cGMP to 5′-noncyclic GMP. The decrease in cGMP closes the gated channels, which stops Na^+ and Ca^{2+} entry and hyperpolarizes the rod. Hyperpolarization stops glutamate's release from the synaptic terminal.

When the light goes off, the rod returns to its dark state as the reaction cascade turns off. Rhodopsin is inactivated by phosphorylation at its C-terminal by rhodopsin kinase, assisted by the binding of arrestin. Transducin is inactivated by the hydrolysis of GTP to GDP by transducin's intrinsic GTPase activity, which inactivates PDE. Guanylate cyclase, the enzyme that synthesizes cGMP from GTP, is activated by the decrease in intracellular Ca^{2+} caused by the channel closure; the enzyme's action is assisted by guanylate cyclase–assisting proteins. As cGMP levels increase, the gated channels close and the rod is re-depolarized. The corresponding rise in intracellular Ca^{2+} restores guanylate cyclase activity to its dark level. Calcium feedback may also regulate rhodopsin phosphorylation by recoverin as well as the sensitivity of the gated channel.

"Rim" proteins

Rod sacs differ from those of cones in that they are disconnected from the outer plasma membrane. The rim of each rod sac has a unique collection of proteins. Two are peripherin and ROM1, which play a role in the development and maintenance of the sac's curvature. Peripherin and ROM1 are also found in cone outer segments. A third protein is a member of a superfamily of ATP-binding cassette (ABC) transporters. These include the cystic fibrosis transmembrane regulator (CFTR); P-glycoprotein, which is involved in multidrug resistance; TAP1 and TAP2, which transport peptides in lymphocytes; prokaryotic permeases; and others. The ABC protein is unique to rod sacs and is not found in cones. It functions as a transporter of all-*trans* retinal.

Biswas-Fiss EE. Functional analysis of genetic mutations in nucleotide binding domain 2 of the human retina specific ABC transporter. *Biochemistry.* 2003;42(36):10683–10696.

Outer-segment energy metabolism

ATP is necessary to drive the reactions that control the ionic current generators as well as the transporters in the outer segment. Because only the inner, and not the outer, segment contains mitochondria, oxidative metabolism is confined to the former. The outer segment is responsible for glycolysis, including the hexose monophosphate pathway and the phosphocreatine shuttle, which produces ATP and GTP and modulates NADPH. NADPH reduces retinal to retinol before it is returned to the RPE for isomerization and reduces glutathione, which protects against oxidative stress.

Cone Phototransduction

Qualitatively, cone phototransduction resembles that of rods. Light-activated cone opsins start an enzymatic cascade that hydrolyzes cGMP and closes cone-specific cGMP-gated cation channels on the outer-segment membrane. Cone phototransduction is comparatively insensitive but fast and capable of adapting enormously to the ambient levels of illumination. The greater the ambient light levels, the faster and more temporally accurate is the response of a cone. Speed and temporal fidelity are important for all aspects of cone vision. This is one reason acuity improves progressively with increased illumination. Because of their ability to adapt, cones are indispensable to good vision. Without cones, one loses the ability to read and see colors and can be legally blind. In comparison, lost rod function is less of a visual handicap.

Several factors contribute to light adaptation. For example, higher levels of illumination bleach away photopigments, making the outer segment less sensitive to light. As light levels increase, so does the noise level, which reduces sensitivity. Biochemical and neural feedback speed up the cone response. This feedback must be increased as light intensity increases and the cone absorbs more and more light. The biochemistry responsible for this speedup has not yet been deciphered. All the processes that turn the rod response off are probably stronger in cones. The life span of activated cone opsin must be shorter, its turn-off and the turn-off of cone transducin (a G protein) faster than they are in rods. In addition, increasing light must enhance the turn-off mechanisms in cones.

Cones also show neurally mediated negative feedback. Horizontal cells of the inner nuclear layer synapse antagonistically back onto cones, releasing γ-aminobutyric acid (GABA), an inhibitory transmitter. When light hyperpolarizes a cone, the cone hyperpolarizes neighboring horizontal cells. This inhibits the horizontal cells, stopping the release of GABA, which depolarizes (disinhibits) the cone by a recurrent synapse. This depolarization antagonizes the hyperpolarization produced by light and tries to put the cone back in the dark. Depolarization occurs with a synaptic delay so that its main effect is on the later response of the cone. Horizontal cell feedback occurs with strong stimuli, undoubtedly preventing the cone from being overloaded. The feedback also turns the cone response off more quickly, enabling the cone to respond more rapidly to a new stimulus. This process thus increases the flicker fusion frequency, which is much higher in cones (about 100 Hz) than in rods (about 30 Hz).

Trivariant color vision

To see colors, mammals must have at least 2 different spectral classes of cones. Most normal humans have 3 types of cones and consequently a 3-variable color vision (3 cone opsins) system. Most mammals have divariant color vision with middle-wavelength-sensitive (M) cones detecting high-resolution achromatic (black and white) contrast and short-wavelength-sensitive (S) cones detecting only color, by comparing their signals with those of the M cones. This mechanism creates blue/yellow color vision. Because the S cones contribute only to color vision, they are much less numerous than M cones.

In primates, a third cone mechanism evolved to enhance color vision by splitting the high-resolution M cones into long (L)- and middle (M)-wavelength cones. This creates red/green color vision. Both L and M cones contribute to achromatic and chromatic contrast. Therefore, both are more numerous than S cones in the human retina.

Most color vision defects involve red/green discrimination and the genes coding for the L- and M-cone opsins. These genes are in tandem on the X chromosome. There is 1 copy of the L-cone opsin gene at the centromeric end of the X chromosome and 1–6 copies of the M-cone gene arranged in a head-to-tail tandem array. Normally, only the most proximal of these 2 genes is expressed. Most color vision abnormalities are caused by unequal crossing over between the L- and M-cone opsin genes. This creates hybrid opsins that have different spectral absorption functions, usually less ideal. Some males have a serine-to-alanine substitution at amino acid 108 on the cone opsin gene, which allows more sensitivity to red light. Therefore, female subjects with both the serine-containing and the alanine-containing opsins could have tetravariant color vision.

Rod-Specific Gene Defects

Rhodopsin

More than 100 different mutations cause autosomal dominant retinitis pigmentosa (ADRP). Mutations occur in different ways; they can alter transduction, protein folding, or localization of the protein. The most common mutation is P23H (responsible for 10% of RP cases in the United States), in which the protein does not fold properly and instead accumulates in the rough endoplasmic reticulum. Generally, mutations affecting the intradiscal area and amino terminal of rhodopsin are less severe than those in the cytoplasmic region and the carboxyl tail. Alterations in the middle of the gene, coding for the transmembrane regions, result in moderately severe defects. Relatively uncommon mutations have been reported in the rhodopsin gene, causing autosomal recessive retinitis pigmentosa (ARRP) and a stationary form of nyctalopia.

Rod transducin

A dominant G38D mutation produces Nougaret disease, the oldest known form of autosomal dominant stationary nyctalopia. With this mutation, transducin becomes continuously activated, an example of constitutively active rods that do not degenerate.

Rod cGMP phosphodiesterase

Defects in either the α- (PDEA) subunit or β- (PDEB) subunit of cGMP phosphodiesterase (rod PDE) cause ARRP. These are nonsense mutations that truncate the catalytic domain of the protein. An H258D mutation in PDEB also causes dominant stationary nyctalopia. This mutation is near the binding site of the γ-subunit of PDE and may lead to constitutively active PDE.

Rod cGMP–gated channel

Null mutations of the rod cGMP-gated channel β-subunit cause ARRP. No degeneration from the α- or γ-subunits has been reported.

Arrestin

A homozygous defect in codon 309 causes Oguchi disease, a form of stationary nyctalopia. It produces a frameshift in and truncation of arrestin. There is genetic heterogeneity because rhodopsin kinase gene defects also cause Oguchi disease.

Rhodopsin kinase

Null mutations of rhodopsin kinase cause Oguchi disease. These mutations also retard activated rhodopsin's turnoff.

Guanylate cyclase

Null mutations of guanylate cyclase cause Leber congenital amaurosis (LCA), a childhood autosomal recessive form of RP. LCA shows genetic heterogeneity.

Rod ABC transporter

Recessive defects of ABC transporter cause Stargardt disease. There is allelic heterogeneity, which reflects the severity of the gene defect. Mild defects cause macular degeneration, intermediate ones cause cone–rod dystrophy, and severe ones cause RP. Heterozygous defects are also found in 4% of age-related macular degeneration.

L-type calcium channel

The L-type calcium channel gene codes for an α-subunit, and defects cause X-linked stationary nyctalopia. The protein seems to determine transmitter release from the rod synaptic terminal and may also affect cones.

Cone- and Rod-Specific Gene Defects

Peripherin (RDS)

There is great allelic heterogeneity in the *peripherin/RDS* gene. Defects cause several dominantly inherited retinal degenerations that range from ADRP to macular degeneration, pattern macular dystrophy, vitelliform macular dystrophy, butterfly macular dystrophy, and fundus flavimaculatus. A null mutation of the homologous murine gene causes a semidominant form of degeneration, with failure of rod outer-segment development and slow degeneration.

ROM1

Double-heterozygotic mutations in both the *ROM1* and the peripherin gene cause "digenic" RP. A *ROM1* gene defect alone has been reported in a patient with a vitelliform macular dystrophy, but this gene is not responsible for Best macular dystrophy (discussed later in the chapter).

Myosin VIIA

A heterozygous null mutation in a form of myosin VIIA, causes Usher syndrome type I. Affected subjects have deafness and vestibular ataxia at birth and develop ARRP.

Oxygen-regulated protein

Homozygous defects in oxygen-regulated protein cause autosomal dominant RP. Expression of this unusual gene is modulated by oxygen.

Cone-Specific Gene Defects

Cone cGMP-gated channel

A homozygous defect in the cone cGMP-gated channel α-subunit causes achromatopsia, loss of all cone function.

L- and M-cone opsins

Two genetic steps involving L- and M-cone opsins lead to "blue-cone achromatopsia." One reduces the tandem array of these genes to 1 gene, and the second eliminates the residual gene. Another defect in a sequence upstream from this tandem array can also cause blue-cone achromatopsia. These defects occur in males because of the gene's location on the X chromosome.

L- or M-cone opsins

Defects in one or the other of the X-linked L- or M-cone opsin genes cause red/green color deficiencies, again almost exclusively in males.

RPE-Specific Gene Defects

RPE 65

Homozygous defects of RPE 65 cause Leber congenital amaurosis, a generalized loss of photoreceptor function. Mice with this defect retain some cone function. The protein influences the formation of 11-*cis*-retinol. Cones may have access to another pool of this isomer.

Bestrophin

Heterozygous missense mutations of the bestrophin gene produce Best disease, a dominantly inherited form of macular degeneration, which involves the entire RPE layer but causes damage only in the macula. The protein is membrane-bound with 4 transmembrane regions.

TIMP3

Heterozygous point mutations of TIMP3 produce Sorsby macular dystrophy. This protein is an inhibitor of a metalloproteinase that regulates the extracellular matrix.

CRALBP

Homozygous defects of CRALBP (cytoplasmic retinal-binding protein) cause retinitis punctata albescens. This protein facilitates 11-*cis*-retinal formation and transport; it is also found in Müller cells.

11-cis-retinol dehydrogenase

Homozygous defects of 11-*cis*-retinol dehydrogenase cause fundus albipunctus, a form of stationary nyctalopia. This enzyme forms 11-*cis*-retinal from 11-*cis*-retinol and may also exist in Müller cells.

EFEMP1

A single heterozygous nonconservative mutation of EFEMP1 (EGF-containing fibrillin-like extracellular matrix protein) causes malattia leventinese (Doyne honeycomb retinal dystrophy), a dominant form of macular degeneration. It is uncertain whether the protein is unique to RPE.

Ubiquitously Expressed Genes Causing Retinal Degenerations

REP-1

REP-1 (Rab escort protein-1) is an X-linked gene that causes choroideremia. The protein is involved in prenylating Rab proteins, a process that facilitates their binding to cytoplasmic membranes and promoting vesicle fusion. Photoreceptors, RPE, and/or the choroid must be uniquely vulnerable for this process to occur.

OAT

Homozygous defects of OAT (ornithine amino transferase) cause gyrate atrophy. The enzyme breaks down ornithine, which, in high concentrations, seems toxic to the RPE.

MTP

Homozygous defects in MTP (microsomal triglyceride transfer protein) cause abetalipoproteinemia, or Bassen-Kornzweig syndrome, a condition characterized by ARRP and the patient's inability to absorb fat. The condition is treatable with fat-soluble vitamins.

PEX1

Homozygous defects in *PEX1* cause infantile Refsum disease, with RP, retardation, and hearing deficits. Infantile Refsum disease represents the least severe disease in a spectrum of familial disorders involving mutations in the *PEX* genes. The *PEX* genes encode for peroxins, proteins needed for peroxisome biogenesis.

PAHX

Homozygous defects of *PAHX* cause Refsum disease, with RP, cerebellar ataxia, and peripheral polyneuropathy. The enzyme degrades phytanic acid and is located in peroxisomes. Patients with Refsum disease may be treated with a phytanic acid–restricted diet.

Inner Nuclear Layer

The inner nuclear layer has 3 classes of neurons (bipolar, horizontal, and amacrine cells) and a glial cell (the Müller cell). There are separate bipolar cells for cones and rods and at least 2 distinctly different types of cone bipolars, *on-bipolars* and *off-bipolars* (Fig 13-2). The former are inhibited, the latter excited by the glutamate transmitter released by cones. Thus, when light hyperpolarizes the cones, the on-bipolar is excited (turned on) and the off-bipolar inhibited (turned off). When a shadow depolarizes the cones, the reverse occurs.

Some cone bipolars synapse only with L cones and others only with M cones, a differentiation that is necessary for color vision. In the fovea, some cone bipolars synapse with a single L or M cone (Fig 13-3), which provides the highest spatial acuity. This cone selectivity is preserved throughout the ganglion cell layer. This selectivity for L- or M-cone inputs is transmitted by a tonic responding system of small ganglion cells. Separate L- and M-cone on-bipolars and off-bipolars transmit a faster, phasic signal to a parallel system of larger ganglion cells. Rods and probably S cones have only on-bipolar cells. Neither rods nor S cones are involved in high spatial resolution. The S cones are involved in color vision and the rods in twilight vision.

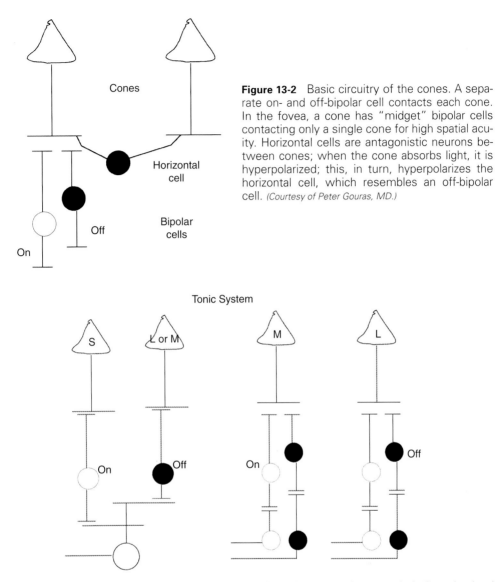

Figure 13-2 Basic circuitry of the cones. A separate on- and off-bipolar cell contacts each cone. In the fovea, a cone has "midget" bipolar cells contacting only a single cone for high spatial acuity. Horizontal cells are antagonistic neurons between cones; when the cone absorbs light, it is hyperpolarized; this, in turn, hyperpolarizes the horizontal cell, which resembles an off-bipolar cell. *(Courtesy of Peter Gouras, MD.)*

Figure 13-3 The tonic system transmits signals from the cones that are relatively maintained for the duration of the light or dark stimulus. This system provides the brain with information about a separate cone system, necessary for color vision. It preserves the polarity of the signal for each cone type. This is best shown here in the S-cone channel, which receives a signal of opposite polarity (off) from the L and M cones. *(Courtesy of Peter Gouras, MD.)*

The horizontal cells are antagonistic interneurons that inhibit photoreceptors (see Fig 13-2) by releasing GABA when depolarized. The dendrites of horizontal cells go to cones. One class of horizontal cells goes to L and M cones. Another class goes mainly to S cones. A thin axon terminal that emanates from the cell body of horizontal cells sends dendrites to rods. The dendrites of horizontal cells receive glutamate from cones and rods and release GABA back onto cones and rods. This provides negative feedback. When light causes the cone to hyperpolarize and stop its transmitter release, the horizontal cell is also hyperpolarized (turned off). This stops the release of GABA from the horizontal cell onto the cone, consequently depolarizing the cone.

Cone amacrine cells mediate antagonistic interactions among on-bipolars, off-bipolars, and ganglion cells. The rods have an unusual amacrine cell that receives the input of rod bipolars and delivers signals to on- and off-bipolar ganglion cells. Thus, rod signals undergo additional synaptic delays before they reach the ganglion cell output.

The retinal ganglion cells can be classified into 2 main types: *on* (center cells excited) and *off* (center cells inhibited by light in the center of their receptive field). A shadow initiates the opposite reaction in these 2 cell types. There are 3 main subgroups of retinal ganglion cells: tonic cells driven by L or M cones, tonic cells driven by S cones, and phasic cells.

Tonic cells driven by either L or M cones include small cells concentrated in the fovea (responsible for high acuity) and others located extrafoveally (see Fig 13-4). They project to the parvocellular layers of the lateral geniculate nucleus (the main relay station to the visual cortex) and mediate both high spatial resolution and color vision.

Tonic cells driven by S cones have a unique physiology designed to detect successive color contrast, blue/yellow or gray/brown borders. These ganglion cells are excited by short waves entering and long waves leaving their receptive fields (see Fig 13-3). The phasic cells are larger, less concentrated in the fovea, and faster-conducting than the ganglion cells (Fig 13-4). They project to the magnocellular layers of the lateral geniculate nucleus and may be more important in movement detection.

Müller cells are the least understood of all the retinal cells. Nonneural, they play a supportive role to the neural tissue extending from the inner segments of the photoreceptors to the ILM, which is formed by their end-feet. They buffer the ionic concentrations

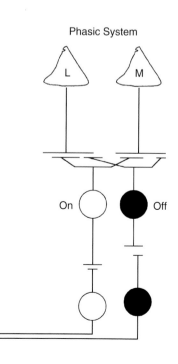

Figure 13-4 The phasic system transmits signals at the beginning or end of a light stimulus. This produces a brief or transient response. L- and M-cone signals of the same polarity mix in driving the phasic system. *(Courtesy of Peter Gouras, MD.)*

in the extracellular space, seal off the subretinal space by forming the external limiting membrane (ELM), and may play a role in the vitamin A metabolism of cones.

The other nonneural, or neuroglial, cells of the retina are *macroglia* (astrocytes, oligodendroglia, and Schwann cells) and *microglia*. These cells provide physical support, respond to retinal cell injury, regulate the ionic and chemical composition of the extracellular milieu, participate in the blood–retina barrier, form the myelination of the optic nerve, guide neuronal migration during development, and exchange metabolites with neurons. Neuroglia have high-affinity transmitter-uptake systems and voltage-dependent and transmitter-gated ion channels; they can release transmitters, but their role in signaling, as in many other functions, is unclear.

In addition, the neural retina contains blood vessels with endothelial cells and pericytes. Pericytes play a role in the autoregulation of retinal blood vessels and are an early target in diabetes. The pathogenesis of diabetic retinopathy seems to be due to defects in the polyol pathway. Aldose reductase, the rate-limiting first enzyme in the conversion of many sugars to their alcohols, has a known role in the formation of diabetic cataracts. Accumulation of sorbitol and its aldose reductase–mediated metabolite, fructose, causes repeated osmotic insults and cataractogenesis. Similar conditions may lead to thickening of the basement membrane and pericyte loss in the blood vessels of the retina.

Retinal Electrophysiology

Changes in the light flux on the retina produce electrical changes in all of the retinal cells, including the RPE and Müller cells, as well as neurons. These electrical changes result from ionic currents that flow when ion-specific channels are opened or closed. These currents reach the vitreous and the cornea, where they can be detected noninvasively by an electroretinogram (ERG). The initiating process of the currents is the ionic response started in the rods and cones that influences the ionic current both *directly* by changes in Na^+ and K^+ fluxes and *indirectly* by synaptically modifying second-order retinal neurons.

The changes in the electrical potentials of the rods and cones are shown in Figure 13-5, which depicts the responses of rods and cones to a pulse of light or a pulse of darkness.

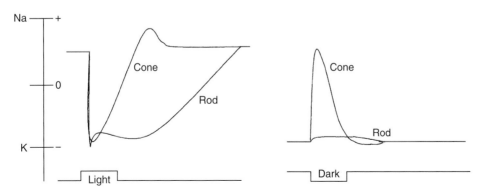

Figure 13-5 The response of a rod and cone to a pulse of light and a pulse of darkness. The light pulse hyperpolarizes both photoreceptors. The rod responses are prolonged. The cone responses turn off quickly even while the pulse of light is on. Darkness depolarizes the cone rapidly but has only a small effect on the slower rod response.

Light hyperpolarizes cones and rods. The cone response is rapid; it turns off while the light is still on and overshoots the dark potential. The rod response is more prolonged and turns off very slowly. Dark depolarizes the cone and has little influence on the rod, which is saturated at high light levels and too slow to respond to the "shadow." The ionic changes are due to the shift in the photoreceptors' conductivity to Na^+ and K^+ ions. The concentration gradients for these ions are reversed across the membrane of the photoreceptors so that changes in the conductivity to these ions move currents in the opposite directions.

Liou GI, Fei Y, Peachey NS, et al. Early onset photoreceptor abnormalities induced by targeted disruption of the interphotoreceptor retinoid-binding protein gene. *J Neurosci.* 1998;18(12): 4511–4520.

Molday RS. Photoreceptor membrane proteins, phototransduction, and retinal degenerative diseases. The Friedenwald Lecture. *Invest Ophthalmol Vis Sci.* 1998;39(13):2491–2513.

CHAPTER 14

Retinal Pigment Epithelium

The retinal pigment epithelium (RPE) is a single layer of cuboidal epithelial cells that constitutes the outermost layer of the retina. The RPE is located between the highly vascular choriocapillaris and the outer segments of photoreceptor cells (Fig 14-1). In humans, there are approximately 4–6 million RPE cells per eye. The ratio of photoreceptor cells to RPE cells is roughly 45:1. The RPE is derived embryologically from the same neural anlage as the sensory retina, but it differentiates into a secretory epithelium. Although it has no photoreceptive or neural function, the RPE is essential to the support and viability of photoreceptor cells.

Anatomical Description

The RPE cells are polarized epithelial cells. They have long microvillous processes on their apical surfaces that interdigitate with outer segments of photoreceptor cells. Their basal surface, which is adjacent to Bruch's membrane (an extracellular matrix between the RPE

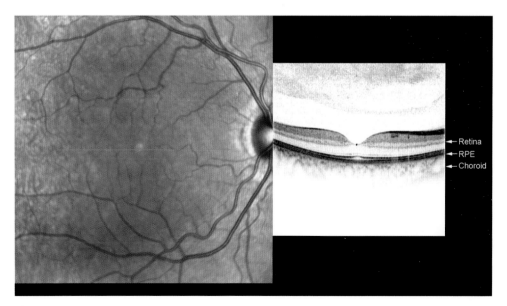

Figure 14-1 A spectral domain optical coherence tomography (OCT) section of retina showing the relationship of RPE to the retina and the choriocapillaris. *(Courtesy of Sandeep Grover, MD.)*

and choriocapillaris), has many infoldings. RPE cells are joined near their apical side by tight junctions that block the passage of water and ions. As such, the RPE contributes to the blood–retina barrier. In addition to the organelles found in most cells (eg, the nucleus, Golgi apparatus, smooth and rough endoplasmic reticulum, and mitochondria), the RPE has melanin granules and phagosomes that reflect 2 of its important roles (discussed shortly). The RPE is particularly rich in microperoxisomes, suggesting that it is quite active in detoxifying the large number of free radicals and oxidized lipids that are generated in this highly oxidative and light-rich environment.

Biochemical Composition

Biochemically, the RPE is a dynamic and complex cell. It must meet demands for its own active metabolism, its extraordinary phagocytic function, and its role as a biological filter for the neurosensory retina. These processes impose a very high energy requirement on the RPE; not surprisingly, the cells contain all the enzymes of the 3 major biochemical pathways: glycolysis, Krebs cycle, and the pentose phosphate pathway. Glucose is the primary carbon source used for energy metabolism and for conversion to protein. Although the RPE does make a minor contribution to the glycosaminoglycan- and proteoglycan-containing interphotoreceptor matrix, glucose is not converted to glycogen in the RPE. Glucosamine, fucose, galactose, and mannose are all metabolized to some extent in the RPE, although mannose seems to be passed on almost directly to the photoreceptors.

Regarding the chemical composition of the RPE, over 80% of wet weight is contributed by water. Proteins, lipids, and nucleic acids contribute most of the remaining weight.

Proteins

Nearly 850 proteins have been identified in the RPE. Up to 200 acidic proteins are present, and approximately 180 plasma-membrane proteins have been identified. Many proteins that are found in other cells are present also in the RPE. For example, hydrolytic enzymes such as glutathione, peroxidase, catalase, and superoxide dismutase, which are important for detoxification, are present in the RPE. The cytoskeletal proteins actin, myosin, α-actinin, fodrin, and vinculin are also present.

Other proteins are present in the RPE but are localized differently from other cells. A well-known example of this is the sodium pump, which uses energy derived from adenosine triphosphate (ATP) hydrolysis to transport Na^+ and K^+ against their electrochemical gradients. Na^+,K^+-ATPase has a unique location in RPE cells. Whereas most polarized epithelial cells localize this protein to their basolateral surface, the RPE places it on its apical surface. It is thought that Na^+,K^+-ATPase is apically located to maintain the balance of Na^+ and K^+ in the subretinal space. Additional proteins have been shown to have a reversed polarity in RPE cells compared with other polarized epithelial cells, including NCAM-140 and folate receptor α. In addition, some proteins are expressed only in the RPE. One such protein, RPE65, is an obligate component of the isomerization of vitamin A, which is required for regeneration of visual pigment (described later in the chapter).

Lipids

Lipids account for approximately 3% of the wet weight of the RPE; about half are phospholipids. Phosphatidylcholine and phosphatidylethanolamine make up more than 80% of the total phospholipid content. In general, levels of saturated fatty acids in the RPE are higher than in the adjacent outer segments. The saturated fatty acids palmitic acid and stearic acid are used for retinol esterification and for energy metabolism by the RPE mitochondria. The level of polyunsaturated fatty acids, such as docosahexaenoic acid (22:6–3), is much lower in the RPE than in the outer segments, although the level of arachidonic acid is relatively high. A number of studies have suggested that the retina may be spared the effects of essential fatty acid deficiency because the RPE efficiently sequesters fatty acids from the blood. The RPE actively conserves and efficiently reuses the fatty acids, thus preventing their loss as waste products.

Nucleic Acids

Approximately 1% of the wet weight of the RPE is contributed by RNA. RNA is synthesized continually by the RPE due to production of the many enzymes needed for cell metabolism, phagocytosis of shed discs, and maintenance of the retinoid pathway and transport functions.

Major Physiologic Roles of the RPE

The RPE has a number of physiologic roles. Critical among these are

- visual pigment regeneration
- phagocytosis of shed photoreceptor outer-segment discs
- transport of necessary nutrients and ions to photoreceptor cells and removal of waste products from photoreceptors
- absorption of scattered and out-of-focus light via pigmentation
- adhesion of the retina

These functions are discussed briefly in the following sections. Other important functions subserved by the RPE include its role in synthesis and remodeling of the interphotoreceptor matrix, formation of the blood–retina barrier, and elaboration of humoral and growth factors.

Visual Pigment Regeneration

Regeneration of the visual pigment rhodopsin, a process that has been studied extensively, involves both photoreceptors and the RPE. The RPE plays a major role in the uptake, storage, and mobilization of vitamin A for use in the visual cycle. Indeed, the RPE is second only to the liver in its concentration of vitamin A.

The basic function of the RPE cell in the visual process is to generate 11-*cis*-retinaldehyde (used in the formation of rhodopsin). As described in detail in Chapter 13, the photoreceptor cell synthesizes opsin, which uses 11-*cis*-retinaldehyde in the regeneration of rhodopsin. In the photoreceptor cell, rhodopsin is photolyzed and undergoes a *cis*-to-*trans* isomerization. All-*trans*-retinaldehyde is released and converted to all-*trans*-retinol by retinoldehydrogenase. The retinol is returned to the RPE in the presence of interphotoreceptor retinoid-binding protein (IRBP). In the RPE, retinol is converted to retinyl ester in the presence of the enzyme lecithin retinol acyltransferase. When needed for regeneration of rhodopsin, the retinyl ester is converted by an isomerohydrolase (isomerase) to 11-*cis*-retinol and is subsequently converted to 11-*cis*-retinal by a dehydrogenase. The 11-*cis*-retinal is returned to the photoreceptor cell along with IRBP. The protein RPE65 is thought to play a role in the isomerization step because RPE65 knockout mice cannot regenerate rhodopsin.

The RPE acquires vitamin A in 3 ways:

1. through release during bleaching of rhodopsin and return via the regeneration process of the visual cycle
2. from circulation, presumably through a receptor-mediated mechanism
3. via phagocytosis of shed photoreceptor outer-segment discs

The aldehyde and alcohol forms of vitamin A are membranolytic; hence, several retinoid-binding proteins mediate both vitamin A metabolism within the RPE and vitamin A's exchange with adjacent outer segments. A number of retinoid-binding proteins have been isolated and characterized in the RPE, in the subretinal space, and in photoreceptors. The RPE esterifies retinol with available fatty acids (predominantly palmitic acid and, to a lesser extent, stearic and oleic acids) and stores retinol as a retinyl ester, a form no longer lytic to cell membranes. In conditions of hypervitaminosis A, toxicity to the RPE is minimal because of vitamin A storage as the ester.

Phagocytosis of Shed Photoreceptor Outer-Segment Discs

The RPE plays a crucial role in turnover of the photosensitive membrane of rod and cone photoreceptors. In the mid-1960s, autoradiography was used to establish that proteins were synthesized in the inner segments of the photoreceptor cells and were transported to the outer segment and incorporated into new discs forming at the base of the outer segment. The band of radioactive protein was displaced toward the apex of the cell over a period of approximately 9–11 days. The vital role of the RPE in phagocytosis of these discs was demonstrated when the radioactive distal tip of the outer segment arrived in the RPE cell and was subsequently phagocytosed.

The shed outer-segment discs are encapsulated in phagosomes, which in turn fuse with lysosomes and are digested. During degradation of the discs, building blocks are recycled into photoreceptors for use in the synthesis and assembly of new discs. The lipofuscin characteristic of the RPE is derived from photosensitive membranes. Each photoreceptor cell sheds approximately 100 outer-segment discs per day. Because many photoreceptors interdigitate with a single RPE cell, each RPE cell ingests/digests more than 4000 discs daily! The shedding event follows a circadian rhythm: in rods, shedding is most vigorous within 2 hours of light onset; in cones, shedding occurs more vigorously at onset of darkness. Recent evidence suggests that the neurotransmitter dopamine acts within the photoreceptor–pigment epithelial complex to control disc shedding. Defects in the phagocytic function of the RPE are seen in Royal College of Surgeons rats; these defects lead to degeneration of the photoreceptor cells.

Transport

The health and integrity of retinal neurons depend on a well-regulated extracellular environment. A critical function of the RPE that contributes to this regulation is control of the volume and composition of fluid in the subretinal space through transport of ions, fluid, and metabolites. The distribution of transport proteins residing in the apical and basolateral membrane domains of the cell is clearly asymmetric, and this difference is what allows the epithelium to carry out vectorial transport. The membrane proteins remain in their proper location because of tight junction proteins. Intercellularly, asymmetry or polarity of the cell is maintained because of the intracellular molecular machinery that synthesizes new proteins and delivers them preferentially to the apical or basolateral cell membranes. Cytoskeletal proteins are fundamental in determining cell polarity and regulating transport.

The aqueous environment of the subretinal space is actively maintained by the ion-transport systems of the RPE. The active transport of a variety of ions (K^+, Ca^{2+}, Na^+, Cl^-, and HCO_3^-) across the RPE has been well documented. This transport is vectorial in most cases; for example, Na^+ is actively transported from the choriocapillaris toward the subretinal space, whereas K^+ is transported in the opposite direction. The apical membrane of the RPE appears to be the major locus of this transport. The ouabain-sensitive Na^+,K^+-ATPase is present at the apical, but not the basal, side. Similarly, an active bicarbonate-transport system appears to be located in this portion of the RPE membrane. High carbonic anhydrase activity seems to be associated with both the apical and basal sides of the cell.

Net ionic fluxes in the RPE are responsible for the transepithelial electrical potential that can be measured across the RPE apical membrane, a potential rapidly modified in the presence of a variety of metabolic inhibitors (eg, ouabain and dinitrophenol). In addition, the RPE apical membrane must be responsive to the changing conditions of phototransduction. For example, light evokes a decrease in K^+ ion concentration in the subretinal space, thus hyperpolarizing the RPE. Because the activity of Na^+,K^+-ATPase is controlled in part by K^+ ion concentration, light can affect the ionic composition of the subretinal space and the transport functions of the RPE. Active vectorial transport systems for other retinal metabolites (eg, taurine, methionine, and folate) have also been demonstrated. The RPE, therefore, appears to be important for maintaining the ionic environment of the subretinal space, which in turn is responsible for maintaining the integrity of the RPE–photoreceptor interface. The trans-RPE potential is the basis for the electro-oculogram (EOG), which is the most common electrophysiologic test for evaluating the RPE.

Pigmentation

A characteristic feature of the RPE is the presence of melanin pigment. Pigment granules are abundant in the cytoplasm of adult RPE cells, predominantly in the apical and mid-portions of the cell. During development, activation of the tyrosinase promoter triggers the onset of melanogenesis in this cell and marks the commitment of the neuroectoderm to become RPE. Although most melanogenesis occurs before birth, melanin production in the RPE does occur throughout life, albeit at a slow rate. As humans age, the melanin granules fuse with lysosomes; thus, the fundus of an older person is less pigmented than that of a young person.

The exact role of melanin inside cells remains speculative. One universally recognized function of melanin is to act as a neutral-density filter in scattering light. In so doing, melanin may have a protective role. In spite of the minimization of light scatter, visual acuity in the minimally pigmented fundus can be normal. Visual problems in individuals with albinism are attributable to foveal aplasia, not optical scatter. Genetic ocular disorders associated with melanin include varying forms of albinism. OCA refers to oculocutaneous albinism, of which there are 10 types. The OCA1 and OCA2 types are due to defects in the tyrosinase gene and the pink-eyed dilution gene, respectively. When melanin levels are below a critical level, there is aberrant neuronal migration in the visual pathway, lack of foveal development, low vision, nystagmus, and strabismus (ocular albinism is characterized by a lack of pigment in the eye but relatively normal pigmentation of skin and hair). Melanin is thought to play a role in retinal development because albino mammals have underdeveloped central retinas, more contralateral projections of ganglion cells, and failure of foveal development. Melanin is a free-radical stabilizer and can bind many toxins. Some regard this feature as protective; others think that it contributes to tissue toxicity.

Retinal Adhesion

None of the aforementioned functions would be possible without another RPE function—namely, maintenance of retinal adhesion. The subretinal space is never bridged by tissue, and yet the neural retina remains rather firmly attached to the RPE throughout life. This adhesion is vital to the retina because detachment of the photoreceptors from the RPE can lead to permanent morphologic change in the tissue.

Multiple systems keep the retina in place. These factors include passive hydrostatic forces, interdigitation of outer segments and RPE microvilli, active transport of subretinal fluid, and the complex structure and binding properties of the interphotoreceptor matrix. In situations of pathology, retinal adhesion can diminish, and detachment of the retina occurs. Detachment does not occur simply because there is a hole in the retina or a leak in the RPE; there must be either positive traction pulling the neural retina or positive forces pushing fluid into the subretinal space.

The RPE in Disease

Clearly, the RPE is vital for normal visual function. Three retinal degenerations in humans appear to be caused by defects unique to the RPE: Sorsby fundus dystrophy and 2 forms of autosomal recessive retinitis pigmentosa (RP). There are 2 generalized retinal degenerations: Usher syndrome (type 1B) and sex-linked RP, in which the defective gene is expressed strongly in the RPE and weakly in neural retina. It has been suggested that some forms of macular degeneration, such as vitelliform macular degeneration (Best disease) and malattia leventinese (dominant drusen), may be due to a primary defect in the RPE. Age-related macular degeneration and Stargardt disease appear to affect the RPE early in their course, although the genetic defect is in the rods. Finally, choroideremia and gyrate atrophy produce blindness by their early impact on the RPE. In certain pathologic situations (including proliferative vitreoretinopathy and subretinal neovascularization), RPE cells detach from the basement membrane and become migratory. Efforts are now under way to determine effective methods of RPE transplantation that may ameliorate the functional deficits in these diseases.

Gallemore RP, Hughes BA, Miller SS. Retinal pigment epithelial transport mechanisms and their contributions to the electroretinogram. *Prog Retin Eye Res.* 1997;16:509–566.

Marmor MF, Wolfensberger TJ, eds. *The Retinal Pigment Epithelium: Function and Disease.* New York: Oxford; 1998:103–134.

CHAPTER 15

Free Radicals and Antioxidants

The adverse effects of reactive forms of oxygen have been repeatedly proposed as causal factors in many types of tissue pathology, including cataract and age-related macular degeneration (AMD). Lipid peroxides are formed when free radicals or singlet oxygen molecules react with unsaturated fatty acids, which are present in cells largely as glycerylesters in phospholipids or triglycerides. It has been hypothesized that the oxidation of membrane phospholipids increases the permeability of cell membranes and/or inhibits membrane ion pumps. This loss of barrier function is thought to lead to edema, disturbances in electrolyte balance, and elevation of intracellular calcium, all of which contribute to cell malfunction.

Cellular Sources of Active Oxygen Species

The term *reactive oxygen intermediates (ROIs)* is used collectively to describe free radicals, hydrogen peroxide (H_2O_2), and singlet oxygen. *Free radicals* are molecules or atoms that possess an unpaired electron. This property makes them highly reactive toward other molecular species. Free radicals consist of superoxide anion (O_2^-), the hydroxyl radical ($OH\cdot$), and the lipid peroxyl radicals. Some free-radical reactions are involved in normal cell functions; others are thought to be important mediators of tissue damage. Oxygen-derived free radicals and their metabolites are generated within aerobic organisms in several ways.

Oxygen necessary for normal metabolism usually undergoes tetravalent (4-electron) reduction by intracellular systems, such as cytochrome oxidase in mitochondria (Fig 15-1), and is finally discarded as water without leakage of ROIs. However, a small percentage of the metabolized oxygen undergoes univalent reduction in four 1-electron steps. Oxygen accepts an electron from a reducing agent in each of these steps, and several ROIs are formed that are highly reactive.

Some of the reactive species leak out of their enzyme-binding sites and may damage other components of tissues, such as proteins, membrane lipids, and DNA, if they are not captured by detoxifying enzymes. Superoxide is not only produced in mitochondrial electron-transport systems but also formed in some enzymatic reactions, such as the xanthine and xanthine oxidase system. Hydrogen peroxide is produced directly in peroxisomes, as well as by enzyme-catalyzed dismutation of superoxide (see Fig 15-1). Any free iron (Fe^{2+}) present may catalyze formation of the hydroxyl radical from superoxide and hydrogen peroxide. Iron and other catalytic metals such as copper may also be involved

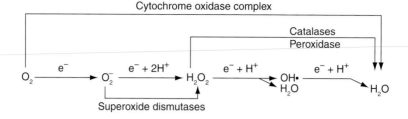

Figure 15-1 Enzymes involved in the metabolism of oxygen and in the detoxification of oxygen radicals generated by the univalent reduction of molecular oxygen. The univalent pathway involves a series of single electron transfers, producing the superoxide free radical (O_2^-), hydrogen peroxide (H_2O_2), water, and the hydroxyl radical (OH•). Superoxide dismutase catalyzes the conversion of superoxide to hydrogen peroxide without oxidizing other molecules. Catalase and peroxidase catalyze the reduction of hydrogen peroxide to water without formation of the toxic hydroxyl radical. These enzyme systems are capable of preventing the buildup of toxic species produced from the univalent reduction of oxygen. The cytochrome oxidase complex appears to catalyze the tetravalent reduction of oxygen to water without leakage of reactive intermediates. *(Courtesy of F. J. G. M. van Kuijk, MD, PhD.)*

in generating these species by accelerating nonenzymatic oxidation of several molecules, including glutathione.

Other sources of activated oxygen species include products from the enzymatic synthesis of prostaglandins, leukotrienes, and thromboxanes (see Chapter 9, Fig 9-1). The NADPH oxidase system of phagocytes yields activated oxygen species, especially during inflammation reactions. Oxygen-radical production is also associated with ionizing radiation and the metabolism of many chemicals and drugs, including carcinogenic compounds. Formation of reactive oxygen species—such as singlet oxygen by a light-mediated mechanism—is considered in the following section.

Superoxide and hydrogen peroxide are relatively stable in biological systems, whereas the hydroxyl radical is extremely reactive and capable of producing broad, nonspecific oxidative damage. However, free radicals and other active oxygen species also are important in many biological reactions that maintain normal cell functions, such as mitochondrial and microsomal electron-transport systems.

Mechanisms of Lipid Peroxidation

The mechanism by which random oxidation of lipids takes place is called *auto-oxidation*. This oxidation is a free-radical chain reaction usually described as a series of 3 processes: initiation, propagation, and termination. During the initiation step, the fatty acid is converted to an intermediate radical after removal of an allylic hydrogen. The propagation step follows immediately, and the fatty-acid radical intermediate reacts with oxygen at either end to produce fatty-acid peroxy radicals. Thus, a new fatty-acid radical is formed, which again can react with oxygen. As long as oxygen is available, a single free radical can lead to oxidation of thousands of fatty acids. A termination reaction, in which 2 radicals form a nonradical product, can interrupt the chain reaction. Auto-oxidation is also inhibited by free-radical scavengers such as vitamin E, which cause termination reactions.

Polyunsaturated fatty acids are susceptible to auto-oxidation because their allylic hydrogens are easily removed by several types of initiating radicals. The primary products of auto-oxidation formed during the propagation step are hydroperoxides (ROOH), which may decompose, especially in the presence of trace amounts of transition metal ions (eg, free iron or copper), to create peroxy radicals (ROO·), hydroxy radicals (HO·), and oxy radicals (RO·).

Photo-oxidation is a process by which oxygen is activated electronically by light to form singlet oxygen, which in turn reacts at a diffusion-controlled rate with unsaturated fatty acids or other cellular constituents. The mechanism of singlet-oxygen generation most widely accepted involves exposure of a photosensitizer to light in the presence of normal triplet oxygen ($^3O_2$). A photosensitizer is excited by absorption of light energy to an excited singlet state, which rapidly relaxes to an excited triplet state. In this state, the sensitizer may react with triplet oxygen ($^3O_2$) to form singlet oxygen ($^1O_2$). Photo-oxidation can be inhibited by singlet-oxygen quenchers such as carotenoids, which are discussed later in this chapter.

Lipid peroxidation not only causes direct damage to the cell membrane but also causes secondary damage in cells through its aldehydic breakdown products. Lipid hydroperoxides are unstable, and they break down to form many aldehydes, such as malondialdehyde and 4-hydroxyalkenals. These aldehydes can react quickly with proteins, inhibiting the proteins' normal functions. Both the lens and the retina are susceptible to such oxidative damage.

Oxidative Damage to the Lens

The lens is susceptible to challenge by various active species of oxygen because it contains low levels of molecular oxygen and trace amounts of transition metals such as copper and iron. It is thought that metal-catalyzed auto-oxidation reactions of various reducing agents in the lens can lead to the production of potentially damaging oxidants, such as oxidized glutathione (GSSG) and dehydroascorbic acid, as well as hydrogen peroxide, which can go on to produce hydroxyl radicals. In addition, ultraviolet radiation entering the lens can generate ROIs. Although most UVB radiation (<320 nm wavelength) striking the human eye is absorbed either by the cornea or by the high level of ascorbic acid in the aqueous humor, a certain proportion is able to reach the lens epithelium, where it can cause damage. UVA light (320–400 nm wavelength) is able to reach more deeply into the lens, where it can react with various chromophores to generate hydrogen peroxide, superoxide anion, and singlet oxygen. Although repair or regeneration mechanisms are active in the lens epithelium and superficial cortex, there are no such mechanisms in the deep cortex and the nucleus, where any damage to lens proteins and membrane lipids is irreversible. One result of this damage can be cross-linking and insolubilization of proteins, leading to loss of transparency (see Chapter 11). Certain types of human cataracts appear to initiate at the site of the fiber cell plasma membrane, possibly because oxygen is 5–7 times more soluble in membrane lipids than in cytoplasm.

To defend against oxidative stress, the young, healthy lens possesses a variety of effective antioxidant systems. These include the enzymes glutathione peroxidase, catalase, and superoxide dismutase (SOD) (Fig 15-2). By means of the glutathione redox cycle, GSSG is reconverted to glutathione (GSH) by glutathione reductase via the pyridine nucleotide NADPH, which is provided by the hexose monophosphate shunt as the reducing pathway. Thus, GSH acts as a major scavenger of active oxygen species in the lens. For reasons that are not well understood, the mammalian lens contains unusually high levels of protein sulfhydryl groups; however, it is clear that the groups must exist nearly completely in the reduced state for the tissue to remain transparent. The young human lens contains a high level of GSH, which is first synthesized in the epithelium and then migrates to the lens cortex and nucleus. With age, levels of GSH decline significantly in the human lens, par- ticularly in the nucleus. Studies have indicated that a cortical–nuclear barrier may exist in the mature human lens, which inhibits the free flow of GSH to the nucleus. The result is that with age, the human lens nucleus becomes more susceptible to oxidative damage and cataract. Nuclear cataracts show high levels of oxidized cysteine and methionine in the lens proteins.

The free-radical scavengers ascorbic acid and vitamin E are also present in the lens. These scavengers work in conjunction with GSH and the glutathione redox cycle to pro- tect against oxidative damage. Carotenoids that can quench singlet oxygen also exist in the lens. Epidemiologic (observational) studies have shown that people with higher levels of plasma antioxidants, particularly vitamin E, have a reduced risk of cataract, particularly nuclear cataract. However, 2 prospective, randomized placebo-controlled clinical trials— the Age-Related Eye Disease Study (AREDS) and the Vitamin E, Cataract and Age-

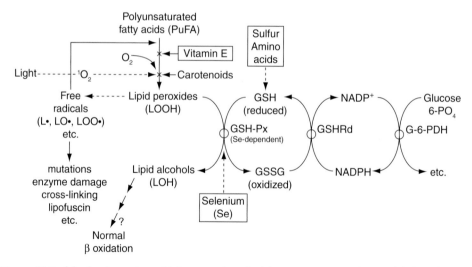

Figure 15-2 Mechanisms by which several antioxidants protect against oxidative damage. *Upper left,* Free radicals lead to the formation of lipid peroxides. Vitamin E inhibits this auto-oxidation process by scavenging free-radical intermediates. Carotenoids inhibit photo-oxidation by quenching singlet oxygen ($^1O_2$). *Center,* If lipid hydroperoxides are formed, they can be re-duced by GSH-Px, which requires selenium as a cofactor. If these protective enzymes are not fully active, more free radicals are formed by breakdown of lipid peroxides, which in turn leads to additional oxidation of polyunsaturated fatty acids. *G-6-PDH* = glucose-6-PO$_4$ dehydroge-nase, *GSH* = glutathione, *GSH-Px* = glutathione peroxidase, *GSHRd* = glutathione reductase, *GSSG* = oxidized glutathione. *(Courtesy of F. J. G. M. van Kuijk, MD, PhD.)*

Related Maculopathy Trial (VECAT)—found that high-dose formulations of vitamin C, vitamin E, and beta carotene (AREDS), as well as vitamin E alone, neither prevented the development nor slowed the progression of age-related cataracts.

Age-Related Eye Disease Study Research Group. A randomized, placebo-controlled clinical trial of high-dose supplementation with vitamins C and E and beta carotene for age-related cataract and vision loss: AREDS report no. 9. *Arch Ophthalmol.* 2001;119(10):1439–1452.

Lyle BJ, Mares-Perlman JA, Klein BE, et al. Serum carotenoids and tocopherols and incidence of age-related nuclear cataract. *Am J Clin Nutr.* 1999;69(2):272–277.

McNeil JJ, Robman L, Tikellis G, Sinclair MI, McCarty CA, Taylor HR. Vitamin E supplementation and cataract: randomized controlled trial. *Ophthalmology.* 2004;111(1):75–84.

Padgaonkar VA, Lin LR, Leverenz VR, Rinke A, Reddy VN, Gblin FJ. Hyperbaric oxygen *in vivo* accelerates the loss of cytoskeletal proteins and MIP26 in guinea pig lens nucleus. *Exp Eye Res.* 1999;68(4):493–504.

Sweeney MH, Truscott RJ. An impediment to glutathione diffusion in older normal human lenses: a possible precondition for nuclear cataract. *Exp Eye Res.* 1998;67(5):587–595.

Vulnerability of the Retina to Free Radicals

Experimental data have shown that retinal photoreceptors degenerate when they are exposed to oxidative challenges such as hyperbaric oxygen, iron overload, or injection of lipid hydroperoxides into the vitreous humor. The retina also degenerates when antioxidative defenses are reduced, which presumably elevates levels of lipid peroxidation in the absence of unusual oxidative stress. The retina is made vulnerable to damage from lipid peroxidation by several distinctive characteristics, 4 of which are considered here:

1. Vertebrate retinal rod outer segments are susceptible to damage by oxygen because of their high content of polyunsaturated fatty acids. Their phospholipids typically contain about 50 mol% docosahexaenoic acid, the most highly polyunsaturated fatty acid that occurs in nature. It is well established that polyunsaturated fatty acids are sensitive to peroxidation in proportion to their number of double bonds.

2. The rod inner segment is very rich in mitochondria, which may leak activated oxygen species.

3. The excellent oxygen supply through the choroid and the retinal vessels elevates the risk of oxidative damage. Vertebrate retinas maintained in vitro showed at least a sevenfold higher rate of oxygen consumption per milligram of protein compared with all other tissues tested (except the adrenal gland). The oxygen tension is highest at the choroid and drops toward the inner segments because of the high metabolic demand of their mitochondria. Oxygen consumption has been reported to decrease when the retina is illuminated.

4. Light exposure may trigger photo-oxidative processes mediated by singlet oxygen, and the RPE may play a key role.

The RPE is tightly packed with endoplasmic reticulum and appears to be rich in antioxidant enzymes in most species tested. The RPE of pigmented animals contains melanin granules, which function as a light trap. Although melanin is commonly assumed to be photoprotective, its role in the prevention of light damage to ocular tissues is not clearly understood. Evidence suggests that the RPE is quite sensitive to dietary antioxidant deficiency, in which light-activated melanin may contribute to phototoxicity. If an RPE cell dies, then the numerous photoreceptors supported by that RPE cell may suffer severe damage or death.

Intense light at levels that may be encountered in daily life is phototoxic to the retina. Even though the cornea absorbs some UV radiation, the retinas of young people are exposed to a substantial amount of light in the range of 350–400 nm (young lenses transmit these wavelengths). The lens yellows with age, and the cutoff wavelength in older people moves up to approximately 430 nm. Because the adult lens absorbs nearly 100% of light below 400 nm, little or no UV light reaches the retina in older people.

In addition to UV light, blue light (400–500 nm) can be harmful to the retina (blue-light hazard). The photoreceptors in the retina are particularly susceptible to damage by blue light, a process that can lead to cell death and retinal disease. This happens due to the formation of the phototoxic compound A2E. A2E (ie, A2E epoxide) specifically targets cytochrome oxidase and induces irreversible DNA damage (apoptosis) of RPE cells. This molecular process is believed to be a precursor to the pathogenesis of AMD. Carotenoids (eg, lutein and zeaxanthin) present in the retina act as a blue-light filter, shielding the photoreceptors in the retina from this radiation, and in vitro studies have suggested that vitamin E and other antioxidants inhibit A2E-epoxide formation.

Shaban H, Richter C. A2E and blue light in the retina: the paradigm of age-related macular degeneration. *Biol Chem.* 2002;383(3–4):537–545.

Sparrow JR, Vollmer-Snarr HR, Zhou J, et al. A2E-epoxides damage DNA in retinal pigment epithelial cells. Vitamin E and other antioxidants inhibit A2E-epoxide formation. *J Biol Chem.* 2003;278(20):18207–18213.

Antioxidants in the Retina and RPE

Several antioxidant mechanisms have been established in biological systems, including free-radical scavenging, quenching of singlet oxygen, and enzymatic reduction of hydroperoxides. Antioxidants found in vertebrates include selenium, GSH, selenium-dependent glutathione peroxidase, non–selenium-dependent glutathione peroxidase (glutathione-S-transferase), vitamin E, and carotenoids. Antioxidants in vertebrates also include SOD and catalase, and antioxidant roles for ascorbate and melanin have also been reported. The relation between some of these antioxidants and the protective mechanisms is shown in Figure 15-2.

Yu BP. Cellular defenses against damage from reactive oxygen species. *Physiol Rev.* 1994;74(1):139–162.

Selenium, Glutathione, Glutathione Peroxidase, and Glutathione-S-Transferase

A number of enzymes have been identified that can provide antioxidant protection by a peroxide-decomposing mechanism. For example, selenium-dependent glutathione peroxidase (GSH-Px) and several enzymes of the glutathione-S-transferase (GSH-S-Ts) group can reduce organic hydroperoxides. GSH-Px is also active with H_2O_2 as a substrate, although the GSH-S-Ts group cannot act on H_2O_2. All of these enzymes require GSH, which is converted to GSSG during the enzymatic reaction. The hexose monophosphate shunt enzymes produce NADPH, which is needed for reduction of GSSG by GSH reductase. Both GSH-Px and GSH-S-Ts activities have been measured in human and in animal retinas. The highest concentration of selenium in the human eye is present in the RPE: 100–400 ng in the RPE cells of a single human eye, up to 10 times more than in the retina (40 ng). In addition, the amount of selenium appears to be similar in both eyes of the same individual. The selenium level in the human retina is constant with age; in the human RPE, however, the level increases with age.

Vitamin E

Vitamin E acts by scavenging free radicals, thus terminating the propagation steps and leading to interruption of the auto-oxidation reaction. Reports on the vitamin E content of the retina of the adult rat raised on normal chow diets show values ranging from 215 to 325 ng. A detailed study on the vitamin E content of microdissected parts of vertebrate eyes showed that the RPE is rich in vitamin E relative to the photoreceptors and that photoreceptors are rich in vitamin E relative to most other cells in the eye. Studies on vitamin E in postmortem human eyes also found that the level of vitamin E is higher in the RPE than in the retina. Furthermore, vitamin E levels in human retinal tissues increase with age until the sixth decade of life and then decrease. This decrease coincides with the age at which the incidence of AMD increases in the population.

> Friedrichson T, Kalbach HL, Buck P, van Kuijk FJ. Vitamin E in macular and peripheral tissues of the human eye. *Curr Eye Res.* 1995;14(8):693–701.

Superoxide Dismutase and Catalase

Superoxide dismutase catalyzes the dismutation of superoxide to hydrogen peroxide, which is further reduced to water by catalase or peroxidase. Two types of SOD are usually isolated from mammalian tissues: *Cu-Zn SOD*, the cytoplasmic enzyme, which is inhibited by cyanide; and *Mn SOD*, the mitochondrial enzyme, which is not inhibited by cyanide.

Catalase catalyzes the reduction of hydrogen peroxide to water. Information on catalase activity in the retina is currently rather limited. Total retinal catalase activity was found to be very low but detectable in the rabbit. A protective role for catalase has been reported in rats with experimental allergic uveitis.

Ascorbate

Ascorbate (vitamin C) is thought to function synergistically with vitamin E to terminate free-radical reactions. It has been proposed that vitamin C can react with the vitamin E radicals formed when vitamin E scavenges free radicals. Vitamin E radicals are then regenerated to native vitamin E. The vitamin C radicals resulting from this regeneration can be reduced by NADH reductase, with NADH as the electron acceptor. Ascorbic acid is found throughout the eye of many species in concentrations that are high relative to those in other tissues.

Delamere NA. Ascorbic acid and the eye. In: Harris JR, ed. *Subcellular Biochemistry,* Vol 25. Ascorbic Acid: Biochemistry and Biomedical Cell Biology. New York: Plenum Press; 1996: 313–329.

Carotenoids

Various roles have been proposed for carotenoids (xanthophylls) in biological systems, including limiting chromatic aberration at the fovea of the retina and the quenching of singlet oxygen. β-Carotene is the precursor of vitamin A and can act as a free-radical trap at low oxygen tension. In postmortem human retinas, carotenoids have been shown to make up the yellow pigment in the macula. A mixture of the 2 carotenoids *lutein* and *zeaxanthin* is present in the macula and located in the Henle fiber layer. It has been demonstrated that in humans, zeaxanthin is concentrated primarily in the fovea, whereas lutein is dispersed in the retina. Interestingly, little β-carotene is present in the human eye. Furthermore, carotenoids are present only in the retina and not at all in the RPE. In the peripheral retina, lutein and zeaxanthin are also concentrated in the photoreceptor outer segments and may act as antioxidants to protect the macula against short-wavelength visible light. Figure 15-3A shows the localization of antioxidants in the human macula and peripheral retina; Figure 15-3B shows their localization in a cross section of the peripheral retina.

Khachik F, Bernstein PS, Garland DL. Identification of lutein and zeaxanthin oxidation products in human and monkey retinas. *Invest Ophthalmol Vis Sci.* 1997;38(9):1802–1811.
Mayne ST. Beta-carotene, carotenoids, and disease prevention in humans. *FASEB J.* 1996;10(7): 690–701.

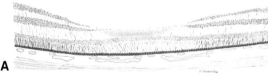

A

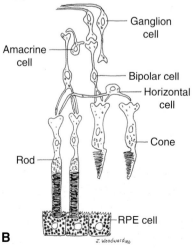

Figure 15-3 **A,** The localization of antioxidants in the human macula and peripheral retina. *Yellow* represents carotenoids, *blue* represents vitamin E, and *red* represents selenium. Vitamin E and selenium are primarily concentrated in the RPE. In the macula, carotenoids are present in the fibers of Henle; in the peripheral retina, they are also present in the rods. **B,** The localization in a cross section of the peripheral retina. Vitamin E and selenium remain primarily concentrated in the RPE but are also enriched in the rod outer segments. Carotenoids have been found in rod outer segments in the peripheral retina. *(Illustrations by J. Woodward, MD; courtesy of F. J. G. M. van Kuijk, MD, PhD.)*

PART V

Ocular Pharmacology

CHAPTER 16

Pharmacologic Principles

Introduction

Ophthalmic medications and distant humoral and local neural transmitters both manipulate the same receptors. The drugs differ from the natural transmitters in not only the mechanism and location of delivery but also the quantity of agent released and the feedback control of the active agent. For example, mydriatic and cycloplegic dilating drops are applied in a location remote from their intended sites of action in enormous quantities that swamp homeostatic mechanisms. In contrast, the intrinsic neurotransmitters controlling the pupil are released in precise locations in minute quantities as part of a delicately balanced system.

Pharmacotherapy depends on a frequently unreliable mechanism—the patient—to deliver agents. These medications are given infrequently in volumes greater than the tear film capacity; the type of medication and the dosing regimen are adjusted based on the clinical response. The more reliable physiologic processes in healthy patients, in contrast, continuously deliver the appropriate quantities of transmitter via precisely controlled feedback mechanisms. Further, pharmacologic agents often produce unwanted side effects, known as *toxicity*, by acting at sites other than the intended location. Drug therapy may also induce counteracting mechanisms, such as up-regulating drug-metabolizing enzymes or down-regulating receptors that alter the therapeutic effect. Occasionally, medications may cause an allergic reaction. These effects all differ from the highly specific physiologic neural and humoral agents, which work in concert with feedback mechanisms and have immune privilege.

In the future, we will be able to model most, if not all, of our pharmacologic interventions on natural physiologic processes. Delivering agents directly to the desired site of action or continuously from a sustained-release device or deposit will improve efficacy and compliance and reduce side effects. Additional areas of future research include

- coupling drug release to feedback-control mechanisms (eg, glaucoma therapy regulated by a pressure-sensing strain gauge)
- achieving higher specificity of action by designing drugs to complement the geometry of receptor sites
- designing medication with structural modifications that eliminate allergenic moieties or minimize side-effect profiles
- recognizing genetic traits that predispose individuals to disease, and devising drugs that repair or modify the defective gene product
- manipulating the genome to effect repair or regeneration

The study of ocular pharmacology begins with a review of some general principles of pharmacology, with particular attention to special features of the eye that facilitate or impede ocular therapy.

Pharmacokinetics

Pharmacokinetics deals with the cycle of a drug through the body, including the absorption, distribution, metabolism, and excretion of that drug. To achieve a therapeutic effect, a drug must reach its site of action in sufficient concentration. The concentration at the site of action is a function of the route of administration, the amount administered, the extent and rate of absorption at the administration site, the distribution and binding in tissues, the movement by bulk flow in circulating fluids, the transport between compartments, biotransformation, and excretion. Pharmacokinetics and dose together determine *bioavailability,* or concentration of the active drug at the therapeutic site.

Pharmacodynamics

Pharmacodynamics refers to the biological activity and clinical effect of drugs. It is the drug action after pharmacokinetics has distributed the active agent to the therapeutic site. Included within the area of pharmacodynamics are the tissue receptor for the drug and the intracellular changes initiated by the binding of the active drug with the receptor. The pharmacodynamic action of a drug is often described using the receptor for that drug, for example an α-adrenergic agonist or β-adrenergic antagonist.

Pharmacotherapeutics

Pharmacotherapeutics is the application of a drug in order to reach a given clinical endpoint, such as the prevention or treatment of disease. The therapeutic dose may vary for any patient, based on the patient's age, gender, race, other currently prescribed medications, and preexisting medical conditions. Pharmacotherapeutics are covered in Chapter 17.

Toxicity

Toxicity refers to the adverse effects of either medication or environmental chemicals, including poisoning. Toxicity may be influenced by pharmacokinetics and/or pharmacodynamics. For example, topically applied ophthalmic medications are readily absorbed through the mucous membranes of the eye and nasopharynx, as well as by absorption through the iris and ciliary body. Topical absorption avoids the first-pass metabolism of the liver and increases systemic bioavailability. The systemic toxicity of these medications may therefore be more than expected relative to the total topical dose. Local toxicity of topical agents is more common than systemic toxicity, however. Local toxicity may be a type I IgE-mediated hypersensitivity reaction or may represent a delayed reaction to either the medication or the preservatives. The older preservatives thimerosal and benzalkonium chloride are frequently implicated in ocular toxicity. New preservatives developed in response to this problem dissipate upon exposure to light or to the ions in the tear film. Two examples of these are oxychloro complex (Purite), which breaks down to sodium chloride and water, and sodium perborate, which breaks down to hydrogen peroxide before becoming oxygen and hydrogen. These "disappearing preservatives" theoretically should have no toxicity to the corneal surface.

These pharmacologic principles apply differently to the elderly. Compared with younger patients, older patients have less lean body mass due to a decrease in muscle bulk, less body water and albumin, and an increase in the relative percentage of adipose tissue. These physiologic differences alter tissue binding and drug distribution. Human renal function decreases 50% with age; both hepatic perfusion and enzymatic activity are variably affected as well. The elderly tend to be on more chronic medications, many of which are processed simultaneously by the same, already compromised, metabolic systems.

The pharmacokinetic processing of drugs in the elderly is therefore significantly altered, extending the effective half-life of most medications. The pharmacodynamic action of a drug is often independently potentiated in the elderly. The increase in both drug effect and side effects occurs even if the dose is decreased in consideration of these pharmacokinetic changes. Thus, the pharmacotherapeutic effects and the toxicity of medication may be altered simply by the aging process, independent of drug dosage. Accordingly, the selection of a specific therapeutic agent should be guided by the general health, age, and concomitant medication taken by a patient.

Pharmacokinetics: The Route of Drug Delivery

Topical Administration

Eyedrops
Most ocular medications are administered topically as drops. This route of administration maximizes the anterior segment concentrations while minimizing systemic toxicity. The drug gradient from the concentrated tear reservoir to the relatively barren corneal and conjunctival epithelium forces a passive route of absorption.

Amount administered   Some features of topical ocular therapy limit its effectiveness. Very little of an administered drop is retained by the eye. When a 50-µL drop is delivered from the usual commercial dispenser, the volume of the tear lake rises from 7 µL to only 10 µL in the blinking eye of an upright patient. Thus, at most, 20% of the administered drug is retained (10 µL/50 µL). A rapid turnover of fluid in the tear lake also occurs, 16% per minute in the undisturbed eye, with even faster turnover if the drop elicits reflex tearing. Consequently, for slowly absorbed drugs, only 50% of the drug that was initially retained in the tear reservoir (50% of the 20% of the delivered medication, or 10%) remains 4 minutes after instillation ($0.84^4 \times 0.50$), and only 17% remains after 10 minutes, or 3.4% of the original dose. The amount of time that a drug remains in the tear reservoir and tear film is called the "residence time" of a medication. It is affected not only by drug formulation but also by the timing of subsequent medication, tear production, and drainage.

Some simple measures have been shown to improve ocular absorption of materials that do not traverse the cornea rapidly. Patients using more than one topical ocular medication should be instructed to allow 5 minutes between drops; otherwise, the second drop may simply wash out the first. Blinking also diminishes a drug's effect by activating the nasal lacrimal pump mechanism, forcing fluid from the lacrimal sac into the nasophar- ynx, and creating a negative sac pressure that empties the tear lake (see BCSC Section 7, *Orbit, Eyelids, and Lacrimal System*). Patients can circumvent this loss of drug reservoir by either compressing the nasolacrimal duct with digital pressure at the medial canthus or closing the eyelids for 5 minutes after instillation of each drop. These 2 measures will prevent emptying of the tear lake and will reduce systemic toxicity by decreasing absorp- tion through the nasal mucosa. Nasolacrimal occlusion will increase the absorption of topically applied materials (Fig 16-1) and decrease the systemic absorption and potential toxicity (Fig 16-2). Tear reservoir retention and drug contact time can also be extended either by increasing the viscosity of the vehicle or by using drug delivery objects such as contact lenses, collagen shields, and inserts.

Topical medications that are absorbed by the nasal mucosa can attain significant lev- els in the blood. One to 2 drops of a topical medication may provide a significant systemic dose of that drug. For example, a 1% solution of atropine has 1 g/100 mL, or 10 mg/1 mL. A simpler way of remembering this is to add a 0 to the drug percentage to change to

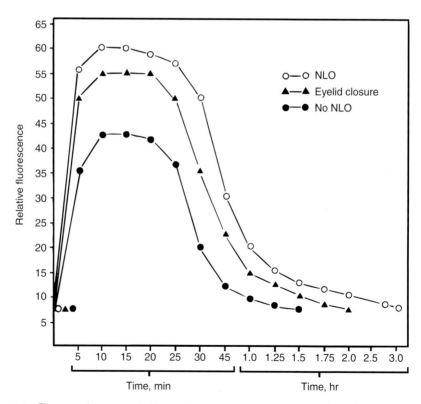

Figure 16-1 Fluorescein concentration in the anterior chamber at various times after applica- tion: with nasolacrimal occlusion (NLO), with 5 minutes of eyelid closure, or with no interven- tion (no NLO).

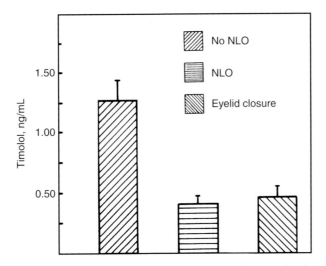

Figure 16-2 Systemic absorption of timolol at various times after application: with nasolacrimal obstruction (NLO), with 5 minutes of eyelid closure, or with no intervention (no NLO).

mg/mL. As there are 20 drops per milliliter (up to 40 in some newer, small-tip dispensers), there is ¼–½ mg per drop. If this drop is given bilaterally, there is up to 1 mg of active agent available for systemic absorption.

Because the contact time of topical medication is short, the rate of transfer from the tear fluid into the cornea is critical. The fenestrated barriers in the vascular endothelium and the mucosa of the stomach allow rapid diffusion of all but large molecules through extracellular passages. In contrast, the corneal epithelium and endothelium have tight intercellular junctions that limit passage of molecules in the extracellular space. Topically applied medication must first pass through hydrophobic/lipophilic cell membranes in the epithelium, then through the hydrophilic/lipophobic corneal stroma, and finally through the hydrophobic/lipophilic cell membranes in the endothelium in order to enter the anterior segment. Topical ophthalmic drug formulations must therefore be both lipophilic and hydrophilic. As nonionic particles are more lipophilic than ionic particles, they pass through the cellular phospholipid membranes more readily. The pH of the medication can be manipulated to increase the percentage of the drug in an uncharged or nonionized form. Mechanical disruption of the epithelial barrier in corneal abrasion or infection also increases the rate of intraocular drug penetration.

Similar considerations apply to the conjunctiva. The permeability of the conjunctiva to small water-soluble molecules is thought to be 20 times that of the cornea. Perilimbal conjunctiva offers an effective transscleral route for delivery of drugs to anterior segment structures.

The factors determining the amount of medication that can penetrate the cornea are concentration and solubility in the delivery vehicle, viscosity, lipid solubility, and the drug's pH, ionic and steric form, molecular size, chemical structure and configuration, vehicle, and surfactants. In addition, reflex tearing and the binding of the active medication to proteins in tears and tissue affect drug bioavailability.

Drug concentration and solubility   It may be necessary to load the tear reservoir with concentrated solutions in order to get a sufficient amount of a drug through the corneal barriers (eg, selecting pilocarpine 4% instead of pilocarpine 1%). A practical limit to exploiting these high concentrations is reached when the high tonicity of the resulting solutions elicits reflex tearing or when drugs that are poorly water-soluble reach their solubility limits and precipitate. A drug with adequate solubility in an aqueous solution can be formulated as a solution, whereas a drug with poor solubility may need to be provided in a suspension. A suspension requires agitation so that the active medication is redistributed prior to administration. Suspensions may be more irritating to the ocular surface than solutions are, a factor that may affect the choice of drug formulation.

Viscosity   The addition of high-viscosity substances such as methylcellulose and polyvinyl alcohol to the drug increases drug retention in the inferior cul-de-sac, aiding drug penetration. There is little correlation between increasing solution viscosity and increasing efficacy, however, thus indicating that these substances may act by altering the barrier function of the corneal epithelium as well as by increasing drug contact time with the cornea.

Lipid solubility   To traverse the cornea, a drug must pass sequentially through the lipid-rich environment of the epithelial cell membranes, through the water-rich environment of the stroma, and finally through the lipid barrier at the endothelium. Studies of the permeability of isolated corneas to families of chemical compounds show that lipid solubility is more important than water solubility in promoting penetration. To determine the solubility of a drug or group of drugs, researchers ascertain the ratio of lipid solubility to water solubility for each compound in the series by (1) measuring the phase separation of a drug between 2 solvents—1 lipid-soluble and 1 water-soluble (eg, octanol and water); and (2) calculating the ratio of the drug concentration in the 2 compartments (partition coefficient). Drugs with greater relative lipid solubility have a higher partition coefficient.

For substituted ethoxzolamides, the permeability coefficient is 70 times higher for compounds of high lipid solubility than for those of low lipid solubility. Drugs with higher lipid solubility and a higher partition coefficient have increased penetration of cell membranes. However, compounds with excessively high partition coefficients are often poorly soluble in tears. Experimental studies of substituted compounds need to account for the effects of the substituents on potency, on solubility, and on the permeability coefficient.

pH and ionic charge   Many eye medications are alkaloids, or weak bases. Such drugs as tropicamide, cyclopentolate, atropine, and epinephrine exist in both charged and uncharged forms at the slightly alkaline pH of tears (pH 7.4). The partition coefficients, and therefore the drug penetration, can be increased by raising the pH of the water phase, thereby increasing the proportion of drug molecules in the more lipid-soluble, uncharged form.

Surfactants   Many preservative agents used in topical drops to prevent bacterial contamination are surface-active agents that alter cell membranes in the cornea as well as in bacteria. They reduce the barrier effect of the corneal epithelium and increase drug permeability. For example, a 0.1% carbachol solution containing 0.03% benzalkonium chloride can elicit the same miotic response as a 2% solution without it.

Reflex tearing   Ocular irritation and secondary tearing wash out the drug reservoir in the tear lake and reduce the contact time of the drug with the cornea. Reflex tearing occurs when topical medications are not isotonic and when they have a nonphysiologic pH or contain irritants.

Tissue binding of medication   Tear and surface proteins, as well as ocular melanin, may bind topical or systemic medication, making the drug unavailable or creating a slow release reservoir. This binding may alter the lag time, or onset of action, of a medication, as well as the peak effect and duration of action, and can cause a delayed local toxicity despite discontinuation of the medication. The retinal toxicity that progresses even after discontinuation of the aminoquinoline antimalarial agents chloroquine and hydroxychloroquine is one example of this effect.

Ointments

Another strategy for increasing the contact time of ocular medications is the use of ointments. Commercial oil-based ointments usually consist of petrolatum and mineral oil. The mineral oil allows the ointment to melt at body temperature. Both ingredients are also effective lipid solvents. However, most water-soluble medications are insoluble in the ointment and are present as microcrystals. Only those microcrystals on the surface of the ointment dissolve in the tears; the rest are trapped until the ointment melts. Such protracted, slow release may prevent the drug from reaching a therapeutic level in the tears. Only if the drug has high lipid solubility (which allows it to diffuse through the ointment) and some water solubility will it escape from the ointment into both the corneal epithelium and the tears. Fluorometholone, chloramphenicol, and tetracycline are examples of drugs that achieve higher aqueous levels when administered as ointment rather than as drops.

Local Administration

Periocular injections

Injection of medication beneath the conjunctiva or the Tenon capsule allows drugs to bypass the conjunctival and corneal epithelial barriers and absorb passively down a concentration gradient into the sclera and intraocular tissues. Subconjunctival, sub-Tenon, and retrobulbar injections all allow medications to reach therapeutic levels behind the lens–iris diaphragm. This approach is especially useful for drugs with low lipid solubility (such as penicillin), which do not penetrate the eye adequately if they are given topically. Injections can also be helpful in delivering medication closer to the local site of action— for example, posterior sub-Tenon injections of steroids for cystoid macular edema (CME) or subconjunctival injection of 5-fluorouracil after trabeculectomy. Retrobulbar and peribulbar anesthesia techniques for ocular surgery are covered in BCSC Section 11, *Lens and Cataract*. Other examples of local, injectable medications are botulinum toxin, which is used in the treatment of benign essential blepharospasm and hemifacial spasm and for cosmesis; and retrobulbar alcohol as therapy for chronic pain in blind eyes.

Intraocular medications

The intraocular injection of drugs instantly delivers effective concentrations at the target site. There are 2 types of intraocular injections: intracameral injections into the anterior chamber and intravitreal injections into the vitreous cavity. Great care must be taken to avoid using preserved medication and to control the concentration of such agents so that the delicate internal structures of the eye are protected from toxicity.

Intraocular injections have been used to treat diabetic diffuse macular edema, persistent CME, and central retinal vein occlusion; they have also been used after vitrectomy for severe proliferative diabetic retinopathy as well as for some ocular neoplasms. Intraoperative use of tissue plasminogen activator (tPA) assists fibrinolysis and subretinal hemorrhage displacement and drainage; silicon oil, intraocular gases, and perfluorooctane facilitate vitreoretinal surgery, decrease postoperative complications, and enhance postoperative outcomes. Intraocular injections of expansile gases are routinely used in pneumatic retinopexy to treat superior retinal detachments, to flatten the posterior pole after vitrectomy for macular holes, and to displace submacular blood.

Intraocular implants allow the slow release of medication over months to years. Ganciclovir implants may be placed into the vitreous cavity for treatment of cytomegalovirus (CMV) retinitis, allowing immediate and sustained therapeutic levels with a prolonged disease remission of 8 to 13 months. Intravitreal antivirals and ganciclovir implants have also been used with limited success in progressive outer retinal necrosis in AIDS patients. Fluocinolone acetonide intravitreal implants (Retisert) are used for the control of chronic posterior uveitis.

Chen SN, Yang TC, Ho CL, Kuo YH, Yip Y, Chao AN. Retinal toxicity of intravitreal tissue plasminogen activator: case report and literature review. *Ophthalmology.* 2003;110(4):704–708.

de Smet MD, Vancs VS, Kohler D, Solomon D, Chan CC. Intravitreal chemotherapy for the treatment of recurrent intraocular lymphoma. *Br J Ophthalmol.* 1999;83(4):448–451.

Jonas JB, Hayler JK, Söfker A, Panda-Jonas S. Intravitreal injection of crystalline cortisone as adjunctive treatment of proliferative diabetic retinopathy. *Am J Ophthalmol.* 2001;131(4): 468–471.

Rahhal FM. Treatment advances for CMV retinitis. *AIDS Read.* 1999;9(1):28–34.

Roig-Melo EA, Macky TA, Heredia-Elizondo ML, Alfaro DV III. Progressive outer retinal necrosis syndrome: successful treatment with a new combination of antiviral drugs. *Eur J Ophthalmol.* 2001;11(2):200–202.

Velez G, Boldt HC, Whitcup SM, Nussenblatt RB, Robinson MR. Local methotrexate and dexamethasone phosphate for the treatment of recurrent primary intraocular lymphoma. *Ophthalmic Surg Lasers.* 2002;33(4):329–333.

Systemic Administration

Just as the intercellular tight junctions of the corneal epithelium and endothelium limit anterior access to the interior of the eye, similar barriers limit access through vascular channels. The vascular endothelium of the retina, like that of the brain, is nonfenestrated and knitted together by tight junctions. Although both the choroid and the ciliary body have fenestrated vascular endothelia, the choroid is effectively sequestered by the RPE; and the ciliary body, by its nonpigmented epithelium.

Drugs with higher lipid solubilities more readily penetrate the blood–ocular barrier. Thus, chloramphenicol, which is highly lipid-soluble, penetrates 20 times better than does penicillin, which has poor lipid solubility.

The ability of systemically administered drugs to gain access to the eye is also influenced by the degree to which they are bound to plasma proteins. Only the unbound form can cross the blood–ocular barrier. Sulfonamides are lipid-soluble but penetrate poorly, because at therapeutic levels, more than 90% of the medication is bound to plasma proteins. Similarly, the greater binding of plasma protein to oxacillin reduces its penetration, compared with that of methicillin. Because bolus administration of a drug exceeds the binding capacity of plasma proteins and leads to higher intraocular drug levels than can be achieved by a slow intravenous drip, this approach is used for the administration of antibiotics in order to attain high peak intraocular levels.

Sustained-release oral preparations

The practical value of sustained-release preparations is significant. For example, a single dose of acetazolamide will reduce IOP for up to 10 hours, whereas a single dose of sustained-release acetazolamide will produce a comparable effect lasting 20 hours. Sustained-release medications offer a more steady blood level of the drug, avoid marked peaks and valleys, and reduce the frequency of administration.

Intravenous injections

Intravenous medication can be administered for either diagnostic or therapeutic effect. Two diagnostic medications, sodium fluorescein and indocyanine green, are used for retinal angiography to diagnose retinal and choroidal disease. Edrophonium chloride is used intravenously in the diagnosis of myasthenia gravis.

Intravenous medications are also used therapeutically in ophthalmology. Although intravitreal injections have replaced intravenous therapy for postoperative endophthalmitis, continuous intravenous administration of an antibiotic is an effective way of maintaining intraocular levels in endogenous infection (see BCSC Section 12, *Retina and Vitreous*).

The barriers and reservoir effects of the eye change the ocular pharmacodynamics of antibiotics such as ampicillin, chloramphenicol, and erythromycin. These agents penetrate the eye with higher initial intraocular levels and maintain comparable bioavailability for 4 hours when given as a single intravenous bolus rather than by continuous infusion. Medication may have better intraocular penetration in the inflamed eye than in the healthy eye due to the disruption of the blood–aqueous and blood–retina barriers. This disruption is demonstrated by the leakage of fluorescein from inflamed retinal vessels into the vitreous during angiography.

Studies of the rabbit eye have found that the bioavailability of intravenous ampicillin, tetracycline, and dexamethasone is different in various structures of the rabbit eye, with the highest levels of these medications found in the sclera and conjunctiva, followed by the iris and ciliary body, and finally the cornea, aqueous humor, choroid, and retina. Very low levels appeared in the lens and vitreous. The drugs showed no marked differences in their vascular distribution, however. The tissue bioavailability is determined by the vascularity of the tissue and the barriers that exist between the blood and that tissue.

Intramuscular agents

In ophthalmology, intramuscular agents are used less frequently than topical, oral, or intravenous agents. Notable exceptions include the use of prostigmine in the diagnosis of myasthenia gravis and the local therapeutic use of botulinum toxin in facial dystonias.

Methods of Ocular Drug Design and Delivery

New ocular drugs are designed with a focus on specificity and safety, with delivery systems aimed at improving convenience and patient compliance. Each of the following new approaches responds to a specific problem in ocular pharmacokinetics.

Prodrugs

Prodrugs are inert compounds that are activated by one of the enzymatic systems within the eye. Dipivefrin HCl (Propine) is a prodrug of epinephrine; it has better lipid solubility than epinephrine and increases corneal penetration 17-fold. Thus, a 0.1% solution can be used in place of epinephrine 1%–2%. Corneal esterases convert dipivefrin to epinephrine, and, as dipivefrin has low intrinsic activity, it is virtually free of the systemic side effects of epinephrine. Another topical prodrug, latanoprost (Xalatan), is converted to prostaglandin F2α by corneal esterases for the treatment of glaucoma. Valacyclovir HCl (Valtrex) is an antiviral prodrug that is easily absorbed through the gastrointestinal system and quickly converted to the active form of acyclovir. Likewise, famciclovir is a prodrug of the active antiviral penciclovir.

Sustained-release devices and gels

Drop therapy involves periodic delivery of relatively large quantities of a drug. A sufficient amount of the drug must bind to receptors to achieve a therapeutic effect. The surrounding tissues often retain additional medication, acting as a local reservoir for sustained release between applications. The high peak drug levels attained in bolus dosing can cause local and systemic side effects, as for example, the miosis and induced accommodation resulting from the use of pilocarpine.

Delivery devices Devices have been developed that deliver an adequate supply of medication at a steady-state level, thus achieving beneficial effects with fewer adverse effects. The Ocusert delivery system, designed to deliver pilocarpine at a steady rate of 40 µg/hr, was the therapeutic equivalent of 2% pilocarpine used 4 times a day. However, because the total daily dose of pilocarpine was only 960 µg (24 hours × 40 µg/hr) when delivered with the device as compared to 4000 µg (4 doses × 2000 mg/100 mL × 0.05 mL/dose) with drops, miosis was less marked, and the induced accommodation was reduced. The Ocusert device was discontinued as the use of pilocarpine decreased, but it remains an interesting example of steady-state drug delivery. This device may be resurrected in the future for use with other medications.

The gel form of timolol maleate (Timoptic-XE) contains a heteropolysaccharide that thickens on contact with the tear film, maintaining therapeutic levels while decreasing the dosing to once daily.

The ganciclovir sustained-release intraocular device (Vitrasert) is surgically implanted and delivers a steady source of ganciclovir for 5–8 months. An ethylene vinyl acetate disc with polyvinyl alcohol coating serves as a drug reservoir. The thickness of the polyvinyl alcohol lid regulates the delivery of ganciclovir to target tissue. Fluocinolone acetonide vitreal implants (Retisert) are likewise used for a slow, targeted delivery of corticosteroids to the vitreous cavity for posterior uveitis.

Collagen cornea shields

Porcine scleral tissue is extracted and molded into contact lens–like shields that are useful as a delivery system to prolong the contact between a drug and the cornea. Drugs can be incorporated into the collagen matrix during the manufacturing process, absorbed into the shield during rehydration, or applied topically while the shield is in the eye. Because the shield dissolves in 12, 24, or 72 hours, depending on the manufacturing process for collagen cross-linking, the drug is released gradually into the tear film, and high concentrations are maintained on the corneal surface and in the conjunctival cul-de-sac.

The shields have been used in the early management of bacterial keratitis, as well as for antibiotic prophylaxis. They have also been used to promote epithelial healing after ocular surgery, trauma, or spontaneous erosion. Despite these therapeutic benefits, collagen shields are poorly tolerated because they are very uncomfortable.

New technology in drug delivery

Liposomes are synthetic lipid microspheres that serve as multipurpose vehicles for the topical delivery of drugs, genetic material, and cosmetics. They are produced when phospholipid molecules interact to form a bilayer lipid membrane in an aqueous environment. The interior of the bilayer consists of the hydrophobic fatty-acid tails of the phospholipid molecule, whereas the outer layer is composed of hydrophilic polar-head groups of the molecule. A water-soluble drug can be dissolved in the aqueous phase of the interior compartment, whereas a hydrophobic drug can be intercalated into the lipid bilayer itself. Biodegradable nanoparticles, such as nanospheres, nanocapsules, and micelles, are also used to transport hydrophobic drugs and genes and are modeled after the molecular structure of viruses.

The physical process of moving charged molecules by an electrical current is called *iontophoresis.* This procedure places a relatively high concentration of the drug locally, where it can achieve maximum benefit with little waste or systemic absorption. Animal studies have demonstrated that iontophoresis increases penetration of various antibiotics and antiviral drugs across ocular surfaces into the cornea and the interior of the eye. However, patient discomfort, ocular tissue damage, and necrosis restrict the popularity of this mode of drug delivery.

Pharmacodynamics: The Mechanism of Drug Action

Most drugs act by binding to and altering the function of regulatory macromolecules, usually neurotransmitter receptors, hormone receptors, or enzymes. Binding may be a reversible association mediated by electrostatic and/or van der Waals forces, or it may involve formation of a covalent intermediate. If the drug–receptor interaction stimulates the receptor's natural function, the drug is termed an *agonist.* Stimulation of an opposing effect characterizes an *antagonist*. Corresponding effectors of enzymes are termed *activators* and *inhibitors*. This terminology is crucial to understanding the next chapter.

The relationship between the initial drug–receptor interaction and the drug's clinical dose-response curve may be simple or complex. In some cases, the drug's clinical effect closely reflects the degree of receptor occupancy on a moment-to-moment basis. Such is usually the case for drugs that affect neural transmission or for drugs that are enzyme inhibitors. In contrast, some drug effects lag hours behind receptor occupancy or persist long after the drug is gone. Such is the case with many drugs acting on hormone receptors, because their effects are often mediated through a series of biochemical events.

In addition to differences in timing of receptor occupancy and drug effects, the degree of receptor occupancy can differ considerably from the corresponding drug effect. For example, because the amount of carbonic anhydrase present in the ciliary processes is 100 times that required to support aqueous secretion, more than 99% of the enzyme must be inhibited before secretion is reduced. On the other hand, some maximal hormone responses occur at concentrations well below that required for receptor saturation, indicating the presence of "inbound receptors."

Bochot A, Couvreur P, Fattal E. Intravitreal administration of antisense oligonucleotides: potential of liposomal delivery. *Prog Retin Eye Res.* 2000;19(2):131–147.

Eller MG, Schoenwald RD, Dixson JA, Segarra T, Barfknecht CF. Topical carbonic anhydrase inhibitors. III: optimization model for corneal penetration of ethoxzolamide analogues. *J Pharm Sci.* 1985;74(2):155–160.

Hsiue GH, Chang RW, Wang CH, Lee SH. Development of in situ thermosensitive drug vehicles for glaucoma therapy. *Biomaterials.* 2003;24(13):2423–2430.

Williams PB, Crouch ER Jr, Sheppard JD Jr, Lattanzio FA Jr, Parker TA, Mitrev PV. The birth of ocular pharmacology in the 20th century. *J Clin Pharmacol.* 2000;40(9):990–1006.

Zimmerman TJ, Kooner KS, Kandarakis AS, Ziegler LP. Improving the therapeutic index of topically applied ocular drugs. *Arch Ophthalmol.* 1984;102(4):551–553.

CHAPTER 17

Ocular Pharmacotherapeutics*

Legal Aspects of Medical Therapy

The US Food and Drug Administration (FDA) has statutory authority both to approve the marketing of prescription drugs and to specify the uses of these drugs. The FDA has created a 3-step process regulating human testing of new drugs before they are approved for marketing. After animal and in vitro studies, *phase 1* testing begins; this involves testing 10–80 people for toxicology and pharmacokinetic data concerning dosage range, absorption, metabolism, and toxicity. *Phase 2* testing involves randomized, controlled clinical trials on a minimum of 50–100 affected people to determine safety and effectiveness. *Phase 3* testing uses controlled and uncontrolled trials to evaluate the overall risk–benefit relationship and to provide an adequate basis for physician labeling. The data gathered from these tests are then submitted as part of a new drug application for marketing. The FDA's approval of each drug and its specific uses is based on documentation submitted by manufacturers that supports the safety and efficacy of specific drug applications.

Once approved for any use, a drug may be prescribed by individual physicians for any indication in all age groups without violating federal law. However, physicians remain liable to malpractice actions. In particular, a nonapproved use that does not adhere to an applicable standard of care places a practitioner in a difficult legal position. If a respectable minority of similarly situated physicians prescribes in the same manner, a standard of care could be met in most jurisdictions. Informed consent in equivocal cases is helpful.

Many common drugs have off-label application in ophthalmology. A limited listing of these includes, but is not limited to, the following drugs:

- bevacizumab (Avastin), an antiangiogenic drug used off-label in intravitreal injection for multiple neovascular ocular diseases
- acetylcysteine (Mucomyst 10% and 20%), used as a mucolytic in filamentary keratopathy and as an anticollagenase agent in severe alkali injuries

*This chapter may include information on pharmaceutical applications that are not considered community standard, that are approved for use only in restricted research settings, or that reflect indications not included in approved FDA labeling ("off-label"). For example, many ophthalmic uses of systemic medications are off-label, including most systemic antibiotics and antifungal agents compounded for treatment of ocular infections such as keratitis or endophthalmitis. Many antifungal agents are used with an off-label application based on in vitro and animal data, because human data for unusual infectious agents are often limited. **The FDA has stated that it is the responsibility of the physician to determine the FDA status of each drug or device he or she wishes to use and to use them with appropriate, informed patient consent in compliance with applicable law.**

- tissue plasminogen activator (Activase), used as an intravitreal injection for thrombolysis and fibrinolysis
- fluorouracil (5-FU), used to improve the outcomes of glaucoma filtration surgery
- mitomycin (Mutamycin), used to improve the outcomes of glaucoma filtration surgery
- cyclosporine A (Sandimmune), used off-label as a 2% compounded solution in high-risk corneal transplants and in severe vernal, ligneous, and autoimmune keratopathies
- doxycycline, used for ocular rosacea
- edetate disodium (EDTA), used for band keratopathy

One of the most commonly used medications, topical prednisolone, has not been approved specifically for postoperative care. When used postoperatively for cataract surgery, it is an off-label usage.

The FDA has established clear guidelines on investigational drugs, and their use must meet specified commercial and investigative requirements.

Cholinergic Agents

A number of commonly used ophthalmic medications affect the activity of acetylcholine receptors in synapses of the somatic and autonomic nervous systems (Fig 17-1). Such receptors are found in

- the motor end plates of the extraocular muscles and levator palpebrae superioris (supplied by somatic motor nerves)
- the cells of the superior cervical ganglion (sympathetic) and the ciliary and sphenopalatine (parasympathetic) ganglia (supplied by preganglionic autonomic nerves)
- parasympathetic effector sites in the iris sphincter and ciliary body and in the lacrimal, accessory lacrimal, and meibomian glands (supplied by postganglionic parasympathetic nerves)

Although all cholinergic receptors are by definition responsive to acetylcholine, they are not homogeneous in their response to other agents, which fall into 2 categories: *Muscarinic agents* are supplied by postganglionic parasympathetic nerves and are responsive to muscarine. *Nicotinic agents* are supplied by somatic motor and preganglionic autonomic nerves and are responsive to nicotine.

Cholinergic agents are further divided into the following groups (Fig 17-2):

- direct-acting agonists, which act on the receptor to elicit an excitatory postsynaptic potential
- indirect-acting agonists, which inhibit the acetylcholinesterase of the synaptic cleft, preventing deactivation of endogenous acetylcholine
- antagonists, which block the action of acetylcholine on the receptor

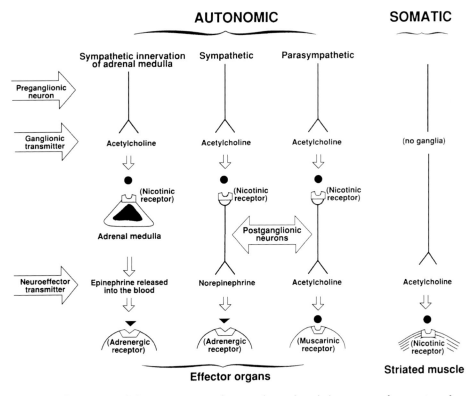

Figure 17-1 Summary of the neurotransmitters released and the types of receptors found within the autonomic and somatic nervous systems. *(Reproduced with permission from Mycek MJ, Harvey RA, Champe PC, eds.* Pharmacology. *2nd ed. Lippincott's Illustrated Reviews. Philadelphia: Lippincott-Raven; 1997:32.)*

Muscarinic Drugs

Direct-acting agonists

Topically applied direct-acting agonists have 3 actions. First, they cause contraction of the iris sphincter, which not only constricts the pupil *(miosis)* but also changes the anatomical relationship of the iris to both the lens and the chamber angle. Second, they cause contraction of the circular fibers of the ciliary muscle, relaxing the zonular tension on the lens equator and allowing the lens to shift forward and assume a more spherical shape *(accommodation)*. Third, they cause contraction of the longitudinal fibers of the ciliary muscle, producing tension on the scleral spur (opening the trabecular meshwork) and facilitating aqueous outflow. Contraction of the ciliary musculature also produces tension on the peripheral retina, occasionally resulting in a retinal tear or even rhegmatogenous detachment.

Acetylcholine does not penetrate the corneal epithelium well, and it is rapidly degraded by acetylcholinesterase (Fig 17-3). Thus, it is not used topically. Acetylcholine 1% (Miochol) and carbachol 0.01% (Miostat) are available for intracameral use in anterior

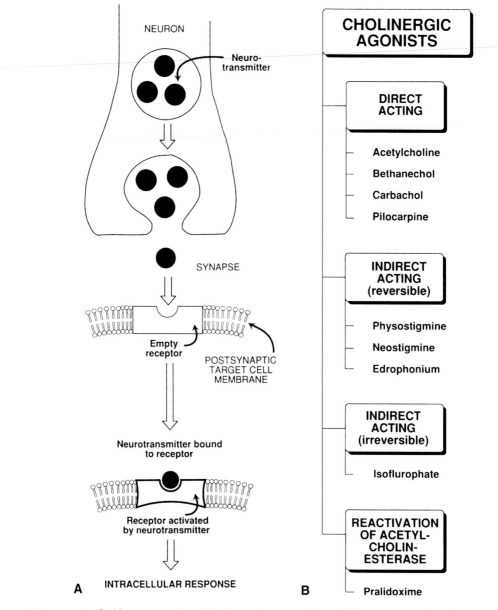

Figure 17-2 A, Neurotransmitter binding triggers an intracellular response. **B,** Summary of cholinergic agonists. *(Part A reproduced with permission from Harvey RA, Champe PC, eds. Pharmacology. Lippin-cott's Illustrated Reviews. Philadelphia: Lippincott; 1992:30. Part B reproduced with permission from Mycek MJ, Harvey RA, Champe PC, eds. Pharmacology. 2nd ed. Lippincott's Illustrated Reviews. Philadelphia: Lippincott-Raven; 1997:35.)*

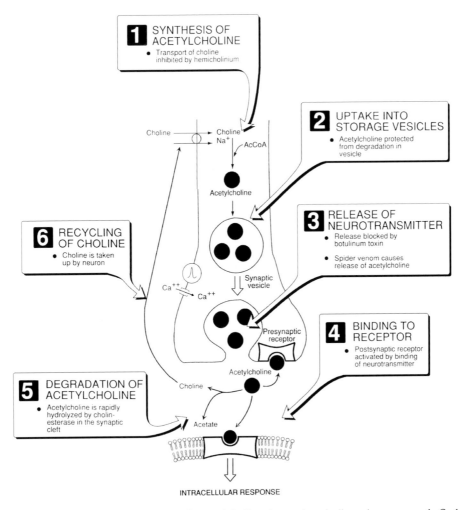

1 SYNTHESIS OF ACETYLCHOLINE
• Transport of choline inhibited by hemicholinium

Choline ⟶ Choline
Na⁺
AcCoA

Acetylcholine

2 UPTAKE INTO STORAGE VESICLES
• Acetylcholine protected from degradation in vesicle

6 RECYCLING OF CHOLINE
• Choline is taken up by neuron

3 RELEASE OF NEUROTRANSMITTER
• Release blocked by botulinum toxin
• Spider venom causes release of acetylcholine

Synaptic vesicle

Ca⁺⁺
Ca⁺⁺

Presynaptic receptor

4 BINDING TO RECEPTOR
• Postsynaptic receptor activated by binding of neurotransmitter

Acetylcholine

5 DEGRADATION OF ACETYLCHOLINE
• Acetylcholine is rapidly hydrolyzed by cholinesterase in the synaptic cleft

Choline

Acetylcholine

Acetate

INTRACELLULAR RESPONSE

Figure 17-3 Synthesis and release of acetylcholine from the cholinergic neuron. *AcCoA =* acetyl coenzyme A. *(Reproduced with permission from Mycek MJ, Harvey RA, Champe PC, eds.* Pharmacology. *2nd ed. Lippincott's Illustrated Reviews. Philadelphia: Lippincott-Raven; 1997:37.)*

segment surgery. These drugs produce prompt and marked miosis, which helps avoid iris capture by the optic of posterior chamber lenses and may prevent iris incarceration in surgical wounds.

Intracameral acetylcholine 1% has a more rapid onset than intracameral carbachol, acting within seconds after instillation, but the effect is short-lived. Acetylcholine is not stable in aqueous form and is rapidly broken down by acetylcholinesterase in the anterior chamber. Intracameral carbachol 0.01% is 100 times more effective and longer lasting than acetylcholine administered similarly. Maximal miosis is achieved within 5 minutes and lasts for 24 hours. In addition, carbachol 0.01% is an effective hypotensive agent and lowers intraocular pressure (IOP) during the critical 24-hour period after surgery.

Pilocarpine 0.12% is used diagnostically to confirm an Adie tonic pupil, a condition in which the parasympathetic innervation of the iris sphincter and ciliary muscle is defective because of the loss of postganglionic fibers. Denervated muscarinic smooth muscle fibers in the affected segments of the iris exhibit supersensitivity and respond well to this weak miotic, whereas the normal iris does not.

Pilocarpine 0.25, 0.5, 1, 2, 3, 4, 6% (qid) and carbachol 1.5, 3% (tid) are used in the treatment of primary open-angle glaucoma (POAG) because they lower IOP by increasing outflow facility (Table 17-1). Use of 4% pilocarpine is contraindicated in acute attacks of angle-closure glaucoma, as this strong miotic may induce intense anterior movement of the lens–iris diaphragm, closing the angle completely. Miotic therapy is not an adequate substitute for laser iridotomy and should not be used for chronic control or prophylaxis of pupillary-block angle-closure glaucoma. (See also BCSC Section 10, *Glaucoma*, Chapter 7.)

Miosis, cataractogenesis, and induced myopia are generally unwelcome side effects of muscarinic therapy. Although the broad range of retinal dark adaptation usually compensates sufficiently for the effect of miosis on vision during daylight hours, patients may be visually incapacitated in dim illumination. In addition, miosis often compounds the effect of axial lenticular opacities; many patients with cataract are unable to tolerate miotics. Older patients with early cataracts have visual difficulty in scotopic conditions; the miosis induced by cholinergic agents may increase the risk of falls.

Younger patients may have difficulty with miotics as well. Induced myopia and induced accommodation occur because of the drug-induced contraction of the ciliary body, which both increases the convexity of the lens and shifts the lens forward. Patients younger than 50 years may manifest disabling myopia and induced accommodation from this side effect. Miotic iris cysts and an increased incidence of retinal detachment due to ciliary body contraction and traction on the pars plana are other complications seen with higher concentrations.

Systemic side effects after ocular use of pilocarpine are rare. They include salivation, diarrhea, vomiting, bronchial spasm, and diaphoresis (Fig 17-4). A slowly dissolving gel (Pilopine HS gel) taken at bedtime minimizes the unwanted side effects of pilocarpine and is useful in younger patients, in patients bothered by variable myopia or intense miosis, in older patients with lens opacities, and in patients who have difficulty complying with more frequent dosing regimens.

Table 17-1 **Miotics**

Generic Name	Trade Name	Strengths
Cholinergic agents		
Carbachol	Isopto Carbachol	1.5, 3%
Pilocarpine HCl	Isopto Carpine	0.25, 1, 2, 4%
	Available generically	0.5, 1, 2, 3, 4, 6%
Pilocarpine HCl ointment	Pilopine HS gel	4%
Cholinesterase inhibitors		
Physostigmine	Available generically	1 mg/mL ampule
Echothiophate iodide	Phospholine Iodide	0.125%

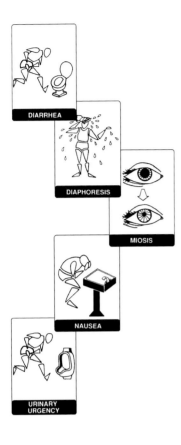

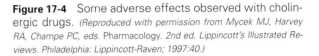

Figure 17-4 Some adverse effects observed with cholinergic drugs. *(Reproduced with permission from Mycek MJ, Harvey RA, Champe PC, eds. Pharmacology. 2nd ed. Lippincott's Illustrated Reviews. Philadelphia: Lippincott-Raven; 1997:40.)*

Ciliary muscle stimulation can be desirable in managing accommodative esotropia. The near response is a synkinesis of accommodation, miosis, and convergence. As discussed previously, muscarinic agonists contract the ciliary body and induce accommodation as a side effect. The patient does not therefore need to accommodate at near, decreasing not only the synkinetic convergence response but also the degree of accommodative esotropia.

Indirect-acting agonists

Topically applied indirect-acting muscarinic agonists (cholinesterase inhibitors) have the same actions as direct-acting muscarinic agonists, although they have a longer duration of action and are frequently more potent. Twice-daily treatment is sufficient. These agents react with the active serine hydroxyl site of cholinesterases, forming a slowly hydrolyzed intermediate. Thus, they render the enzyme unavailable for hydrolyzing spontaneously released acetylcholine. There are 2 classes of cholinesterase inhibitors:

1. *reversible inhibitors,* such as physostigmine (previously marketed as Eserine ointment; available as powder for compounding and as solution for injection) and carbamylate acetylcholinesterase
2. *irreversible inhibitors,* such as echothiophate (Phospholine Iodide) and diisopropyl phosphorofluoridate (DFP; no longer available for ophthalmic use in the United

States), which phosphorylate both the acetylcholinesterase of the synaptic cleft and the butyrylcholinesterase (pseudocholinesterase) of plasma

One carbamylating agent, demecarium bromide (previously marketed as Humorsol; no longer available for ophthalmic use in the United States), is also irreversible; it contains 2 carbamyl groups and cross-links units of the enzyme. Carbamylenzyme is regenerated by hydrolysis of the carbamyl–ester linkage over 3–4 hours. Regeneration of dialkylphosphorylated enzyme is so slow, however, that recovery of activity depends primarily on new enzyme synthesis.

The action of phosphorylating cholinesterase inhibitors can be reversed acutely by treatment with oxime-containing compounds that remove the dialkylphosphate moiety from the enzyme. This treatment must take place rapidly, before the spontaneous elimination of 1 of the alkyl residues (T½ = 20 minutes for butyrylcholinesterase, 270 minutes for acetylcholinesterase), which makes the monoalkylphosphate intermediate no longer susceptible to regeneration by oxime. Thus, the oxime pralidoxime (2-PAM)—although useful in the treatment of acute organophosphate poisoning (eg, insecticide exposure)—is of little value in reversing the marked reduction of plasma butyrylcholinesterase activity that occurs with chronic irreversible cholinesterase-inhibitor therapy.

Patients on chronic, irreversible cholinesterase-inhibitor therapy such as echothiophate may experience toxic reactions from systemic absorption of local anesthetics containing ester groups (eg, procaine) that are normally inactivated by plasma cholinesterase. Administration of the muscle relaxant succinylcholine during induction of general anesthesia is also hazardous in such patients, because the drug would not be metabolized and would result in prolonged respiratory paralysis.

Phosphorylating cholinesterase inhibitors also have local ocular toxicities. Children may develop cystlike proliferations of the iris pigment epithelium at the pupil margin that can block the pupil. For unknown reasons, cyst development can be minimized by concomitant use of phenylephrine (2.5%) drops. In adults, cataracts may develop or preexisting opacities may progress. Interestingly, children rarely if ever develop such cataracts, and adults rarely if ever develop significant epithelial cysts.

Therapy with cholinesterase inhibitors should not be combined with direct-acting cholinergic agonists, because the combination is less effective than either drug given alone.

Because cholinesterase inhibitors are potent insecticides, they were used in the past as treatment for lice infestations of the eyelashes. The adult louse may be smothered with bland ophthalmic ointment or removed mechanically. Nits, however, must be mechanically removed, because they are resistant to suffocation or any medication. Physostigmine, diisopropyl phosphorofluoridate, and demecarium bromide are no longer commercially available for ophthalmic use in the United States.

Antagonists

Topically applied muscarinic antagonists, such as atropine, react with postsynaptic muscarinic receptors and block the action of acetylcholine. Paralysis of the iris sphincter, coupled with the unopposed action of the dilator muscle, causes pupillary dilation, or mydriasis (Table 17-2). Mydriasis facilitates examination of the peripheral lens, ciliary body, and retina and is approved for use therapeutically in the treatment of iritis in adults, as it reduces contact between the posterior iris surface and the anterior lens capsule, thereby preventing the formation of iris–lens adhesions, or posterior synechiae. Atropine and cyclopentolate are FDA approved for use in pediatric patients but not for all indications.

Muscarinic antagonists also paralyze the ciliary muscles, which helps to relieve pain associated with iridocyclitis, inhibit accommodation for accurate refraction in children (cyclopentolate, atropine), and treat ciliary block (malignant) glaucoma. However, use of cycloplegic agents to dilate the pupils of patients with POAG may elevate the IOP, especially in patients requiring miotics for pressure control. It is advisable, therefore, to use short-acting agents and to consider monitoring the pressure in patients with severe optic nerve damage.

Table 17-2 Mydriatics and Cycloplegics

Generic Name	Trade Name	Strengths	Onset	Duration of Action
Phenylephrine HCl*	AK-Dilate	Soln, 2.5%, 10%	30–60 min	3–5 h
	Altafrin	Soln, 2.5%, 10%		
	Mydfrin	Soln, 2.5%		
	Neofrin	Soln, 2.5%		
	Available generically	Soln, 2.5%, 10%		
Hydroxyamphetamine hydrobromide 1%†		Available as powder for compounding		
Atropine sulfate	Atropine-Care	Soln, 1%	45–120 min	7–14 days
	Isopto Atropine	Soln, 1%		
	Available generically	Soln, 1% Ointment, 1%		
Cyclopentolate HCl*	AK-Pentolate	Soln, 1%	30–60 min	2 days
	Cyclogyl	Soln, 0.5%–2%		
	Cylate	Soln, 1%		
	Available generically	Soln, 1%, 2%		
Homatropine hydrobromide	Isopto Homatropine	Soln, 2%, 5%	30–60 min	3 days
	Homatropaire	Soln, 5%		
Scopolamine hydrobromide	Isopto Hyoscine	Soln, 0.25%	30–60 min	4–7 days
Tropicamide	Mydral	Soln, 0.5%, 1%	20–40 min	4–6 h
	Mydriacyl	Soln, 1%		
	Tropicalyl	Soln, 0.5%, 1%		
	Available generically	Soln, 0.5%, 1%		
Cyclopentolate HCl/ phenylephrine HCl	Cyclomydril	Soln, 0.2%, 1%		

* A dilute combination agent, Cyclomydril (cyclopentolate HCl 0.2%/phenylephrine HCl 1%), is available for infant exams.
† Hydroxyamphetamine hydrobromide, in combination with tropicamide, is available commercially as Paremyd 1%; however, it is used for dilating the pupil and cannot be used to test for Horner syndrome.

In situations requiring complete cycloplegia, such as the treatment of iridocyclitis (adults: scopolamine, homatropine, atropine) or the full refractive correction of accommodative esotropia, more potent agents are preferred. Although a single drop of atropine has some cycloplegic effect lasting for days, 2 or 3 instillations a day may be required to maintain full cycloplegia to relieve pain in iritis. It may become necessary to change medications if atropine elicits a characteristic local irritation with swelling and maceration of the eyelids and conjunctival hyperemia. When mydriasis alone is necessary to facilitate examination or refraction, agents with shorter residual effect are preferred, because they allow quicker return of pupil response and reading ability.

Systemic absorption of topically administered muscarinic antagonists can produce dose-related toxicity, especially in children, whose dose is distributed in a smaller body mass. Flushing, fever, tachycardia, and even delirium can result from a combination of central and peripheral effects (Fig 17-5). Mild cases may require only discontinuation of the drug, but severe cases can be treated with intravenous physostigmine (approved in adults and children), slowly titrated, until the symptoms subside. Physostigmine is used because it is a tertiary amine (uncharged), and it is able to cross the blood–brain barrier.

Systemic administration of atropine blocks the oculocardiac reflex, a reflex bradycardia sometimes elicited during ocular surgery by manipulation of the conjunctiva, the globe, or the extraocular muscles. The reflex can also be prevented at the afferent end by retrobulbar anesthesia, although it can occur during administration of the retrobulbar block.

Nicotinic Drugs

Indirect-acting agonists

The only cholinesterase inhibitor that ophthalmologists administer in a dose sufficient to allow it to work as an indirect-acting nicotinic agonist is edrophonium (Enlon; previously marketed as Tensilon). This is a short-acting competitive inhibitor of acetylcholinesterase that binds to the enzyme's active site but does not form a covalent link with it.

Edrophonium (Enlon) is used in the diagnosis of myasthenia gravis, a neuromuscular disease caused by an autoimmunity to acetylcholine receptors in the neuromuscular junction and characterized by muscle weakness and marked fatigability of skeletal muscles. This disease may manifest primarily as ptosis and diplopia. The diagnosis is confirmed by first administering a 2-mg test dose of rapidly injected intravenous edrophonium, followed 60 seconds later by an additional 8 mg if the first dose has no effect. The test dose is given to confirm the patient is not prone to side effects of the medication, including nausea, vomiting, and bradycardia. The patient is then examined for improvement in muscle function. BCSC Section 5, *Neuro-Ophthalmology,* discusses myasthenia gravis and the use of edrophonium in detail. Neostigmine methylsulfate (Prostigmin) is a longer-acting intramuscular agent that is also used in the diagnosis of myasthenia gravis. The longer duration of activity allows the examiner time to specifically assess a complex endpoint, such as orthoptic measurements.

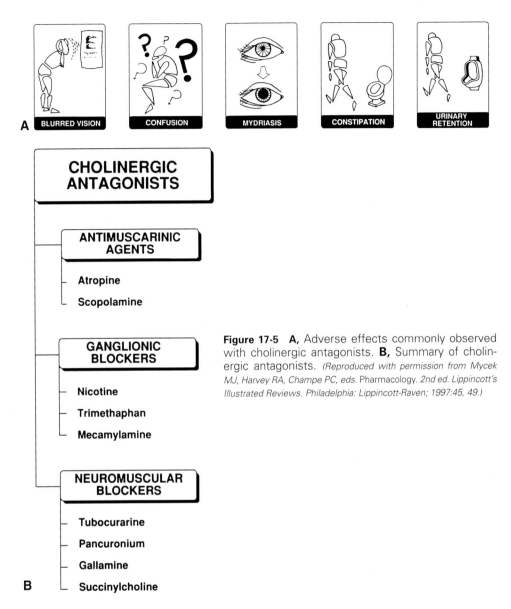

Figure 17-5 **A,** Adverse effects commonly observed with cholinergic antagonists. **B,** Summary of cholinergic antagonists. *(Reproduced with permission from Mycek MJ, Harvey RA, Champe PC, eds.* Pharmacology. *2nd ed. Lippincott's Illustrated Reviews. Philadelphia: Lippincott-Raven; 1997:45, 49.)*

In patients with myasthenia gravis, the inhibition of acetylcholinesterase by edrophonium allows acetylcholine released into the synaptic cleft to accumulate to levels adequate to act through the reduced number of acetylcholine receptors. Because edrophonium also augments muscarinic transmission, muscarinic side effects (vomiting, diarrhea, urination, and bradycardia) may occur unless atropine, 0.4–0.6 mg, is coadministered intravenously.

Antagonists

Nicotinic antagonists are administered as neuromuscular blocking agents to facilitate intubation for general anesthesia. They are of 2 types:

1. *nondepolarizing agents,* including curare-like drugs such as gallamine and pancuronium, which bind competitively to nicotinic receptors on striated muscle but do not cause contraction
2. *depolarizing agents,* such as succinylcholine and decamethonium, which bind competitively to nicotinic receptors and cause an initial receptor depolarization and muscle contraction

In singly innervated (en plaque) muscle fibers, this depolarization–contraction is followed by a prolonged unresponsiveness and flaccidity. However, these drugs produce sustained contractions of multiply innervated fibers, which make up one fifth of the muscle fibers of extraocular muscles. Such contractions of extraocular muscles (a nicotinic agonist action) exert force on the globe, an undesirable effect in cases in which the IOP is to be measured. The use of these agents in the induction of general anesthesia should be avoided in operations on lacerated eyes, because the force of the muscles on the globe could expel intraocular contents.

Adrenergic Agents

Several ophthalmic medications affect the activity of adrenergic receptors in synapses of the peripheral nervous system. Such receptors are found in the following locations:

- the cell membranes of the iris dilator muscle, the superior palpebral smooth muscle of Müller, the ciliary epithelium and processes, the trabecular meshwork, and the smooth muscle of ocular blood vessels (supplied by postganglionic autonomic fibers from the superior cervical ganglion)
- the presynaptic terminals of some sympathetic and parasympathetic nerves, where they have feedback inhibitory actions

Although adrenergic receptors were originally defined by their response to epinephrine (adrenaline), the transmitter of most sympathetic postganglionic fibers is actually norepinephrine. Adrenergic receptors are subclassified into 4 categories—α_1, α_2, β_1, and β_2—based on their profile of responses to natural and synthetic catecholamines (Fig 17-6). The α_1-receptors generally mediate smooth-muscle contraction, whereas α_2-receptors mediate feedback inhibition of presynaptic sympathetic (and sometimes parasympathetic) nerve terminals. The β_1-receptors are found predominantly in the heart, where they mediate stimulatory effects; β_2-receptors mediate relaxation of smooth muscle in most blood vessels and in the bronchi.

Systemic absorption of ocular adrenergic agents is frequently sufficient to cause systemic effects, which are manifested in the cardiovascular system, the bronchial airways, and the brain. Adrenergic agents may be direct-acting agonists, indirect-acting agonists, or antagonists at 1 or more of the 4 types of receptors.

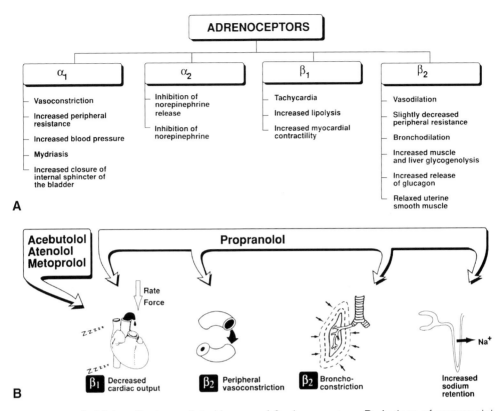

Figure 17-6 A, Major effects mediated by α- and β-adrenoceptors. **B,** Actions of propranolol and β₁ blockers. *(Reproduced with permission from Mycek MJ, Harvey RA, Champe PC, eds. Pharmacology. 2nd ed. Lippincott's Illustrated Reviews. Philadelphia: Lippincott-Raven; 1997:60, 75.)*

α-Adrenergic Agents

Direct-acting α₁-adrenergic agonists

The primary clinical use of direct-acting α₁-adrenergic agonists such as phenylephrine is stimulation of the iris dilator muscle to produce mydriasis. Because the parasympathetically innervated iris sphincter muscle is much stronger than the dilator muscle, the dilation achieved with phenylephrine alone is largely overcome by the pupillary light reflex during ophthalmoscopy. Coadministration of a cycloplegic agent allows sustained dilation.

Systemic absorption of phenylephrine may elevate systemic blood pressure. This effect is of clinical significance if the patient is an infant or has an abnormally increased sensitivity to α-agonists, which occurs with orthostatic hypotension and in association with the use of drugs that accentuate adrenergic effects (eg, reserpine, tricyclic antidepressants, cocaine, monoamine oxidase [MAO] inhibitors—discussed later). Even with lower doses of phenylephrine (2.5%), infants may exhibit a transient rise in blood pressure, because the dose received in an eyedrop is large for them on a per-weight basis. Phenylephrine 10% should be used cautiously, particularly in pledget application and in patients with vasculopathic risk factors. A 10% solution contains 5 mg of drug per drop, and ocular medications passing through the canalicular system are available for systemic absorption through the vascular nasal mucosa (see Chapter 16). In contrast, the typical systemic dose of phenylephrine for hypotension is 50–100 μg given at a time. The ophthalmic use of 10% phenylephrine has been associated with stroke, myocardial infarction, and cardiac arrest. Vascular baroreceptors are particularly sensitive to phenylephrine. An increase in blood pressure after topical application may therefore cause a significant drop in pulse rate that can be particularly dangerous in a vasculopathic individual already on a β-blocking systemic medication.

Indirect-acting adrenergic agonists

Indirect-acting adrenergic agonists are used to test for and localize defects in sympathetic innervation to the iris dilator muscle. Normally, pupil response fibers originating in the hypothalamus pass down the spinal cord to synapse with cells in the intermediolateral columns. In turn, preganglionic fibers exit the cord through the anterior spinal roots in the upper thorax to synapse in the superior cervical ganglion in the neck. Finally, postganglionic adrenergic fibers terminate in a neuroeffector junction with the iris dilator muscle. The norepinephrine released is inactivated primarily by reuptake into secretory granules in the nerve terminal (Fig 17-7). Approximately 70% of released norepinephrine is recaptured.

The testing to confirm and localize a sympathetic lesion is twofold. To confirm a lesion, 4% cocaine is given and the pupil size is measured at 1 hour. Cocaine blocks reuptake of norepinephrine into the presynaptic vesicles in an intact neuron, causing synaptic accumulation and pupillary dilation. The injured side will have less accumulation and show less dilation. Through the use of hydroxyamphetamine, currently available only through compounding pharmacies, the site of the lesion can then be determined to be either preganglionic or postganglionic. Hydroxyamphetamine releases stored norepinephrine from an intact neuron, resulting in pupillary dilation. (See also BCSC Section 5, *Neuro-Ophthalmology*).

Apraclonidine hydrochloride (para-aminoclonidine; Iopidine) is an α_2-adrenergic agonist and a clonidine derivative that prevents release of norepinephrine at nerve terminals (Table 17-3). It decreases aqueous production as well as episcleral venous pressure and improves trabecular outflow. However, its true ocular hypotensive mechanism is not fully understood. When administered pre- and postoperatively, the drug is effective in diminishing the acute IOP rise that follows argon laser iridectomy, argon laser trabeculoplasty, Nd:YAG laser capsulotomy, and cataract extraction. Apraclonidine hydrochloride may be effective for the short-term lowering of IOP, but the development of topical sensitivity and tachyphylaxis often limits long-term use.

Brimonidine tartrate causes less tachyphylaxis than apraclonidine in long-term use; the rate of allergic reactions, such as follicular conjunctivitis and contact blepharodermatitis, is also lower (less than 15% for brimonidine but up to 40% for apraclonidine). Cross-sensitivity to brimonidine in patients with known hypersensitivity to apraclonidine is minimal. Brimonidine's mechanism of lowering IOP is thought to involve both decreased aqueous production and increased uveoscleral outflow. Similar to the case with β-blockers, a central mechanism may account for part of the IOP reduction from brimonidine 0.2%: a 1-week trial of treatment for a single eye caused a statistically significant

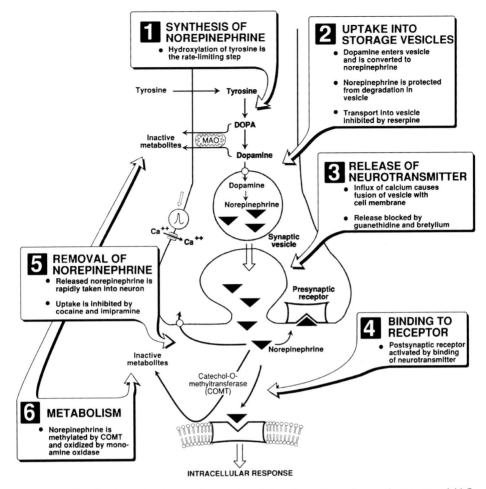

Figure 17-7 Synthesis and release of norepinephrine from the adrenergic neuron. *MAO =* monoamine oxidase inhibitor. *(Reproduced with permission from Mycek MJ, Harvey RA, Champe PC, eds. Pharmacology. 2nd ed. Lippincott's Illustrated Reviews. Philadelphia: Lippincott-Raven; 1997:57.)*

Table 17-3 Adrenergic Agonists

Generic Name	Trade Name	Strengths
β_2-Adrenergic agonists		
Dipivefrin HCl	Propine	0.1%
	Available generically	0.1%
Epinephrine HCl	Not available in US	0.5%, 1%, 2%
α_2-Selective agonists		
Apraclonidine HCl	Iopidine	0.5%, 1% (single-use container)
Brimonidine tartrate	Alphagan P	0.1%, 0.15%
	Available generically	0.2%
Brimonidine tartrate and timolol maleate	Combigan	0.2%, 0.5%

reduction of 1.2 mm Hg in the fellow eye. Brimonidine is now available in a generic 0.2% solution and in a 0.1% and 0.15% solution with the new preservative Purite as Alphagan P. Studies have shown brimonidine tartrate 0.15% (Alphagan P) to be comparable to Alphagan 0.2% (now discontinued) when given 3 times daily.

Brimonidine's peak IOP reduction is approximately 26% (2 hours postdose). At peak, it is comparable to a nonselective β-blocker and superior to the selective β-blocker betaxolol, although at trough (12 hours postdose), the reduction is only 14%–15%, which makes brimonidine at trough less effective than the nonselective β-blockers but comparable to betaxolol. Brimonidine may also have potential neuroprotective properties, as shown in animal models of optic nerve and retinal injury that are independent of IOP reduction. The proposed mechanism of neuroprotection is up-regulation of a neurotrophin, basic fibroblast growth factor, and cellular regulatory genes.

Caution is recommended when using apraclonidine or brimonidine in patients on an MAO inhibitor or tricyclic antidepressant therapy and in patients with severe cardiovascular disease. Use of these drugs concomitantly with β-blockers, antihypertensives, and cardiac glycosides (ophthalmic and systemic) also requires prudence. Although effective in acutely lowering the IOP in angle-closure glaucoma, these drugs may also induce vasoconstriction that can prolong iris-sphincter ischemia and reduce the efficacy of concurrent miotics. Apraclonidine has much greater affinity for α_1-receptors than does brimonidine and is therefore more likely to produce vasoconstriction in the eye. Brimonidine has been shown to not induce vasoconstriction in the posterior segment or optic nerve.

Ligand binding to α_2-receptors in other systems has been shown to mediate inhibition of the enzyme adenylate cyclase. Adenylate cyclase is present in the ciliary epithelium and is thought to have a role in aqueous production.

Antagonists

Thymoxamine hydrochloride (moxisylyte), an α_1-adrenergic blocking agent, acts by competitive inhibition of norepinephrine at the receptor site. Thymoxamine inhibits α-adrenergic receptors of the dilator muscle of the iris and results in pupil constriction but does not have any significant effect on ciliary muscle contraction and therefore does not induce a significant change in anterior chamber depth, facility of outflow, IOP, or accommodation. It is useful for differentiating angle-closure glaucoma from POAG with closed angles and to reverse the pupil dilation caused by phenylephrine. Thymoxamine is not available commercially in the United States even though it has been widely used in Europe for years.

Dapiprazole hydrochloride (previously marketed as Rev-Eyes 0.5%; no longer available in the United States) is an α-adrenergic blocking agent that reverses, in 30 minutes, the mydriasis produced by phenylephrine and tropicamide but not cycloplegics. It affects the dilator muscle but not ciliary muscle contraction (anterior chamber depth, facility of outflow, or accommodation).

β-Adrenergic Agents

β₂-Adrenergic agonists

β_2-Adrenergic agonists lower IOP by increasing uveoscleral outflow and perhaps also by increasing outflow through the trabecular meshwork. The beneficial effect on outflow more than compensates for a small increase in aqueous inflow as detected by fluorophotometry.

β_2-Receptors linked to adenylate cyclase are present in the ciliary epithelium and processes as well as in the trabecular meshwork. Treatment with L-epinephrine, an α- and β-agonist, increases intracellular levels of cyclic adenosine monophosphate (cAMP) in these tissues and in the aqueous humor. In other tissues, β-receptor–mediated generation of cAMP in turn activates cAMP-dependent enzymes, which results in responses such as glycogenolysis and gluconeogenesis in the liver and lipolysis in adipose tissue. However, the biochemical mechanisms responsible for lowering IOP remain to be determined.

L-Epinephrine is no longer commercially available in the United States (see Table 17-3). Local allergic and irritative manifestations as well as systemic adverse effects (headache, palpitations, and cardiac arrhythmias) are common causes of intolerance of long-term epinephrine therapy. Oxidation products of epinephrine may produce black deposits in the conjunctiva. Although such deposits are harmless, they have been mistaken for foreign bodies or even melanomas. Epinephrine therapy has also been associated with a reversible cystoid maculopathy that occurs in approximately 25% of chronically treated aphakic eyes that lack a posterior lens capsule. Although epinephrine maculopathy does not occur in phakic eyes, it has not yet been established whether an intact posterior lens capsule, hyaloid membrane, and/or the presence of an intraocular lens retards the development of the condition.

The prodrug dipivefrin HCl (Propine) 0.1% is therapeutically equivalent to epinephrine compounds of 1%–2%, because the presence of 2 pivalyl residues (see Chapter 16 for more information on prodrugs) increases its lipid solubility and corneal penetration by a factor of 17. The drug has little adrenergic activity until the pivalyl groups are cleaved by corneal esterases. The reductions in both intrinsic activity and concentration employed virtually eliminate the systemic side effects of epinephrine. Extraocular irritation is also reduced because of either the lower concentration or the reduction in auto-oxidation of the phenolic hydroxyls. However, because epinephrine is liberated from the prodrug inside the eye, the risk of epinephrine maculopathy should be unchanged.

Chronic therapy with epinephrine has been shown in an animal model to result in a down-regulation of the number of β-receptors. This phenomenon may underlie the loss of some of its therapeutic effectiveness over time (tachyphylaxis).

β-Adrenergic antagonists

β-Adrenergic antagonists, also known as β-blockers, lower IOP by reducing aqueous humor production as much as 50% (Table 17-4). Six agents are approved for use in the treatment of glaucoma: betaxolol, carteolol, levobunolol, metipranolol, timolol maleate, and timolol hemihydrate. Although it is likely that the site of action resides in the ciliary body, it is not known which is primarily affected: the vasculature of the ciliary processes or the pumping mechanism of the ciliary epithelium. One possible mechanism may be an effect on the β-adrenergic receptor–coupled adenylate cyclase of the ciliary epithelium. Although systemic administration of β-blockers has been reported to elevate blood lipid, such elevation has not been demonstrated with topical β-blockers such as timolol. All β-blockers can inhibit the increase in pulse and blood pressure that is exhibited in response to exertion. For this reason, they may be poorly tolerated in elderly patients

Table 17-4 β-Adrenergic Antagonists

Generic Name	Trade Name	Strengths
Betaxolol HCl	Betoptic S	0.25%
	Available generically	0.5%
Carteolol HCl	Ocupress	1%
	Available generically	1%
Levobunolol HCl	Betagan	0.25%, 0.5%
	Available generically	0.25%, 0.5%
Metipranolol HCl	OptiPranolol	0.3%
	Available generically	0.3%
Timolol maleate	Istalol	0.5%
	Timoptic Ocumeter	0.25%, 0.5%
	Timoptic Ocumeter Plus	0.25%, 0.5%
	Available generically	0.25%, 0.5%
	Timoptic-XE Ocumeter (gel)	0.25%, 0.5%
	Timoptic-XE Ocumeter Plus (gel)	0.5%
	Available generically (gel)	0.25%, 0.5%
Timolol hemihydrate	Betimol	0.25%, 0.5%
Timolol maleate (preservative free)	Timoptic in OcuDose	0.25%, 0.5%
Timolol maleate and dorzolamide HCl	Cosopt Ocumeter Plus	Timolol 0.5%; Dorzolamide 2%
Timolol maleate and brimonidine tartrate	Combigan	Timolol maleate 0.5%; brimonidine tartrate 0.2%

during routine activities, as well as in young, physically active individuals. Nonselective β-blockers inhibit the pulmonary β_2-receptors that dilate the respiratory tree. The induced bronchospasm may be significant in patients with asthma and chronic obstructive lung disease. In patients with heart failure, bradycardia, and second-degree or third-degree atrioventricular block, the underlying cardiac condition may be exacerbated with use of these agents.

Timolol maleate 0.25% or 0.5% (Timoptic) and levobunolol (Betagan) 0.25% or 0.5% are mixed β_1/β_2-antagonists. Tests of more specific β-blockers suggest that β_2-antagonists have a greater effect on aqueous secretion than β_1-antagonists. For example, comparative studies have shown that the specific β_1-antagonist betaxolol 0.5% is approximately 85% as effective in lowering IOP as timolol.

Metipranolol hydrochloride (OptiPranolol) is a nonselective β_1- and β_2-adrenergic receptor–blocking agent. As a 0.3% topical solution, it is similar in effect to other topical nonselective beta-blockers and is efficacious in reducing IOP.

Carteolol hydrochloride (Ocupress) demonstrates intrinsic sympathomimetic activity, which means that, while acting as a competitive antagonist, it also causes a slight to moderate activation of receptors. Thus, even though carteolol produces β-blocking effects, these may be tempered, reducing the effect on cardiovascular and respiratory systems. Carteolol may also be less likely to adversely affect the systemic lipid profile compared with other β-blockers.

Betaxolol is a selective β_1-antagonist that is significantly safer than the nonselective β-blockers when pulmonary, cardiac, central nervous system, or other systemic conditions are considered. Betaxolol may be useful in patients with a history of bronchospastic disorders, although other therapies should be tried in lieu of betaxolol (β selectivity is only relative and not absolute, and some β_2 effect can therefore remain). In general, the IOP-lowering effect of betaxolol is less than that of the nonselective β-adrenergic antagonists. Betaxolol is available as a generic 0.5% solution, as well as a 0.25% solution (Betoptic S). Betoptic S causes less irritation on instillation yet maintains its clinical efficacy when compared with Betoptic 0.5% (now discontinued), a finding that is generally extrapolated to the generic 0.5% solution currently available.

Prodrugs of nonselective β-blockers are being developed, and they may offer the benefit of the higher potency of β_1/β_2-blocking agents while reducing their potential systemic side effects.

It is curious that both β-agonist and β-antagonist drugs can lower IOP. This paradox is compounded by the observation that β-agonist and β-antagonist drugs have slightly additive effects in lowering IOP.

Carbonic Anhydrase Inhibitors

Aqueous humor is secreted into the posterior chamber by the nonpigmented epithelium of the ciliary processes. Although the physiologic mechanisms of secretion are not fully understood, secretion is known to depend largely on active transport of sodium by Na^+,K^+-ATPase on the surface of nonpigmented epithelial cells. Inhibition of that enzyme by ouabain injected into the vitreous cavity of experimental animals reduces secretion markedly. Unfortunately, ouabain and other cardiac glycosides cannot be used clinically to treat glaucoma because effective doses for the eye would require systemic doses toxic to the heart.

However, Na^+ transport and coupled aqueous secretion can be inhibited indirectly. Na^+ transport and fluid flow seem to be partially linked to HCO_3^- formation in the ciliary epithelium, and HCO_3^- formation can be substantially reduced by inhibition of the enzyme carbonic anhydrase (Table 17-5). The linkage between HCO_3^- and Na^+ transport is demonstrated by the fact that the effect on aqueous flow is no greater when ouabain and a *carbonic anhydrase inhibitor (CAI)* are given together than when each drug is given alone.

Carbonic anhydrase catalyzes the hydration of dissolved CO_2 to H_2CO_3, which ionizes into HCO_3^- and H^+. The HCO_3^- is then available to accompany secreted Na^+. When the enzyme is inhibited, the transport of radiolabeled HCO_3^- into the posterior chamber is reduced by up to 60%. That portion (60%) of Na^+ transport accompanied by Cl^- is unaffected by inhibition of carbonic anhydrase and, curiously, is unaffected by coadministration of ouabain. The mechanism(s) of the residual secretion and the means of inhibiting it are yet to be determined. CAIs such as acetazolamide and methazolamide are approved for the treatment of glaucoma in adults, and some preparations of acetazolamide are approved for this use in children. These CAIs may also be effective in treating cystoid macular edema (CME) and pseudotumor cerebri.

Table 17-5 **Carbonic Anhydrase Inhibitors**

Generic Name	Trade Name	Strengths	Onset	Duration of Action
Systemic				
Acetazolamide	Diamox Sequels	500 mg (time-release)	1–1.5 h; 2 h	8–12 h; 18–24 h
	Available generically	125, 250 mg	1–1.5 h	8–12 h
Acetazolamide sodium	Available generically	500 mg, 5–10 mg/kg^3	2 min	4–5 h
Methazolamide	Available generically	25, 50 mg	2–4 h	10–18 h
Topical				
Dorzolamide HCl	Trusopt Ocumeter Plus	2% solution	5 min	8 h
Brinzolamide	Azopt	1% suspension	2 h	8–12 h
Combination Agent				
Dorzolamide HCl and timolol maleate	Cosopt Ocumeter Plus	Dorzolamide HCl 2% and timolol 0.5%	2 h	1 h

The concentration of carbonic anhydrase in the ciliary epithelium of rabbits is one tenth the concentration of that found in the kidney and the choroid plexus of the brain. Carbonic anhydrase is present in considerable excess of what is needed to supply the amount of HCO_3^- transported. Calculations based on the K_{cat} (catalysis constant) and K_m (apparent affinity constant) of the enzyme and the concentrations of substrates and product indicate that 100 times as much enzyme is present as is needed in the ciliary body. Correspondingly, in clinical use, the enzyme must be more than 99% inhibited to significantly reduce aqueous flow. The enzyme in the kidney, present in 1000-fold excess, must be more than 99.9% inhibited to affect the usual pathway for HCO_3^- reabsorption. With the inhibitor methazolamide, the difference in concentration of carbonic anhydrase in the ciliary body and the kidney can be exploited to lower IOP without incurring renal HCO_3^- loss, and an unpleasant metabolic acidosis can be avoided. Even though renal stone formation has been reported with use of methazolamide, it is significantly less than with other agents because of this specific property. In contrast, acetazolamide is actively secreted into the renal tubules, and renal effects are unavoidable.

The topical forms of CAIs—dorzolamide (Trusopt Ocumeter Plus) and brinzolamide (Azopt)—are agents that are also available for chronic treatment of glaucoma. They penetrate the cornea easily, and they are water-soluble and specially formulated for topical ophthalmic use. When administered as solution 3 times a day, they effectively inhibit carbonic anhydrase II and avoid the systemic side effects of oral administration. Both agents are equally effective and reduce IOP by 14%–17%. The concomitant administration of dorzolamide and oral CAIs is not recommended because of potentially additive side effects. Adverse effects of topical CAIs include burning on instillation, punctate keratitis, local allergy, and bitter taste. Dorzolamide hydrochloride and timolol maleate are available as a combination agent, Cosopt, which provides superior antihypertensive action compared with either drug administered alone, but it has slightly less efficacy than both drugs administered concomitantly in clinical trials. However, the use of a single combined medication may improve patient compliance and therefore lead to an equivalent efficacy in clinical practice.

The systemic CAIs are administered orally and/or parenterally. The longer half-life of methazolamide allows it to be used twice daily; acetazolamide is also available in a sustained-release, 500-mg form (Diamox Sequels) used twice a day. None of the compounds has the ideal combination of high potency (low K_i), good ocular penetration (high percentage in the nonionized form and high lipid solubility to facilitate passage through the blood–ocular barrier), high proportion of the drug present in the blood in the unbound form, and long plasma half-life. In addition to lowering IOP by inhibiting ciliary body carbonic anhydrase, each of the agents at high doses further lowers IOP by causing renal metabolic acidosis. The mechanism by which acidosis lowers secretion is uncertain, but it plausibly involves reduction in HCO_3^- formation.

At the onset of acidosis, the renal effects cause alkaline diuresis, with loss of Na^+, K^+, and HCO_3^-. In patients receiving CAI therapy concurrently with diuretics, steroids, or adrenocorticotropic hormone (ACTH), severe hypokalemia can result. This situation may be dangerous for patients using digitalis, in whom hypokalemia may elicit arrhythmias. Such patients on chronic CAI therapy should have potassium levels checked at regular intervals, preferably by their primary care physician.

The acidosis prompts a renal mechanism for HCO_3^- reabsorption unrelated to carbonic anhydrase; this mechanism limits the degree of acidosis and halts both the diuresis and K^+ loss after the first few days of treatment. However, dichlorphenamide (Daranide) also acts as a chloruretic agent and may cause continued K^+ loss; dichlorphenamide is no longer available in the United States.

CAI therapy may interact unfavorably with certain systemic conditions. The alkalinization of the urine present during initial CAI treatment prevents excretion of NH_4^+, a factor to consider in patients with cirrhosis of the liver. Metabolic acidosis may exacerbate diabetic ketoacidosis. In patients with severe chronic obstructive pulmonary disease, respiratory acidosis may be caused by impairment of CO_2 transfer from the pulmonary vasculature to the alveoli. Elderly patients have a physiologically reduced renal function, which predisposes them to severe metabolic acidosis with the use of systemic CAIs.

The use of acetazolamide has been linked to the formation of stones in the urinary tract. In a retrospective case-control series, the incidence of stones was 11 times higher in patients using this drug. The increased risk occurred primarily during the first year of therapy. Continued use after occurrence of a stone was associated with a high risk of recurrent stone formation. However, a history of spontaneous stone formation more than 5 years prior to acetazolamide therapy did not appear to be associated with a special risk. The mechanisms responsible for such stone formation may be related to metabolic acidosis and associated pH changes, as well as to decreased excretion of citrate.

Nearly 50% of patients are intolerant of systemic CAIs because of distressing central nervous system and gastrointestinal side effects, which include numbness and tingling of the hands, feet, and lips; malaise; metallic taste when drinking carbonated beverages; anorexia and weight loss; nausea; somnolence; impotence and loss of libido; and depression. Whenever the clinical situation allows, it is wise to begin therapy at low doses (eg, 125 mg acetazolamide qid or 25–50 mg methazolamide bid), because side effects will be less severe and weaning may actually reduce their incidence. Patients should be informed of the potential side effects of these agents; otherwise, many patients may fail to associate their systemic symptoms with the use of a medication prescribed by the ophthalmologist.

Rare adverse effects from this class of drugs, including the topical agents, comprise those common to other members of the sulfonamide family, such as transient myopia, hypersensitive nephropathy, skin rash, and thrombocytopenia. One potential side effect, aplastic anemia, is idiosyncratic. White blood cell counts do not detect susceptible patients. CAIs have been associated with teratogenic effects (forelimb deformity) in rodents, and their use is not advised during pregnancy.

Prostaglandin Analogues

Prostaglandin (PG) analogues are the newest class of ocular hypotensive agents (Table 17-6). Currently, 4 PG analogues have been approved for clinical use. Latanoprost (Xalatan), bimatoprost (Lumigan), and travoprost (Travatan, Travatan Z) are used once daily, with nighttime dosing; unoprostone (Rescula), used twice daily, has been discontinued in the United States.

Latanoprost is a prodrug of prostaglandin $F_{2\alpha}$ ($PGF_{2\alpha}$); it penetrates the cornea and becomes biologically active after being hydrolyzed by corneal tissue esterase. It appears to lower IOP by enhancing uveoscleral outflow and may reduce the pressure by 6–9 mm Hg (25%–35%). One potential advantage of this agent is once-daily dosing. Other advantages include the lack of cardiopulmonary side effects and the additivity to other antiglaucoma medications.

An ocular side effect unusual to this class of drugs is the darkening of the iris and periocular skin as a result of increased numbers of melanosomes (increased melanin content, or melanogenesis) within the melanocytes. The risk of iris pigmentation correlates with baseline iris pigmentation. Light-colored irides may experience increased pigmentation in 10%–20% of eyes in the initial 18–24 months of therapy, whereas nearly 60% of eyes that are light brown or 2-toned may experience increased pigmentation over the same time period. The long-term sequelae of this side effect are unknown. Other side effects reported in association with the use of a topical PG analogue include conjunctival hyperemia, hypertrichosis of the eyelashes, CME, and uveitis. The 2 latter side effects are more common in eyes with preexisting risk factors for either macular edema or uveitis. Reported systemic reactions include flulike symptoms, skin rash, and possible uterine

Table 17-6 **Prostaglandin Analogues**

Generic Name	Trade Name	Strengths
Bimatoprost	Lumigan	0.03%
Latanoprost	Xalatan	0.005%
Travoprost	Travatan	0.004%
	Travatan Z	0.004%
Unoprostone isopropyl	Rescula	Discontinued in US

bleeding in postmenopausal women. Reactivation of herpetic keratitis has been reported with use of latanoprost.

Combined Medications

Medications that are combined and placed in a single bottle have the potential benefits of improved efficacy, convenience, and compliance, as well as reduced cost. FDA guidelines require the fixed combination to be more efficacious than either agent given alone. The advantage of combined therapy is the convenience and lessened confusion of 1 bottle rather than 2, which may increase the potential for greater compliance and thus improved efficacy in clinical practice. The ocular side effects are the same, whether the drugs are administered in the combined form or individually. It is important to prove that each component has an effect on IOP before using the combined medication. Cosopt, the combination of a β-blocker (timolol maleate 0.5%) and topical CAI (dorzolamide 2%), is more efficacious than either agent administered alone, although it has slightly less efficacy than both agents given concomitantly. If Cosopt is used as monotherapy, a monocular trial of timolol should be tried first. If timolol is effective in significantly lowering the IOP, dorzolamide should be used with timolol in a monocular trial. An alternative trial could involve Cosopt in 1 eye twice daily and timolol in the opposite eye. A formulation of brimonidine 0.2% and timolol 0.5% (Combigan) is approved for the reduction of elevated IOP in patients with glaucoma or ocular hypertension who require adjunctive or replacement therapy due to inadequately controlled IOP. Each agent should be similarly proven effective in a given patient before the combined agent is prescribed.

Osmotic Agents

Actions and Uses

Increased serum osmolarity reduces IOP and vitreous volume by drawing fluid out of the eye across vascular barriers. The osmotic activity of an agent depends on the number of particles in solution and the maintenance of an osmotic gradient between the plasma and the intraocular fluids. It is independent of the molecular weight. Low-molecular-weight agents such as urea that penetrate the blood–ocular barriers produce a small rebound in IOP after an initial lowering because of a reversal of the osmotic gradient when the kidneys clear the blood of excess urea. Osmotic agents are approved for the short-term management of acute glaucoma in adults and may be used in the reduction of vitreous volume prior to cataract surgery.

Agents

Osmotic agents should be used with care in patients in whom cardiovascular overload might occur with moderate vascular volume expansion, such as patients with a history of congestive heart failure, angina, systemic hypertension, or recent myocardial infarct. The osmotic agents glycerin, mannitol, and urea are currently available for ophthalmic use in the United States (Table 17-7).

Table 17-7 Hyperosmotic Agents

Generic Name	Trade Name	Strengths	Dose	Route	Onset	Duration of Action
Glycerin	Available generically		1–1.5 g/kg	Oral	10–30 min	5 h
Mannitol	Osmitrol	5%–20%	0.5–2 g/kg	IV	30–60 min	4–8 h
	Available generically	5%–25%				
Urea	Available generically	Powder	0.5–2 g/kg	IV	30–45 min	5–6 h

Intravenous agents

Mannitol (Osmitrol) must be given intravenously because it is not absorbed from the gastrointestinal tract. Urea is unpalatable and thus is used intravenously. Use of urea is out of favor because of rebound (see the previous section Actions and Uses) and because of its tendency to cause tissue necrosis if it extravasates during administration. Intravenous (IV) administration produces a rapid onset of action, which is usually desirable, but both mannitol and urea have been associated with subarachnoid hemorrhage attributed to rapid volume overload of the blood vessels and/or rapid shrinkage of the brain with traction of the subarachnoid vessels. This shrinkage is of particular concern in the elderly, who already have brain shrinkage from microischemic disease and are therefore at increased risk of bleeding.

These agents are cleared by the kidneys and produce a marked osmotic diuresis that may be troublesome in the operating room. The conscious patient should void shortly before surgery, and a urinal should be available. If general anesthesia is employed, an indwelling urethral catheter may be required to prevent bladder distension.

Oral agents

Glycerin 50%, discontinued in 2004, can be compounded by diluting the 100% solution. This frequently used oral osmotic agent is given over cracked ice to minimize the nauseating sweet taste. The nonmetabolized sugar isosorbide (Ismotic) was preferred in diabetic patients but has been discontinued in the United States.

Cunliffe I. New drugs in glaucoma therapy. *Hosp Med (London).* 2003;64(3):156–160.

Ingram CJ, Brubaker RF. Effect of brinzolamide and dorzolamide on aqueous humor flow in human eyes. *Am J Ophthalmol.* 1999;128(3):292–296.

Lichter PR. Glaucoma clinical trials and what they mean for our patients. *Am J Ophthalmol.* 2003;136(1):136–145.

Moroi SE, Gottfredsdottir MS, Schteingart MT, et al. Cystoid macular edema associated with latanoprost therapy in a case series of patients with glaucoma and ocular hypertension. *Ophthalmology.* 1999;106(5):1024–1029.

Netland PA, Allen RC. *Glaucoma Medical Therapy: Principles and Management.* Ophthalmology Monograph 13. San Francisco: American Academy of Ophthalmology; 1999.

Anti-Inflammatory Agents

Ocular inflammation can be treated with drugs administered topically, by local injection, by ocular implantation, or systemically. These drugs may be classified as glucocorticoids, nonsteroidal anti-inflammatory agents, mast-cell stabilizers, antihistamines, or antifibrotics.

Glucocorticoids

Corticosteroids, or *steroids,* are applied topically to prevent or suppress ocular inflammation in trauma and uveitis, as well as after most ocular surgical procedures (Table 17-8). Subconjunctival and retrobulbar injections of steroids are used to treat more severe cases of ocular inflammation. Systemic steroid therapy is used to treat systemic immune diseases such as giant cell arteritis, vision-threatening capillary hemangiomas in childhood, and severe ocular inflammations that are resistant to topical therapy. Intravenous methylprednisolone is an option in the treatment of demyelinating optic neuritis; BCSC Section 5, *Neuro-Ophthalmology,* discusses this issue in depth.

Glucocorticoids induce cell-specific effects on lymphocytes, macrophages, polymorphonuclear leukocytes, vascular endothelial cells, fibroblasts, and other cells. In each of these types of cells, glucocorticoids must

- penetrate the cell membrane
- bind to soluble receptors in the cytosol

Table 17-8 Topical Anti-Inflammatory Agents

Generic Name	Trade Name	Strengths
Corticosteroids		
Dexamethasone	Maxidex	Ophthalmic susp, 0.1%
Dexamethasone sodium phosphate	Available generically	Ophthalmic soln, 0.1%
Fluorometholone	FML S.O.P.	Ophthalmic ointment, 0.1%
	FML Liquifilm	Ophthalmic susp, 0.1%
	FML Forte Liquifilm	Ophthalmic susp, 0.25%
	Available generically	Ophthalmic susp, 0.1%
Fluorometholone acetate	Flarex	Ophthalmic susp, 0.1%
Loteprednol etabonate	Alrex	Ophthalmic susp, 0.2%
	Lotemax	Ophthalmic susp, 0.5%
Prednisolone acetate	Econopred Plus	Ophthalmic susp, 1%
	Pred Forte	Ophthalmic susp, 1%
	Available generically	Ophthalmic susp, 1%
	Pred Mild	Ophthalmic susp, 0.12%
Prednisolone sodium phosphate	Inflamase Forte	Ophthalmic soln, 1%
	Prednisol	Ophthalmic soln, 1%
	Available generically	Ophthalmic soln, 1%, 0.125%
Rimexolone	Vexol	Ophthalmic susp, 1%
Nonsteroidal Anti-Inflammatory Drugs		
Diclofenac sodium	Voltaren	Ophthalmic soln, 0.1%
Flurbiprofen sodium	Ocufen	Ophthalmic soln*, 0.03%
	Available generically	Ophthalmic soln, 0.03%
Ketorolac tromethamine	Acular	Ophthalmic soln, 0.5%
	Acular PF	Ophthalmic soln, 0.5%
	Acular LS	Ophthalmic soln, 0.4%
Nepafenac	Nevanac	Ophthalmic susp, 0.1%
Bromfenac sodium	Xibrom	Ophthalmic soln, 0.09%

* Indicated for intraoperative miosis only.

- allow the translocation of the glucocorticoid receptor complex to nuclear binding sites for gene transcription
- induce or suppress the transcription of specific mRNAs

The proteins produced in the eye under the control of these mRNAs are not known, and only resultant effects have been described.

At the tissue level, glucocorticoids prevent or suppress the local hyperthermia, vascular congestion, edema, and pain of initial inflammatory responses, whether the cause is traumatic (radiant, mechanical, or chemical), infectious, or immunologic. They also suppress the late inflammatory responses of capillary proliferation, fibroblast proliferation, collagen deposition, and scarring.

At the biochemical level, the most important effect of anti-inflammatories may be the inhibition of arachidonic acid release from phospholipids (see Part IV, Biochemistry). Liberated arachidonic acid is otherwise converted into PGs, PG endoperoxides, leukotrienes, and thromboxanes, which are potent mediators of inflammation. Glucocorticoids also suppress the liberation of lytic enzymes from lysozymes.

The effects of glucocorticoids on immune-mediated inflammation are complicated. Glucocorticoids do not affect the titers of either IgE, which mediates allergic mechanisms, or IgG, which mediates autoimmune mechanisms. Nor do glucocorticoids appear to interfere with the normal processes in the afferent limb of cell-mediated immunity, as in graft rejection. They interfere instead with the efferent limb of the immune response. For example, glucocorticoids prevent macrophages from being attracted to sites of inflammation by interfering with the macrophages' response to lymphocyte-released migration-inhibiting factor. Systemically administered glucocorticoids cause sequestration of lymphocytes, especially the T lymphocytes that mediate cellular immunity. However, the posttranscriptional molecular mechanisms of these responses are as yet unknown. BCSC Section 9, *Intraocular Inflammation and Uveitis,* discusses immune responses in detail.

Adverse effects

Glucocorticoids may cause a number of adverse effects in the eye and elsewhere in the body. Complications in the eye include the following:

- glaucoma
- posterior subcapsular cataracts
- exacerbation of bacterial and viral (especially herpetic) infections through suppression of protective immune mechanisms
- ptosis
- mydriasis
- scleral melting
- eyelid skin atrophy

In the body, oral doses can cause the following:

- suppression of the pituitary–adrenal axis
- gluconeogenesis resulting from hyperglycemia, muscle wasting, osteoporosis

- redistribution of fat from the periphery to the trunk
- central nervous system effects, such as euphoria
- insomnia
- aseptic necrosis of the hip
- peptic ulcer
- diabetes
- occasionally, psychosis

Elderly patients have particular difficulty taking long-term systemic steroids. For example, one side effect, proximal muscle wasting, may make it difficult for these patients to climb stairs. Another adverse effect of glucocorticoids, osteoporosis, exacerbates the risk of falls and fractures for the elderly, who are generally at an increased risk of both. Elderly patients with inflammatory disease may require a steroid-sparing regimen with methotrexate due to steroid-induced complications. The systemic side effects of steroids, as well as the benefits and limitations of alternate-day therapy, are discussed in BCSC Section 1, *Update on General Medicine.*

Steroid-induced elevation in IOP may occur with topical, periocular, nasal, and systemic glucocorticoid therapy. Individuals differ in their responsiveness: approximately 4% develop pressures higher than 31 mm Hg after 6 weeks of therapy with topical dexamethasone. High levels of response are generally reproducible. The mechanism by which steroids decrease the facility of aqueous outflow through the trabecular meshwork remains unknown. IOP response to topical prednisolone in a normotensive cat model is comparable to that with topical dexamethasone.

Individual response to steroids is highly dependent on the duration, strength, and frequency of therapy and the potency of the agent used. Steroid-induced IOP elevation almost never occurs in less than 5 days and rarely in less than 2 weeks. It is not generally appreciated that late responses to therapy are common and that failure of the IOP to rise after 6 weeks of therapy does not ensure that the patient will maintain normal IOP after several months of therapy. For this reason, IOP monitoring is required at periodic intervals during the entire course of chronic steroid therapy to prevent iatrogenic glaucomatous nerve damage. Steroid-induced IOP rises are usually reversible by discontinuance of therapy if the drug has not been used for more than 1 year, but permanent elevations of pressure are common if therapy has continued for 18 months or more.

The anti-inflammatory and pressure-elevating potencies of 6 steroids used in ophthalmic therapy are given in Table 17-9. The anti-inflammatory potency was determined by an in vitro assay of inhibition of lymphocyte transformation, and the IOP effects were determined by testing in individuals already known to be highly responsive to topical dexamethasone. However, until all these agents are compared in a model of ocular inflammation relevant to human disease, no conclusion can be reached about the observed dissociation of effects. The lower-than-expected effect on pressure of some of these agents may be explained by more rapid metabolism of fluorometholone in the eye compared with dexamethasone and by the relatively poor penetration of medrysone. The efficacy of these agents for intraocular inflammation may be similarly reduced.

Table 17-9 Comparison of Anti-Inflammatory* and IOP-Elevating† Potencies

Glucocorticoid	Relative Potency	Rise in IOP (mm Hg)
Dexamethasone 0.1%	24	22
Fluorometholone 0.1%‡	21	6
Prednisolone 1%	2.3	10
Medrysone 1%§	1.7	1
Tetrahydrotriamcinolone 0.25%	1.4	2
Hydrocortisone 0.5%	1.0	3

* Anti-inflammatory potency determined by in vitro assay of inhibition of lymphocyte transformation
† IOP effects determined in topical dexamethasone responders
‡ Rapid metabolism of fluorometholone in the eye compared with dexamethasone
§ Relatively poor ocular penetration of medrysone

When a steroid-induced pressure rise is suspected but continued steroid therapy is warranted, the physician faces the following choices:

- Continue the same treatment and closely monitor the status of the optic nerve.
- Attempt to offset the pressure rise with other agents.
- Reduce the potency, concentration, or frequency of the steroid used, while monitoring both pressure and inflammation.

When alternative classes of anti-inflammatory agents can be employed, a change may be advisable.

Agents and regimens

Choice of available corticosteroid agents and dosage regimens remains somewhat empirical. Steroids can be used topically (iritis), intravenously (optic neuritis), intravitreally (endophthalmitis), or in a periocular fashion (uveitis) (Table 17-10). All corticosteroids may exacerbate bacterial, viral, mycobacterial, and fungal diseases of the eye and should be used with caution in these settings. Prolonged use may result in secondary glaucoma, cataract formation, and secondary ocular infections following suppression of the host response and/or perforation of the globe.

Table 17-10 Usual Route of Corticosteroid Administration in Ocular Inflammation

Condition	Route
Blepharitis	Topical
Conjunctivitis	Topical
Episcleritis	Topical
Scleritis	Systemic
Keratitis	Topical
Anterior uveitis	Topical and/or periocular, systemic
Posterior uveitis	Systemic and/or periocular, intravitreal injection or implant
Endophthalmitis	Systemic/periocular, intravitreal
Macular edema, diabetic	Periocular, intravitreal
Macular edema, cystoid	Topical, periocular, intravitreal
Optic neuritis	Systemic
Temporal arteritis	Systemic
Sympathetic ophthalmia	Systemic and topical, intravitreal implant

Recent developments in corticosteroids are aimed at developing agents with less IOP effect and agents that can be used intraocularly and periocularly.

Rimexolone 1% (Vexol) is a synthetic topical steroid designed to minimize IOP elevations, similar to fluorinated steroids. Common side effects still include visual field defects and posterior subcapsular cataracts. Elevated IOP has been reported, but it is rare. Systemic side effects, including headache, hypotension, rhinitis, pharyngitis, and taste perversion, occur in fewer than 2% of patients.

Loteprednol etabonate 0.5% (Lotemax) is structurally similar to other steroids but lacks a ketone group at position 20. In corticosteroid responders, studies show that patients treated with loteprednol demonstrate a low incidence of clinically significant, increased IOP. Loteprednol etabonate 0.2% (Alrex) is marketed for the temporary treatment of allergic conjunctivitis. Loteprednol etabonate 0.5% with tobramycin 0.3% (Zylet) is approved for superficial bacterial infection of the eye with inflammation.

The fluocinolone acetonide implant (Retisert) was approved for intraocular implantation in the vitreous cavity for chronic, noninfectious uveitis in 2005.

Triesence, a 40 mg/mL, preservative-free triamcinolone acetonide injectable suspension was approved for intraocular use in 2007. FDA-approved indications include visualization during vitrectomy and treatment of sympathetic ophthalmia, temporal arteritis, uveitis, and ocular inflammatory conditions unresponsive to topical corticosteroids.

Armaly MF. Effect of corticosteroids on intraocular pressure and fluid dynamics II. The effect of dexamethasone in the glaucomatous eye. *Arch Ophthalmol.* 1963;70:492–499.

Armaly MF. Effect of corticosteroids on the intraocular pressure and fluid dynamics. The effect of dexamethasone in the normal eye. *Arch Ophthalmol.* 1963;70:482–491.

Becker B, Mills DW. Corticosteroids and intraocular pressure. *Arch Ophthalmol.* 1963;70: 500–507.

Burk SE, Da Mata AP, Snyder ME, Schneider S, Osher RH, Cionni RJ. Visualizing vitreous using Kenalog suspension. *J Cataract Refract Surg.* 2003;29(4):645–651.

Foster CS, Forstot SL, Wilson LA. Mortality rate in rheumatoid arthritis patients developing necrotizing scleritis or peripheral ulcerative keratitis. Effects of systemic immunosuppression. *Ophthalmology.* 1984;91(10):1253–1263.

Leibowitz HM, Bartlett JD, Rich R, McQuirter H, Stewart R, Assil K. Intraocular pressure-raising potential of 1.0% rimexolone in patients responding to corticosteroids. *Arch Ophthalmol.* 1996;114(8):933–937.

Zhan GL, Miranda OC, Bito LZ. Steroid glaucoma: corticosteroid-induced ocular hypertension in cats. *Exp Eye Res.* 1992;54(2):211–218.

Nonsteroidal Anti-Inflammatory Drugs

Derivatives

Derivatives of arachidonic acid, a 20-carbon essential fatty acid, have been shown to be mediators of a wide variety of biological functions, including regulation of smooth muscle tone (in blood vessels, bronchi, uterus, and gut), platelet aggregation, hormone release (growth hormone, ACTH, insulin, renin, and progesterone), and inflammation.

The synthetic cascade that results in the production of a wide variety of derivatives (depending on the stimulus and tissue) begins with stimulation of phospholipase A_2, the enzyme that liberates arachidonic acid from phospholipids of the cell membrane. (Phospholipase A_2 is inhibited by corticosteroids.) Arachidonic acid is then converted either into cyclic endoperoxides by cyclooxygenase (PG synthase) or into hydroperoxides by lipoxygenase. Among the subsequent products of the endoperoxides are the PGs, which mediate inflammation and other responses; prostacyclin, a vasodilator and platelet antiaggregant; and thromboxane, a vasoconstrictor and platelet aggregant. The hydroperoxides form a chemotactic agent and the leukotrienes C_4, D_4, and E_4, previously known as the slow-reacting substance of anaphylaxis.

Classification

The currently available nonsteroidal anti-inflammatory drugs (NSAIDs) inhibit the production and, thus, the inflammation-inducing effects of PGs through the cyclooxygenase pathway. On the basis of chemical structures, NSAIDs can be classified as

- salicylates: acetylsalicylic acid (aspirin), etofenamic acid, flufenamic acid, meclofenamate, mefenamic acid, tolfenamic acid
- indoles: indomethacin, sulindac, tolmetin
- phenylalkanoic acids: diclofenac, fenoprofen, flurbiprofen, ibuprofen, ketoprofen, ketorolac tromethamine, naproxen, piroxicam, sutoprofen
- pyrazolones: oxyphenbutazone, phenylbutazone

Agents

Table 17-11 lists a number of NSAID agents, with their starting doses. Aspirin and other NSAIDs inhibit the local signs of inflammation (local heat, vasodilation, edema, swelling) as well as pain and fever. They have complex effects on clotting. At low doses (300 mg every other day), aspirin permanently inhibits the cyclooxygenase in platelets that is essential for the conversion of arachidonic acid to PGG_2 and thromboxane. Inhibition of thromboxane production in turn prevents coagulation. Whereas nucleated cells can replenish their cyclooxygenase, anucleate platelets cannot. The anticoagulant effect of aspirin therefore lasts for 7–10 days, mirroring the life span of the inhibited platelets, despite the discontinuation of aspirin therapy. Other NSAIDs inhibit clotting in a reversible fashion, and their use does not need to be discontinued as far in advance before elective surgery.

Table 17-11 Nonsteroidal Anti-Inflammatory Drugs

Drug	Starting Dosage
Aspirin	650 mg qid
Fenoprofen (Nalfon)	600 mg qid
Ibuprofen (Motrin, IBU, Advil)	400 mg qid
Indomethacin (Indocin)	25 mg tid
Ketoprofen (Orudis)	75 mg tid
Naproxen (Naprosyn, Naprelan)	250 mg bid
Piroxicam (Feldene)	20 mg qid
Sulindac (Clinoril)	150 mg bid
Tolmetin	400 mg tid

The relative risks and benefits of aspirin therapy should be assessed specifically for each patient. Aspirin therapy for postoperative pain or for pain associated with traumatic hyphema may increase the risk of hemorrhage because of the antiaggregant effect on platelets. This same side effect may benefit those patients having platelet emboli, as in some cases of amaurosis fugax. Diversion of arachidonic acid to the lipoxygenase pathway by inhibition of cyclooxygenase may explain why aspirin use can be associated with asthma attacks and hypersensitivity reactions (mediated by leukotrienes C_4, D_4, and E_4) in susceptible people.

High doses of aspirin, such as those employed in the treatment of arthritis, may occasionally have toxic effects such as headache, dizziness, tinnitus, dimmed vision, mental confusion, drowsiness, hyperventilation, nausea, and vomiting. These effects may be potentiated by the concomitant use of CAIs at doses sufficient to cause systemic acidosis. During metabolic acidosis, a higher proportion of aspirin molecules is shifted into the more lipid-soluble un-ionized form, which more readily penetrates the blood–brain barrier.

Aspirin and other cyclooxygenase inhibitors are less effective than steroids in the treatment of scleritis and uveitis. NSAIDs such as indomethacin can be effective in treating orbital inflammatory diseases. The prophylactic use of indomethacin in patients with cataract has been reported to reduce the incidence of angiographically detected CME, but its effect on visually significant CME has yet to be reported. Topical NSAIDs have been used to treat ocular inflammation and to prevent and treat postoperative CME.

Flurbiprofen sodium (Ocufen) was the first commercially available topical ocular NSAID. When applied preoperatively, it reduces PG-mediated intraoperative miosis.

Topical diclofenac sodium (Voltaren) (see Table 17-8) is FDA-approved for the postoperative prophylaxis and treatment of ocular inflammation and has also been used successfully to prevent and treat CME.

Ketorolac tromethamine (Acular, Acular PF, Acular LS) is approved for the treatment of postoperative inflammation and allergic conjunctivitis. Ketorolac blocks the metabolism of arachidonic acid by cyclooxygenase. Arachidonic acid metabolites are present in higher quantities in the tears of ocular allergic disease patients. Two double-masked studies have revealed that patients with ocular allergies who were treated with ketorolac tromethamine had significantly less conjunctival inflammation, ocular itching, and tearing than those given placebo. Ketorolac does not have a decongestant effect and does not relieve redness. The recommended dose of ketorolac is 1 drop (0.25 mg) 4 times per day. The most common side effects are stinging and burning on instillation (40%).

Nepafenac (Nevanac) was approved in 2005 for tid dosing for pain and inflammation 1 day before and 2 weeks after cataract surgery.

Bromfenac sodium (Xibrom) was approved in 2006 for twice-daily dosing from 24 hours to 2 weeks post–cataract surgery for pain and inflammation.

Topical NSAIDs may be used for their topical analgesic properties after corneal abrasion and after anterior segment surgery and refractive surgical procedures. All agents are associated with corneal complications, including melting and corneal perforation, seen both in postoperative patients as well as in cases of uveitis, most often in patients with preexisting diabetes and ocular surface disorders. The preponderance of these patients was found to be on generic diclofenac, and this product was subsequently removed from the United States market.

Congdon NG, Schein OD, von Kulajta P, Lubomski LH, Gilbert D, Katz J. Corneal complications associated with topical ophthalmic use of nonsteroidal antiinflammatory drugs. *J Cataract Refract Surg.* 2001;27(4):622–631.

Flach AJ. Corneal melts associated with topically applied nonsteroidal anti-inflammatory drugs. *Trans Am Ophthalmol Soc.* 2001;99:205–210.

Guidera AC, Luchs JI, Udell IJ. Keratitis, ulceration, and perforation associated with topical nonsteroidal anti-inflammatory drugs. *Ophthalmology.* 2001;108(5):936–944.

Noble AG, Tripathi RC, Levine RA. Indomethacin for the treatment of idiopathic orbital myositis. *Am J Ophthalmol.* 1989;108(3):336–338.

Mast-Cell Stabilizers and Antihistamines

The human eye has approximately 50 million mast cells. Each cell contains several hundred granules that in turn contain preformed chemical mediators. Allergic conjunctivitis is an immediate hypersensitivity reaction in which triggering antigens couple to reaginic antibodies (IgE) on the cell surface of mast cells and basophils, leading to the release of histamine PG, leukotrienes, and chemotactic factors from secretory granules. The released histamine causes capillary dilatation and increased permeability and thus conjunctival injection and swelling. It also stimulates nerve endings, causing pain and itching. Agents that interfere at different points along this pathway can treat ocular allergy. Corticosteroids are very effective, but ocular side effects limit their application for this chronic condition. Mast-cell stabilizers, NSAIDs, antihistamines, and decongestants have fewer and less dangerous ocular side effects and can be used singly or in combination. Table 17-12 lists agents for the relief of allergic conjunctivitis.

Short-term relief for mild allergic symptoms may be achieved with over-the-counter preparations of topical antihistamines such as antazoline and pheniramine, usually combined with the decongestant naphazoline (Vasocon-A and Naphcon-A, respectively). Specific H_1-antagonists have been developed, such as emedastine (Emadine), levocabastine (Livostin), and azelastine (Optivar).

Emedastine difumarate 0.05% (Emadine) is a relatively selective H_1-receptor antagonist indicated for the temporary relief of the signs and symptoms of allergic conjunctivitis. Recommended dosing is 1 drop up to 4 times per day. The most common side effect reported is headache (11%). Bad taste, blurred vision, burning or stinging, corneal infiltrates, dry eye, rhinitis, and sinusitis are other noted side effects.

Levocabastine HCl has an onset of action that occurs within minutes and lasts for at least 4 hours; it is as effective as cromolyn sodium. The usual dosage of levocabastine 0.05% is 1 drop 4 times per day for up to 2 weeks. This drug has been discontinued in the United States.

Azelastine HCl (Optivar) is effective and well tolerated at a dose of 0.05%. This drug is also available as a nasal spray for the treatment of allergic rhinitis.

Ketorolac tromethamine (Acular), a topical NSAID, is used to prevent itching and provides a rapid onset but does not relieve conjunctival hyperemia.

Table 17-12 Agents for Relief of Allergic Conjunctivitis

Generic Name	Trade Name	Class
Azelastine HCl	Optivar	H₁-antagonist/mast-cell inhibitor
Cromolyn sodium	Crolom, available generically	Mast-cell inhibitor
Emedastine difumarate	Emadine	H₁-antagonist
Epinastine HCl	Elestat	H₁-antagonist/mast-cell inhibitor
Ketorolac tromethamine	Acular, Acular PF, Acular LS	NSAID
Ketotifen fumarate	Zaditor (OTC) Alaway (OTC) Available generically	H₁-antagonist/mast-cell inhibitor
Levocabastine HCl	Discontinued in US	H₁-antagonist
Lodoxamide tromethamine	Alomide	Mast-cell inhibitor
Loteprednol etabonate	Alrex	Corticosteroid
Naphazoline HCl	Ak-Con, Albalon, available generically	Antihistamine
Naphazoline HCl/antazoline phosphate	Vasocon-A	Antihistamine/decongestant
Naphazoline HCl/pheniramine maleate	Naphcon-A, Opcon-A	Antihistamine/decongestant
Nedocromil sodium	Alocril	H₁-antagonist/mast-cell inhibitor
Olopatadine HCl	Patanol, Pataday	H₁-antagonist/mast-cell inhibitor
Pemirolast potassium	Alamast	Mast-cell inhibitor

Mast-cell stabilizers have previously been viewed as preventing calcium influx across mast-cell membranes, thereby preventing mast-cell degranulation and mediator release. Cromolyn sodium (Crolom) inhibits neutrophil, eosinophil, and monocyte activation in vitro. Traditional mast-cell stabilizers such as cromolyn sodium, lodoxamide (Alomide), and pemirolast (Alamast) prevent mast-cell degranulation but take days to weeks to reach their peak efficacy. They have little or no antihistamine effect and do not provide immediate relief from allergic symptoms. They are used for allergic, vernal, and atopic conjunctivitis.

Lodoxamide has been shown to produce stabilization of the mast-cell membrane 2500 times greater than does cromolyn sodium. In treating allergic conjunctivitis, its onset of action is quicker, with less stinging, than that seen with cromolyn sodium. One recent multicenter, double-masked study showed that lodoxamide was superior to cromolyn sodium in treating vernal keratoconjunctivitis. However, as with all mast-cell stabilizers, lodoxamide does not become clinically effective for several weeks. It may therefore be necessary to use topical steroids or H₁-antagonists concurrently with mast-cell stabilizers for the first several weeks, until these agents are fully effective. The usual dose of lodoxamide 0.1% for adults and children older than 2 years is 1–2 drops in the affected eye 4 times daily for up to 3 months. The most frequently reported adverse reactions were burning, stinging, and discomfort upon instillation (15%).

Pemirolast potassium 0.1% (Alamast) is used for the prevention of itchy eyes due to allergic conjunctivitis. In clinical studies, the most common side effects were headache, rhinitis, and cold and flu symptoms, which were generally mild.

Some agents, including olopatadine (Patanol), ketotifen (Zaditor), nedocromil (Alocril), epinastine (Elestat), and azelastine (Optivar), have a mast-cell stabilizing effect as well as H_1-antagonism. These agents provide immediate relief against released histamine and also prevent the future degranulation of mast cells. Olopatadine HCl 0.1% (Patanol) has a rapid onset and at least an 8-hour duration of action. Recommended dosing is 1–2 drops in the affected eye 2 times a day at an interval of 6–8 hours. This drug is now also available for once-a-day dosing as olopatadine 0.2% (Pataday). Adverse reactions of ocular burning, stinging, dry eye, foreign-body sensation, hyperemia, keratitis, eyelid edema, pruritus, asthenia, cold syndrome, pharyngitis, rhinitis, sinusitis, and taste perversion were all reported at an incidence of less than 5%. For ketotifen fumarate 0.025% (Zaditor, Alaway), recommended dosing is 1 drop every 8–12 hours. This medication is now available without a prescription. Side effects of conjunctival injection, headaches, and rhinitis were reported at an incidence of 10%–25%. Nedocromil sodium 2% (Alocril) is a mast-cell stabilizer with a twice-daily dosing regimen.

Corticosteroids are very effective at treating ocular allergies but are prone to abuse and have a more dangerous side-effect profile. Loteprednol etabonate 0.2% (Alrex) is a steroid designed to cause less IOP elevation that can be used for the temporary treatment of ocular allergies. Recalcitrant cases of severe allergic, vernal, and atopic conjunctivitis may require the short-term use of stronger topical steroids, but these cases should be carefully monitored and patients switched to one of the previously mentioned agents as soon as clinically prudent.

Giede-Tuch C, Westhoff M, Zarth A. Azelastine eye-drops in seasonal allergic conjunctivitis or rhinoconjunctivitis. A double-blind, randomized, placebo-controlled study. *Allergy.* 1998;53(9):857–862.

Hingorani M, Moodaley L, Calder VL, Buckley RJ, Lightman S. A randomized, placebo-controlled trial of topical cyclosporin A in steroid-dependent atopic keratoconjunctivitis. *Ophthalmology.* 1998;105(9):1715–1720.

Verin P. Treating severe eye allergy. *Clin Exp Allergy.* 1998;28(suppl 6):44–48.

Antifibrotic Agents

Antiproliferative agents, also known as *antimetabolites,* are occasionally required in the treatment of severe ocular inflammatory diseases, such as Behçet syndrome and sympathetic ophthalmia, or for ocular diseases that are part of a systemic vasculitis. Systemic therapy with such agents is best carried out in consultation with a chemotherapist. The uses and side effects of these agents are discussed in BCSC Section 9, *Intraocular Inflammation and Uveitis.*

Fluorouracil is a fluorinated pyrimidine nucleoside analogue that blocks production of thymidylate synthase and interrupts normal cellular DNA and RNA synthesis. Its primary action may be to cause cellular thymine deficiency and resultant cell death. The effect of fluorouracil is most pronounced on rapidly growing cells, and its use as an antiviral agent is primarily related to destruction of infected cells (eg, warts) by topical application.

Intravitreal injection of 5-fluorouracil has been reported to be beneficial in preventing recurrent proliferative vitreoretinopathy after surgery for complex retinal detachments in an experimental model. Fluorouracil is used postoperatively as a subconjunctival injection and intraoperatively as a topical application to the trabeculectomy site. The drug is thought to inhibit the cellular proliferation that could otherwise occur in response to inflammation. In high-risk patients, including young glaucoma patients ($\leq$40 years), the initial trabeculectomy with adjunctive 5-fluorouracil had a higher success rate than surgery without the adjunct.

Mitomycin C is a compound isolated from the fungus *Streptomyces caespitosus*. The parent compound becomes a bifunctional alkylating agent after enzymatic alteration within the cell; it then inhibits DNA synthesis and cross-links DNA. Mitomycin's immunosuppressive properties are fairly weak; however, it is a potent inhibitor of fibroblast proliferation.

Like fluorouracil, topical mitomycin C has been used in filtering surgery. However, unlike 5-fluorouracil, which requires repeated postoperative injections, it has the advantage of functioning with a single intraoperative application. Randomized comparative studies of mitomycin C with 5-fluorouracil in high-risk patients show lower average pressures with fewer corneal-surface and hypotony-related complications in the groups treated with mitomycin C than in those treated with 5-fluorouracil. Mitomycin C is used as a single topical application during glaucoma filtering operations to impede scarring and prevent surgical failure. Complications of therapy are wound leakage, hypotony, and localized scleral melting. Severe toxicity has been reported in an animal model with intraocular instillation of mitomycin C, resulting in irreversible progressive bullous keratopathy in 3 of 4 rabbits.

Both mitomycin and fluorouracil have been used in the treatment of conjunctival intraepithelial neoplasia. Topical mitomycin C has also been recommended both as a single-dose therapy and as postoperative drops for use in the prevention of recurrence of pterygia after pterygium excision. Recommended dosage is 0.02%–0.04% 4 times daily for 1–2 weeks after surgery. The recurrence rate with such therapy has been reported to be as low as 0%–11%. Unfortunately, several adverse effects—such as corneal edema, corneal and scleral perforation, corectopia, iritis, cataract, and intractable pain—have been reported. A primary conjunctival graft after pterygium removal may offer similar low recurrence rates without these serious complications. Both mitomycin and thiotepa have been used to reduce haze in photorefractive keratectomy (PRK) patients.

Allinson RW. Adjuvant 5-FU and heparin prevent PVR. *Ophthalmology.* 2002;109(5):829–830.

Anderson Penno E, Braun DA, Kamal A, Hamilton WK, Gimbel HV. Topical thiotepa treatment for recurrent corneal haze after photorefractive keratectomy. *J Cataract Refract Surg.* 2003;29(8):1537–1542.

Asaria RH, Kon CH, Bunce C, et al. Adjuvant 5-fluorouracil and heparin prevents proliferative vitreoretinopathy: results from a randomized, double-blind, controlled clinical trial. *Ophthalmology.* 2001;108(7):1179–1183.

Jolimaître P, Malet-Martino M, Martino R. Fluorouracil prodrugs for the treatment of proliferative vitreoretinopathy: formulation in silicone oil and in vitro release of fluorouracil. *Int J Pharm.* 2003;259(1–2):181–192.

Khaw PT. Advances in glaucoma surgery: evolution of antimetabolite adjunctive therapy. *J Glaucoma.* 2001;10(5 suppl 1):S81–S84.

Wormald R, Wilkins MR, Bunce C. Post-operative 5-fluorouracil for glaucoma surgery. Cochrane Database Syst Rev. 2000;(2):CD001132. Review. [Update in Cochrane Database Syst Rev. 2001;(3):CD001132.]

Yamamoto N, Ohmura T, Suzuki H, Shirasawa H. Successful treatment with 5-fluorouracil of conjunctival intraepithelial neoplasia refractive to mitomycin-C. *Ophthalmology.* 2002; 109(2):249–252.

Antibiotics

Penicillins and Cephalosporins

The penicillins and cephalosporins are β-lactam–containing antibacterial agents that react with and inactivate a particular bacterial transpeptidase that is essential for bacterial cell-wall synthesis (Table 17-13). The amide bond of the β-lactam group is surrounded

Table 17-13 Principal Antibiotic Agents

Drug Name	Topical	Subconjunctival	Intravitreal	Intravenous (Adult)
Amikacin sulfate	10 mg/mL	25 mg	400 µg	15 mg/kg daily in 2–3 doses
Ampicillin sodium	50 mg/mL	50–150 mg	500 µg	4–12 g daily in 4 doses
Bacitracin zinc	10,000 units/mL	5000 units		
Carbenicillin disodium	4–6 mg/mL	100 mg	250–2000 µg	8–24 g daily in 4–6 doses
Cefazolin sodium	50 mg/mL	100 mg	2250 µg	2–4 g daily in 3–4 doses
Ceftazidime		200 mg	2200 µg	1 g daily in 2–3 doses
Clindamycin	50 mg/mL	15–50 mg	1000 µg	900–1800 mg daily in 2 doses
Colistimethate sodium	10 mg/mL	15–25 mg	100 µg	2.5–5.0 mg/kg daily in 2–4 doses
Erythromycin	50 mg/mL	100 mg	500 µg	
Gentamicin sulfate	8–15 mg/mL	10–20 mg	100–200 µg	3–5 mg/kg daily in 2–3 doses
Imipenem/cilastatin sodium	5 mg/mL			2 g daily in 3–4 doses
Kanamycin sulfate	30–50 mg/mL	30 mg		
Methicillin sodium	50 mg/mL	50–100 mg	1000–2000 µg	6–10 g daily in 4 doses
Neomycin sulfate	5–8 mg/mL	125–250 mg		
Penicillin G	100,000 units/mL	0.5–1.0 million units		12–24 million units daily in 4 doses
Polymyxin B sulfate	10,000 units/mL	100,000 units		
Ticarcillin disodium	6 mg/mL	100 mg		200–300 mg/kg daily
Tobramycin sulfate	8–15 mg/mL	10–20 mg	100–200 µg	3–5 mg/kg daily in 2–3 doses
Vancomycin HCl	20–50 mg/mL	25 mg	1000 µg	15–30 mg/kg daily in 1–2 doses

by structural features in the antibiotic molecule that resemble the portion of the natural substrate with which the transpeptidase reacts. The peptidase reacts with the antibiotic, forming an inactive acyl intermediate.

Some bacteria are resistant to the action of penicillins and cephalosporins. The lipopolysaccharide outer coat of many gram-negative bacteria may prevent certain hydrophilic antibiotics from reaching their cytoplasmic membrane site of action. Furthermore, some bacteria produce β-lactamases (penicillinase), enzymes capable of cleaving the critical amide bond within these antibiotics. The different penicillins and cephalosporins vary in susceptibility to the β-lactamases produced by different bacterial species.

The penicillins and cephalosporins penetrate the blood–ocular and blood–brain barriers poorly and are actively transported out of the eye by the organic-acid transport system of the ciliary body. However, their penetration into the eye increases with inflammation and with coadministration of probenecid.

Serious and occasionally fatal hypersensitivity (anaphylactoid) reactions can occur in association with penicillin and cephalosporin therapy. Penicillin hypersensitivity affects 0.7%–4% of all treatment courses and has an overall incidence between 0.7% and 10%. Reactions to drugs in the penicillin family may be the most common drug allergy. Although anaphylaxis is more frequent following parenteral administration, it can occur with oral therapy. Such reactions are more likely to occur in individuals with a history of sensitivity to multiple allergens. A history of immediate allergic response (anaphylaxis or rapid onset of hives) to any penicillin is a strong contraindication to the use of any other penicillin. Approximately 10% of people allergic to a penicillin will have cross-reactivity to cephalosporins.

Kelkar PS, Li JT. Cephalosporin allergy. *N Engl J Med.* 2001;345(11):804–809.

Penicillins

There are 5 classes of penicillins, which differ in their spectrum of antibiotic activity and in their resistance to penicillinase:

1. Penicillin G, penicillin V, and phenethicillin are highly effective against most gram-positive and gram-negative cocci, many anaerobes, and *Listeria, Actinomyces, Leptospira,* and *Treponema* organisms. However, most strains of *Staphylococcus aureus* and many strains of *S epidermidis,* anaerobes, and *Neisseria gonorrhoeae* are now resistant, often through production of penicillinase. Resistance by enterococci is often from altered penicillin-binding proteins. Penicillin V and phenethicillin are absorbed well orally, whereas penicillin G is better given intravenously because it is inactivated by stomach acid. These penicillins are excreted rapidly by the kidneys and have short half-lives unless they are given in depot forms (ie, procaine penicillin G) or administered with probenecid, which competitively inhibits excretion by the kidneys.

2. The penicillinase-resistant penicillins include methicillin sodium, nafcillin, oxacillin sodium, cloxacillin sodium, dicloxacillin sodium, and floxacillin. They are less potent than penicillin G against susceptible organisms but are the drugs of choice for infections that are caused by penicillinase-producing *S aureus* and that

are not methicillin resistant. Methicillin and nafcillin are acid-labile and are therefore given either parenterally or by subconjunctival injection. The other agents in this group have reasonable oral absorption. When they are given systemically, coadministration of probenecid reduces renal excretion and outward transport from the eye.

3. The broad-spectrum penicillins such as ampicillin, amoxicillin, and bacampicillin HCl have antibacterial activity that extends to such gram-negative organisms as *Haemophilus influenzae*, *Escherichia coli*, *Salmonella* and *Shigella* species, and *Proteus mirabilis*. Resistant strains of *H influenzae* are becoming more common. These drugs are stable in acid and may be given orally. They are not resistant to penicillinase or to the broader-spectrum β-lactamases that are increasingly common among gram-negative bacteria.

4. Carbenicillin and ticarcillin have antimicrobial activity that extends to *Pseudomonas* and *Enterobacter* species and indole-positive strains of *Proteus*. These drugs are given parenterally or subconjunctivally, although the indanyl ester of carbenicillin may be given orally. They are not resistant to penicillinase and are less active against gram-positive bacteria and *Listeria* species.

5. Piperacillin sodium, mezlocillin sodium, and azlocillin are particularly potent against *Pseudomonas* and *Klebsiella* species and retain a strong gram-positive coverage and activity against *Listeria* species. They are administered parenterally or subconjunctivally, and they are not resistant to penicillinase.

Cephalosporins

Bacterial susceptibility patterns and resistance to β-lactamases have determined the classification of the cephalosporins as first-, second-, third-, or fourth-generation, although fifth- and sixth-generation agents are under development.

- *First-generation.* Cephalothin, cefazolin, cephalexin, cefadroxil, and cephradine have strong antimicrobial activity against gram-positive organisms, especially *Streptococci* species and *S aureus*. They retain moderate activity against gram-negative organisms. Cephalothin is the most resistant of these agents to staphylococcal β-lactamase and is used in severe staphylococcal infections. Because cephalothin is painful when given intramuscularly, it is used only intravenously. In contrast, cefazolin is more sensitive to β-lactamase but has somewhat greater activity against *Klebsiella* species and *E coli*. Cefazolin has a longer half-life and is tolerated both intramuscularly and intravenously; thus it is used more frequently than the other first-generation cephalosporins. Cephalexin, cefadroxil, and cephradine are stable in gastric acid and available in oral forms.

- *Second-generation.* These agents were developed to expand the activity against gram-negative organisms while retaining much of their gram-positive spectrum of activity. Cefamandole, cefoxitin, and cefuroxime display greater activity against *H influenzae*, *Enterobacter aerogenes*, and *Neisseria* species. Cefamandole has increased activity against *Enterobacter* and indole-positive *Proteus* species, *H influenzae*, and *Bacteroides* species. Cefoxitin is active against indole-positive *Proteus* and *Serratia* organisms, as well as against *Bacteroides fragilis*. Cefuroxime is valuable in the treatment of penicillinase-producing *N gonorrhoeae* and ampicillin-resistant *H influenzae,* and its penetration of the blood–brain barrier is adequate for initial treatment of suspected pneumococcal, meningococcal, or *H influenzae* meningitis.

- *Third-generation.* The third-generation cephalosporins have further enhanced activity against gram-negative bacilli, specifically the β-lactamase–producing members of the Enterobacteriaceae family, but they are inferior to first-generation cephalosporins with regard to their activity against gram-positive cocci. Commonly used agents include cefotaxime, cefoperazone sodium, ceftriaxone sodium, ceftazidime, and ceftizoxime sodium. These agents have a similar spectrum of activity against gram-positive and gram-negative organisms; anaerobes; *Neisseria, Serratia,* and *Proteus* species; and some *Pseudomonas* isolates. Cefoperazone and ceftazidime are particularly effective against *Pseudomonas* but lose more coverage of the gram-positive cocci. Cefotaxime penetrates the blood–brain barrier better than the other cephalosporins can, and it presumably also penetrates the blood–ocular barrier.
- *Fourth-generation.* Cefepime HCl and cefpirome have a spectrum of gram-negative coverage similar to that of the third-generation cephalosporins, but these agents are more resistant to some β-lactamases.

No cephalosporin provides coverage for enterococci, *Listeria* and *Legionella* species, or methicillin-resistant *S aureus.*

Other Antibacterial Agents

See Tables 17-14 and 17-15.

Fluoroquinolones

Fluoroquinolones are fluorinated derivatives of nalidixic acid and are available in a variety of chemical structures. The most commonly used ophthalmic agents are ofloxacin, levofloxacin, ciprofloxacin, moxifloxacin, and gatifloxacin. These agents are highly effective, broad-spectrum antimicrobials with potent activity against common gram-positive and gram-negative ocular pathogens. Their mechanism of action targets bacterial DNA supercoiling through the inhibition of DNA gyrase and topoisomerase IV, 2 of the enzymes responsible for replication, genetic recombination, and DNA repair. Mutations in the bacterial genes for these enzymes allow the development of resistance to fluoroquinolone agents. There has been an increased incidence of resistance to these agents, as well as evidence of cross-resistance among agents. Fluoroquinolone resistance has been reported in *Mycobacterium chelonae, S aureus,* coagulase-negative *Staphylococcus* species, *Pseudomonas aeruginosa, Clostridium difficile, Salmonella enterica, E coli,* and *Helicobacter pylori.*

Studies in vitro have demonstrated that the fluoroquinolones, especially ciprofloxacin and temafloxacin, inhibit 90% of common bacterial corneal pathogens and have a lower minimum inhibitory concentration than the aminoglycosides gentamicin and tobramycin and the cephalosporin cefazolin. They are also less toxic to the corneal epithelium than are the aminoglycosides.

Five fluoroquinolones currently available are ofloxacin ophthalmic solution 0.3% (Ocuflox), ciprofloxacin 0.3% (Ciloxan), levofloxacin 0.5% (Quixin), gatifloxacin 0.3%

Table 17-14 Ophthalmic Antibacterial Agents

Generic Name	Trade Name	Solution Strength
Individual Agents		
Azithromycin	AzaSite	1%
Bacitracin zinc	Ak-Tracin; available generically	Ointment (500 units/g)
Chloramphenicol	Powder available for compounding	0.5%, ointment (1%)
Ciprofloxacin HCl	Ciloxan; available generically	0.3%, ointment (0.3%)
Erythromycin	Romycin; available generically	Not available; ointment (0.5%)
Gatifloxacin	Zymar	0.3%
Gentamicin sulfate	Garamycin	0.3%; ointment (0.3%)
	Genoptic	0.3%
	Gentasol	0.3%
	Gentak	0.3%, ointment (0.3%)
	Available generically	0.3%, ointment (0.3%)
Levofloxacin	Quixin	0.5%
Moxifloxacin HCl	Vigamox	0.5%
Ofloxacin	Ocuflox	0.3%
	Available generically	0.3%
Sulfacetamide sodium	Bleph-10	10%
	Available generically	10%, ointment (10%)
Tobramycin sulfate	Ak-Tob	0.3%
	Tobrasol	0.3%
	Tobrex	0.3%, ointment (0.3%)
	Available generically	0.3%
Mixtures		
Polymyxin B sulfate/bacitracin zinc	Ak-Poly-Bac	Not available; ointment (10,000 units/g, 500 units/g)
	Polycin-B	Not available; ointment (10,000 units/g, 500 units/g)
	Available generically	Not available; ointment (10,000 units/g, 500 units/g)
Polymyxin B sulfate/neomycin sulfate/bacitracin zinc	Available generically	Not available; ointment (10,000 units/g, 3.5 mg/base, 400 units/g)
Polymyxin B sulfate/neomycin sulfate/gramicidin	Neosporin; available generically	10,000 units/mL, 1.75 mg/base mL, 0.025 mg/mL
Polymyxin B sulfate/oxytetracycline	Terak	Not available; ointment (10,000 units/g, EQ 5 mg base/g)
Polymyxin B sulfate/trimethoprim sulfate	Polytrim; available generically	10,000 units/mL, EQ 1 mg base/mL

(Zymar), and moxifloxacin 0.5% (Vigamox). They are used in the treatment of corneal ulcers caused by susceptible strains of *S aureus, S epidermidis, Streptococcus pneumoniae, P aeruginosa, Serratia marcescens* (efficacy studied in fewer than 10 infections), and *Propionibacterium acnes*. They are also indicated for bacterial conjunctivitis due to susceptible strains of *S aureus, S epidermidis, S pneumoniae, Enterobacter cloacae, H influenzae, P mirabilis,* and *P aeruginosa*.

Table 17-15 Combination Ocular Anti-Inflammatory and Antibiotic Agents

Generic Name	Trade Name	Preparation and Concentration
Dexamethasone/neomycin sulfate/ polymyxin B sulfate	Ak-Trol, Poly-Dex, Dexacidin, Maxitrol, available generically	Susp, 0.1%; EQ 3.5 mg base/mL; 10,000 units/mL
	Maxitrol Available generically	Ointment, 0.1%; EQ 3.5 mg base/g; 10,000 units/g
Dexamethasone/tobramycin	Tobradex	Susp, 0.1%, 0.3%
	Available generically	Susp, 0.1%, 0.3%
	Tobradex	Ointment, 0.1%, 0.3%
Hydrocortisone/neomycin sulfate/ polymyxin B sulfate	Cortisporin, available generically	Susp, 1%; EQ 3.5 mg base/mL; 10,000 units/mL
Hydrocortisone/neomycin sulfate/ polymyxin B sulfate/bacitracin zinc	Ak-Spore, Cortisporin, available generically	Ointment, 1%; EQ 3.5 mg base/g; 5000 units/g; 400 units/g
Loteprednol etabonate/tobramycin	Zylet	Susp, 0.5%, 0.3%
Prednisolone acetate/gentamicin sulfate	Pred-G	Susp; EQ 0.3% base; 1%
	Pred-G S.O.P.	Ointment; EQ 0.3% base; 0.6%
Neomycin sulfate/polymyxin B sulfate/prednisolone acetate	Poly-Pred	Susp; EQ 0.35% base; 10,000 units/mL; 0.5%
Prednisolone acetate/sulfacetamide sodium	Blephamide, available generically	Susp, 0.2%, 10%
	Blephamide S.O.P.	Ointment, 0.2%, 10%
Prednisolone sodium phosphate/ sulfacetamide sodium	Vasocidin, available generically	Soln, 0.25%, 10%
	Ak-Cide	Ointment, 0.5%, 10%

These fluoroquinolones have a high rate of penetration into ocular tissue. Their sustained tear concentration levels exceed the minimum inhibitory concentrations of key ocular pathogens for up to 12 hours or more after 1 dose. They also deliver excellent susceptibility kill rates, with one in vitro study confirming eradication of 87%–100% of indicated pathogenic bacteria, including P aeruginosa. In addition, ofloxacin provides patient comfort and prevents precipitates from forming. Ofloxacin has a high intrinsic solubility that enables it to be formulated at a near-neutral 6.4 pH. Ciprofloxacin is formulated at a pH of 4.5, gatifloxacin at a pH of 6.0, and moxifloxacin at a pH of 6.8. The combination of high efficacy and safety has made fluoroquinolones the most prescribed anti-infectives for the treatment of ocular pathogens.

The most frequently reported drug-related adverse reaction is transient ocular burning or discomfort. Other reported reactions include stinging, redness, itching, chemical conjunctivitis/keratitis, periocular/facial edema, foreign-body sensation, photophobia, blurred vision, tearing, dry eye, and eye pain. Although rare, reports of dizziness have also been received. Both norfloxacin and ciprofloxacin have been reported to cause white, crystalline corneal deposits of medication, which resolve after discontinuation of the drug.

Sulfonamides

Sulfonamides are derivatives of para-aminobenzenesulfonamide. They are structural analogues and competitive antagonists of para-aminobenzoic acid for the bacterial synthesis of folic acid. These drugs affect only the bacteria that must synthesize their own folic acid. Mammalian cells are not affected, because they are unable to synthesize folic acid. Sulfonamides are bacteriostatic only. They are more effective when administered with trimethoprim, a potent inhibitor of bacterial dihydrofolate reductase; together, they block successive steps in the synthesis of tetrahydrofolic acid. Systemic pyrimethamine, sulfadiazine, and folinic acid are used in the treatment of toxoplasmosis. Chlamydia requires a 3-week course of systemic sulfonamide therapy.

Sulfacetamide ophthalmic solution (10%–30%) and ointment (10%) penetrate the cornea well but may sensitize the patient to sulfonamide medication. Susceptible organisms include *S pneumoniae, Corynebacterium diphtheriae, H influenzae, Actinomyces* species, and *Chlamydia trachomatis.* Local irritation, itching, periorbital edema, and transient stinging are some of the common adverse effects from topical administration. As with all sulfonamide preparations, severe sensitivity reactions such as toxic epidermal necrolysis and Stevens-Johnson syndrome have been reported. The incidence of adverse reactions to all sulfonamides is approximately 5%.

Tetracyclines

The tetracycline family includes agents produced by *Streptomyces* species (chlortetracycline, oxytetracycline, demeclocycline), as well as the semisynthetically produced agents tetracycline, doxycycline, and minocycline. Tetracyclines enter bacteria by an active transport across the cytoplasmic membrane. They inhibit protein synthesis by binding to the 30S ribosomal subunit, thus preventing access of aminoacyl tRNA to the acceptor site on the mRNA–ribosome complex. Host cells are less affected because they lack an active-transport system. Doxycycline and minocycline are more lipophilic and thus more active by weight. Doxycycline is the most commonly used tetracycline for ophthalmic conditions, as well as the most commonly used parenteral tetracycline in the United States. The tetracyclines may depress prothrombin, thus prolonging the bleeding in patients on anticoagulation medication. As bacteriostatic drugs, tetracyclines may inhibit bactericidal medication such as the penicillins and therefore should not be used concurrently. The use of tetracyclines may decrease the efficacy of oral contraceptives. Patients should be instructed to use an additional form of birth control during administration of tetracyclines and for 1 month after discontinuation of their use.

Tetracyclines are broad-spectrum bacteriostatic antibiotics, active against many gram-positive and gram-negative bacteria and also against *Rickettsia* species, *Mycoplasma pneumoniae,* and *Chlamydia* species. However, many strains of *Klebsiella* and *H influenzae* and nearly all strains of *Proteus vulgaris* and *P aeruginosa* are resistant. These agents demonstrate cross-resistance. Tetracycline is poorly water-soluble but is soluble in eyedrops containing mineral oil; it readily penetrates the corneal epithelium. Chlortetracycline has also been used previously in ophthalmic preparation, but neither chlortetracycline nor tetracycline is currently available for ophthalmic use in the United States. Oxytetracycline is available in combination with polymyxin as an ophthalmic ointment.

Systemic therapy with the tetracyclines is used for chlamydial infections; because these drugs are excreted into oil glands, they are also used for staphylococcal infections of the meibomian glands. They chelate to calcium in milk and antacids and are best taken on an empty stomach. As tetracyclines may cause gastric irritation, they can be taken with nondairy agents to improve compliance. Tetracyclines should not be given to children or pregnant women, because they can be deposited in growing teeth, causing permanent discoloration of the enamel, and may also deposit in bone and inhibit bone growth. Tetracyclines depress plasma prothrombin activity and thereby potentiate warfarin (Coumadin). They have been implicated as a cause of pseudotumor cerebri, a condition discussed in BCSC Section 5, *Neuro-Ophthalmology*. The use of tetracyclines also causes photosensitivity; consequently, patients taking tetracycline should avoid extended exposure to sunlight. Degraded or expired tetracyclines may cause renal toxicity, also called Fanconi syndrome.

Chloramphenicol

Chloramphenicol, a broad-spectrum bacteriostatic agent, inhibits bacterial protein synthesis by binding reversibly to the 50S ribosomal subunit, preventing aminoacyl tRNA from binding to the ribosome. Chloramphenicol is effective against most *H influenzae, Neisseria meningitidis,* and *N gonorrhoeae,* as well as all anaerobic bacteria. It has some activity against *S pneumoniae, S aureus, Klebsiella pneumoniae, Enterobacter* and *Serratia* species, and *P mirabilis. P aeruginosa* is resistant.

Chloramphenicol penetrates the corneal epithelium well during topical therapy and penetrates the blood–ocular barriers readily when given systemically. However, the use of this agent is limited because it has been implicated in an idiosyncratic and potentially lethal aplastic anemia. Although most cases of this anemia have occurred after oral administration, some have been associated with parenteral and even topical ocular therapy. Chloramphenicol is available as a powder for compounding, but it should not be used if an alternative agent with less potential toxicity is available.

Aminoglycosides

The aminoglycosides consist of amino sugars in glycosidic linkage. They are bactericidal agents that are transported across the cell membrane into bacteria, where they bind to the 30S and 50S ribosomal subunits, interfering with initiation of protein synthesis. The antibacterial spectrum of these agents is determined primarily by the efficiency of their transport into bacterial cells. Such transport is energy-dependent and may be reduced in the anaerobic environment of an abscess. Resistance to aminoglycosides may be caused by failure of transport, low affinity for the ribosome, or plasmid-transmitted ability to enzymatically inactivate the drug. The coadministration of drugs such as penicillin that alter bacterial cell-wall structure can markedly increase aminoglycoside penetration, resulting in a synergism of antibiotic activity against gram-positive cocci, especially enterococci. One such aminoglycoside, amikacin, is remarkably resistant to enzymatic inactivation.

Gentamicin, tobramycin, kanamycin, and amikacin have antibacterial activity against aerobic, gram-negative bacilli such as *P mirabilis*; *P aeruginosa*; and *Klebsiella, Enterobacter,* and *Serratia* species. Gentamicin and tobramycin are also active against gram-positive *S aureus* and *S epidermidis*. Kanamycin is generally less effective than the others against gram-negative bacilli. Resistance to gentamicin and tobramycin has gradually increased as a result of a plasmid-transmitted ability to synthesize inactivating enzymes. Thus, amikacin, which is generally impervious to these enzymes, is particularly valuable in treating such resistant organisms. It is effective against tuberculosis, as well as atypical mycobacteria, and can be compounded for topical use against mycobacterial infection.

Aminoglycosides are not absorbed well orally but are given systemically by intramuscular or intravenous routes. They do not readily penetrate the blood–ocular barrier but may be administered as eyedrops, ointments, or periocular injections. Gentamicin and carbenicillin should not be mixed for IV administration because the carbenicillin inactivates the gentamicin over several hours. Similar incompatibilities exist in vitro between gentamicin and other penicillins and cephalosporins.

Use of streptomycin is now limited to *Streptococcus viridans* bacterial endocarditis, tularemia, plague, and brucellosis. Neomycin is a broad-spectrum antibiotic, effective against *Enterobacter* species, *K pneumoniae, H influenzae, N meningitidis, C diphtheriae,* and *S aureus.* It is given topically in ophthalmology and orally as a bowel preparation for surgery. Neomycin is too toxic to be used intravenously but can be given orally because it is not absorbed from the gut. Topical allergy to ocular use of neomycin occurs in approximately 8% of cases. Neomycin can cause punctate epitheliopathy and retard re-epithelialization of abrasions.

All aminoglycosides can cause dose-related vestibular and auditory dysfunction and nephrotoxicity when they are given systemically. Systemic use of aminoglycosides should be limited to serious infections, and the plasma concentration of drug and blood urea nitrogen should be monitored to avoid overdosing.

Miscellaneous antibiotics

Vancomycin is a tricyclic glycopeptide derived from cultures of *Nocardia orientalis.* It is bactericidal for most gram-positive organisms through the inhibition of glycopeptide polymerization in the cell wall. It is useful in the treatment of staphylococcal infections in patients who are allergic to or have not responded to the penicillins and cephalosporins. It can also be used in combination with aminoglycosides to treat *S viridans* or *Streptococcus bovis* endocarditis. Oral vancomycin is poorly absorbed but is effective in the treatment of pseudomembranous colitis that is caused by *C difficile.* Vancomycin resistance has increased in isolates of *Enterococcus* and *Staphylococcus,* and antibiotic resistance is transmitted between pathogens by a conjugative plasmid.

Vancomycin may be used topically or intraocularly to treat sight-threatening infections of the eye, including infectious keratitis and endophthalmitis caused by methicillin-resistant staphylococci or streptococci. It has been used within the irrigating fluid of balanced salt solution during intraocular surgery. There is controversy concerning the contribution of this prophylactic use of vancomycin to the emergence of resistant bacteria, as well as to an increased risk of postoperative CME. Vancomycin is a preferred substitute for a cephalosporin used in combination with an aminoglycoside in the empirical treatment of endophthalmitis. See BCSC Section 8, *External Disease and Cornea,* and Section 9, *Intraocular Inflammation and Uveitis,* for further discussion.

The IV dosage of vancomycin in adults with normal renal function is 500 mg every 6 hours or 1 g every 12 hours. Dosing must be adjusted in subjects who have renal impairment. Topical vancomycin may be compounded and given in a concentration of 50 mg/mL in the treatment of infectious keratitis. Intravitreal vancomycin combined with an aminoglycoside may be used for initial empirical therapy for exogenous bacterial endophthalmitis. A dose of 1 mg/0.1 mL establishes intraocular levels significantly higher than the minimum inhibitory concentration for most gram-positive organisms.

Unlike systemic treatment, topical vancomycin and intraocular vancomycin have not been associated with ototoxicity or nephrotoxicity. Hourly use of 50 mg of vancomycin per milliliter delivers a dose of 36 mg/day, which is well below the recommended systemic dose. In addition to the ototoxicity and nephrotoxicity associated with systemic therapy, chills, rash, fever, and anaphylaxis are other possible complications. Further, rapid IV infusion may cause "red-man syndrome" due to flushing.

Erythromycin is a macrolide (many-membered lactone ring attached to deoxy sugars) antibiotic that binds to the 50S subunit of bacterial ribosomes and interferes with protein synthesis. It is bacteriostatic against gram-positive cocci such as S pyogenes and S pneumoniae, gram-positive bacilli such as C diphtheriae and Listeria monocytogenes, and a few gram-negative organisms such as N gonorrhoeae. It may be bactericidal, in sufficient dosing, against susceptible organisms.

Drug resistance is rising and is as high as 40% among streptococcus isolates. There are 4 mechanisms of resistance:

1. esterases from Enterobacteriaceae
2. mutations that alter the 50S ribosome
3. enzyme modification of the ribosomal binding site
4. active pumping to extrude the drug

Macrolide antibiotics such as erythromycin are the treatment of choice for Legionella pneumophila, the agent of legionnaires' disease, as well as for M pneumoniae. Erythromycin is administered orally as enteric-coated tablets or in esterified forms to avoid inactivation by stomach acid. It can also be administered parenterally or topically as an ophthalmic ointment. The drug penetrates the blood–ocular and blood–brain barriers poorly.

Clarithromycin and azithromycin are semisynthetic macrolides with spectrums of activity similar to that of erythromycin. Clarithromycin is more effective against staphylococci, streptococci, and M leprae and azithromycin is more active against H influenzae, N gonorrhoeae, and Chlamydia species. Both agents have enhanced activity against Mycobacterium avium-intracellulare, atypical mycobacteria, and Toxoplasma gondii. Azithromycin 1% (AzaSite) was recently FDA approved for bacterial conjunctivitis caused by CDC coryneform group G, H influenzae, S aureus, S mitis group, and S pneumoniae.

Polymyxin B sulfate is a mixture of basic peptides that function as cationic detergents to dissolve phospholipids of bacterial cell membranes, thus disrupting cells. It is used topically or by local injection to treat corneal ulcers. Gram-negative bacteria are susceptible, including Enterobacter and Klebsiella species and P aeruginosa; bacterial sensitivity is related to phospholipid content of the cell membrane, and resistance may occur if a cell wall prevents access to the pathogen cell membrane. Topical hypersensitivity is an uncommon occurrence. Systemic use of this medication was abandoned due to severe nephrotoxicity.

Bacitracin is a mixture of polypeptides that inhibit bacterial cell-wall synthesis. It is active against *Neisseria* and *Actinomyces* species and *H influenzae* and most gram-positive bacilli and cocci. It is available as an ophthalmic ointment either alone or in various combinations with polymyxin, neomycin, and hydrocortisone. The primary side effect is local hypersensitivity, although this is not commonly seen.

Topical povidone-iodine solution (Betadine 5%) exhibits broad-spectrum antimicrobial activity when used to prepare the surgical field and to rinse the ocular surface and has FDA approval for this purpose. It is the only agent that has been shown to have a significant effect on postsurgical endophthalmitis. It is contraindicated in patients with hypersensitivity to iodine or to intravenous contrast dye. Povidone-iodine scrub may be used periocularly, but it is contraindicated in the eye because it is damaging to the corneal epithelium.

Castillo A, Benitez del Castillo JM, Toledano N, Diaz-Valle D, Sayaques O, Garcia-Sanchez J. Deposits of topical norfloxacin in the treatment of bacterial keratitis. *Cornea.* 1997;16(4): 420–423.

Ciulla TA, Starr MB, Masket S. Bacterial endophthalmitis prophylaxis for cataract surgery: an evidence-based update. *Ophthalmology.* 2002;109(1):13–24.

Goll C, Balmer P, Schwab F, Rüden H, Eckmanns T. Different trends of MRSA and VRE in a German hospital, 1999-2005. *Infection.* 2007;35(4):245–249.

Han DP, Wisniewski SR, Wilson LA, et al. Spectrum and susceptibilities of microbiologic isolates in the Endophthalmitis Vitrectomy Study. *Am J Ophthalmol.* 1996;122(1):1–17. [Erratum appears in *Am J Ophthalmol.* 1996;122(6):920.]

Kollef MH. Limitations of vancomycin in the management of resistant staphylococcal infections. *Clin Infect Dis.* 2007;45(suppl 3):S191–S195.

Liesegang TJ. Use of antimicrobials to prevent postoperative infection in patients with cataracts. *Curr Opin Ophthalmol.* 2001;12(1):68–74.

Werner G, Klare I, Fleige C, Witte W. Increasing rates of vancomycin resistance among *Enterococcus faecium* isolated from German hospitals between 2004 and 2006 are due to wide clonal dissemination of vancomycin-resistant enterococci and horizontal spread of vanA clusters. *Int J Med Microbiol.* 2008;298(5–6):515–527.

Antifungal Agents

See Table 17-16.

Polyenes

The polyene antibiotics are named for a component sequence of 4 to 7 conjugated double bonds. That lipophilic region allows them to bind to sterols in the cell membrane of susceptible fungi, an interaction that results in damage to the membrane and leakage of essential nutrients. Other antifungals (such as flucytosine and the imidazoles) and even other antibiotics (such as tetracycline and rifampin) can enter through the damaged membrane, yielding synergistic effects.

Natamycin and amphotericin B are 2 examples of polyene macrolide antibiotics. Natamycin is available as a 5% suspension for topical ophthalmic use (once an hour).

Table 17-16 Antifungal Agents

Generic (Trade) Name	Route	Dosage	Indication/ (additional reports of use)
Polyenes			
Amphotericin B (Fungizone; available generically)	Topical	0.1%–0.5% solution; dilute with water for injection or dextrose 5% in water	*Aspergillus* *Candida* *Cryptococcus* *(Blastomyces)* *(Coccidioides)* *(Colletotrichum)* *(Histoplasma)*
	Subconjunctival Intravitreal IV	0.8–1.0 mg 5 µg Because of possible side effects and toxicity, dose needs to be carefully adjusted.	
Natamycin (Natacyn)	Topical	5% suspension	*Fusarium* *(Aspergillus)* *(Candida)* *(Cephalosporium)* *(Curvularia)* *(Penicillium)*
Imidazoles			
Ketoconazole (Nizoral; available generically)	Oral	200 mg daily, up to 400 mg for severe or incomplete response	*Blastomyces* *Candida* *Coccidioides* *Histoplasma*
Miconazole nitrate (available as powder for compounding)	Topical Subconjunctival Intravitreal	1% solution 5 mg 10 µg	*Candida* *Cryptococcus* *Aspergillus*
Triazoles			
Fluconazole (Diflucan)	Oral	200 mg daily	*Candida* *Cryptococcus* *(Acremonium)*
Itraconazole (Sporanox)	Oral IV	200 mg daily	*Aspergillus* *Blastomyces* *Histoplasma* *(Candida)* *(Curvularia)* (nonsevere *Fusarium*)
Fluorinated Pyrimidine			
Flucytosine (Ancobon)	Oral	50–150 mg/kg daily divided every 6 h	*Candida* *Cryptococcus* *(Aspergillus)*
	Topical	1% solution	

Local hypersensitivity reactions of the conjunctiva and eyelid and corneal epithelial toxicity may occur. Amphotericin B may be reconstituted at 0.25%–0.5% in sterile water (with deoxycholate to improve solubility) for topical use (every 30 minutes). It may also be administered systemically for disseminated disease, although careful monitoring for renal and other toxicities is required. Both of these agents penetrate the cornea poorly. They have been used topically against a variety of filamentous fungi, including species of

Aspergillus, Cephalosporium, Curvularia, Fusarium, and *Penicillium,* as well as the yeast *Candida albicans.* Systemic amphotericin B has been reported as useful in the treatment of systemic *Aspergillus, Blastomyces, Candida, Coccidioides, Cryptococcus,* and *Histoplasma* infections.

Imidazoles and triazoles

The imidazole- and triazole-derived antifungal agents also increase fungal cell-membrane permeability and interrupt membrane-bound enzyme systems. The triazoles have less effect on human sterol synthesis, as well as a longer half-life, than the imidazoles, and they are being more actively developed. The imidazole miconazole is available in a 1% solution that may be injected subconjunctivally (5 mg/0.5 mL, once or twice daily) or applied topically. Miconazole penetrates the cornea poorly.

Ketoconazole is available in 200-mg tablets for oral therapy (once or twice daily). Ketoconazole normally penetrates the blood–brain barrier and, presumably, the blood–ocular barrier poorly, but therapeutic levels can be achieved in inflamed eyes. The triazole itraconazole, with an expanded antifungal spectrum and less systemic toxicity, has largely replaced ketoconazole. However, there is an extensive and growing list of potentially dangerous drug interactions with itraconazole, and this list should be consulted prior to instituting systemic therapy. Fluconazole, another triazole, may also increase the plasma concentrations of other medications. The imidazole and triazole antifungals act against various species of *Aspergillus, Coccidioides, Cryptococcus,* and *Candida.*

Flucytosine

Flucytosine (5-fluorocytosine) is converted by some species of fungal cells to 5-fluorouracil by cytosine deaminase, and then to 5-fluorodeoxyuridylate. This last compound inhibits thymidylate synthase, an important enzyme in DNA synthesis. Host cells lack cytosine deaminase activity and are less affected. Only fungi that have both a permease to facilitate flucytosine penetration and a cytosine deaminase are sensitive to flucytosine. Flucytosine is taken orally at 50–150 mg/kg daily, divided every 6 hours. Although the drug is well absorbed and penetrates the blood–ocular barrier well, the majority of *Aspergillus* and half of *Candida* isolates are resistant. Flucytosine is used primarily as an adjunct to systemic amphotericin B therapy.

Antiviral Agents

See Table 17-17.

Topical antiviral agents

Three agents that compete with natural nucleotides for incorporation into viral and mammalian DNA have been used to treat herpes simplex virus (HSV) keratitis. Idoxuridine (5-iodo-2′-deoxyuridine) and trifluridine (Viroptic) are structural analogues of thymidine and work in a similar manner; vidarabine is an analogue of adenine. Trifluridine (1% drops, every 2–4 hours) is more soluble than the other agents and can be used in drop form, providing adequate penetration of diseased corneas to treat herpetic iritis. Trifluridine is currently marketed in the United States; idoxuridine and vidarabine powder are available for compounding. Vidarabine can be used if an agent with a different mechanism of action is required. Cross-resistance does not seem to occur among these agents.

Table 17-17 Antiviral Agents

Generic Name	Trade Name	Topical Concentration/ Ophthalmic Solution	Systemic Dosage
Trifluridine	Viroptic; available generically	1%	
Idoxuridine	Available as powder for compounding	0.1%	
Vidarabine monohydrate	Available as powder for compounding	3% (ophth ointment)	
Acyclovir sodium*	Zovirax; available generically		*Oral:* Herpes simplex keratitis (HSV) 200 mg 5 times daily for 7–10 days *Oral:* Herpes zoster ophthalmicus (HZV) 600–800 mg 5 times daily for 10 days; IV if patient is immunocompromised
Azidothymidine (AZT)/zidovudine	Retrovir; available generically		Dosage variable per source consulted; dosing per internal medicine consultation recommended
Cidofovir*†	Vistide		*IV induction:* 5 mg/kg constant infusion over 1 h once weekly for 2 consecutive weeks *Maintenance:* 5 mg/kg constant infusion over 1 h administered every 2 weeks
Famciclovir*†	Famvir HZV		500 mg 3 times daily for 7 days
Foscarnet sodium	Foscavir; available generically		*IV induction:* By controlled infusion only, either by central vein or by peripheral vein induction: 60 mg/kg (adjusted for renal function) given over 1 h every 8 h for 14–21 days *Maintenance:* 90–120 mg/kg given over 2 h once daily
Ganciclovir	Vitrasert		*Intravitreal:* 4.5 mg sterile intravitreal insert designed to release the drug over a 5–8 mo period
Ganciclovir sodium*†	Cytovene IV		*IV induction:* 5 mg/kg every 12 h for 14–21 days *Maintenance:* 5 mg/kg daily for 7 days
Valacyclovir HCl*‡	Valtrex HZV		1 g 3 times daily for 7–14 days

* Dose adjustment is recommended for geriatric and renal patients or with concomitant nephrotoxic medications.
† Because of potential side and toxic effects with systemic dosage, the possible dosage adjustments and warnings should be followed properly.
‡ At high doses, valacyclovir has been associated with thrombotic thrombocytopenic purpura/hemolytic uremic syndrome (TTP/HUS) in immunocompromised patients.

Systemic antiviral agents

Acyclovir is a synthetic guanosine analogue that requires phosphorylation to become active. It undergoes monophosphorylation by viral thymidine kinase. Because the viral thymidine kinase in HSV types 1 and 2 has many times more affinity to acyclovir than does host thymidine kinase, high concentrations of acyclovir monophosphate accumulate in infected cells. Acyclovir monophosphate is then further phosphorylated to the active compound acyclovir triphosphate. The triphosphate cannot cross cell membranes and accumulates further. This increased concentration of acyclovir triphosphate is 50–100 times greater in infected cells than in uninfected cells.

Acyclovir triphosphate inhibits virus growth in 3 ways:

1. It can function as a competitive inhibitor of DNA polymerases, with viral DNA polymerases being significantly more susceptible to acyclovir triphosphate than are human DNA polymerases.
2. It can be a DNA chain terminator.
3. It can produce irreversible binding between viral DNA polymerase and the interrupted chain, causing permanent inactivation.

The result is a several-hundred-fold inhibition of HSV growth, with minimal toxicity to uninfected cells.

Acyclovir-resistant thymidine kinase HSVs have evolved. They occur primarily in patients receiving multiple courses of therapy or in patients with AIDS. Thymidine kinase mutants are susceptible to vidarabine and foscarnet. Changes in viral DNA polymerase structures can also mediate resistance to acyclovir.

Acyclovir can be used topically (this product has been discontinued in the United States), orally, or intravenously. Oral acyclovir is only 15%–30% bioavailable, and food does not affect absorption. For unknown reasons, bioavailability is lower in patients with transplants. Acyclovir is minimally protein-bound (10%–30%), and drug interactions through binding displacement have not been reported. The drug is well distributed, with cerebrospinal fluid (CSF) and brain concentrations equaling approximately 50% of serum values. Concentrations of acyclovir in zoster vesicle fluid are equivalent to those in plasma. Aqueous humor concentrations are 35% that of plasma; and salivary concentrations, 15%. Vaginal concentrations are equivalent to those of plasma, and breast-milk concentrations exceed them.

The percutaneous absorption of topical acyclovir is low and occurs primarily when large areas are treated. Plasma concentrations of 0.3 µg/mL were noted in patients treated topically with this drug for herpes zoster (HZV). Peak serum concentrations after oral ingestion of acyclovir average 0.6 mg/mL and occur 90 minutes after dosing, but peak serum concentrations after IV administration reach approximately 10 mg/mL.

The plasma half-life for normal adults and neonates is 3.3 and 3.8 hours, respectively. It increases to 20 hours in anuric patients. In the urine, 60%–90% of acyclovir is excreted unchanged through both glomerular filtration and tubular secretion. As a result, acyclovir may interfere with the renal excretion of drugs that are eliminated through the renal tubules (eg, methotrexate); probenecid significantly decreases the renal excretion of acyclovir. A major metabolite of acyclovir, carboxymethoxymethylguanine, accounts for

10%–20% of the total administered dose and is excreted in urine. Acyclovir is effectively removed by hemodialysis (60%) but only minimally removed by peritoneal dialysis. A commonly used intravenous dosage for acyclovir is 1500 mg/m²/day.

Acyclovir is off-label for HSV and HZV ophthalmicus but has proven to be effective in preventing the recurrence of HSV epithelial and stromal keratitis in oral doses of 400 mg twice a day. Although this prophylactic dosage was originally studied over a 1-year treatment period, clinicians are now using this dosage indefinitely to decrease the likelihood of disease recurrence. Similar dosing of acyclovir has proven beneficial in reducing the likelihood of recurrent herpetic eye disease after corneal transplantation. However, oral acyclovir was not found to be of benefit when used with topical steroids and trifluridine in the treatment of active HSV stromal keratitis. The addition of oral acyclovir to a regimen of topical antiviral agents may be considered in patients with HSV iridocyclitis. Although the benefit of this drug did not reach statistical significance, study enrollment was halted due to inadequate numbers of patients. Although well tolerated in oral form, parenteral acyclovir can cause renal toxicity due to crystalline nephropathy. Neurotoxicity may also occur with intravenous use.

Valacyclovir is currently approved for management of HZV infections in immunocompetent persons but not for HSV. It is an amino acid ester prodrug of acyclovir; its bioavailability is much higher than that of acyclovir (54% vs 20%). The recommended dosage is 1 g 3 times a day for 7–14 days. Valacyclovir has been associated with nephrotoxicity and thrombocytopenia in immunocompromised patients.

Famciclovir is the prodrug of penciclovir and is currently approved for the management of uncomplicated acute HZV. It has demonstrated efficacy in relieving acute zoster signs and symptoms and reducing the duration of postherpetic neuralgia when administered during acute zoster. The recommended dosage for the management of acute HZV is 500 mg 3 times a day for 7 days.

Ganciclovir (9-2-hydroxypropoxymethylguanine) is a synthetic guanosine analogue active against many herpesviruses. It is approved for cytomegalovirus (CMV) retinitis and for CMV prophylaxis in advanced HIV and in transplant patients. As with acyclovir, it must be phosphorylated to become active. Infection-induced kinases, viral thymidine kinase, or deoxyguanosine kinase of various herpesviruses can catalyze this reaction. After monophosphorylation, cellular enzymes convert ganciclovir to the triphosphorylated form, and the triphosphate inhibits viral DNA polymerase rather than cellular DNA polymerase. Ganciclovir triphosphate competitively inhibits the incorporation of guanosine triphosphate into DNA. Because of its toxicity and the availability of acyclovir for treatment of many herpesvirus infections, its use is currently restricted to treatment of CMV retinitis, predominantly as an intraocular implant.

Systemic ganciclovir is used primarily intravenously, because less than 5% of an oral dose is absorbed. The intravenous induction dose is 5 mg/kg every 12 hours for 14–21 days. Once the infection is under control, a daily dose of 6 mg/kg is required for maintenance of the virus-free state. CSF concentrations are approximately 50% those of plasma, with peak plasma concentrations reaching 4–6 sLg/mL. The plasma half-life is 3–4 hours in people with normal renal function, increasing to over 24 hours in patients with severe renal insufficiency. Over 90% of systemic ganciclovir is eliminated unchanged in urine, and dose modifications are necessary for individuals with compromised renal function. Ganciclovir is approximately 50% removed by hemodialysis. Bone marrow suppression is the primary side effect of systemic therapy. Oral ganciclovir may be used in the suppression of CMV retinitis after initial control is obtained with parenteral therapy. Ganciclovir can be administered intravitreally or as a sustained-release intraocular device (Vitrasert). Because of the long duration of remission and the low side-effect profile, the ganciclovir implant has become the preferred treatment for CMV retinitis, specifically in isolated ocular infection.

Foscarnet (phosphonoformic acid) inhibits DNA polymerases, RNA polymerases, and reverse transcriptases. In vitro, it is active against herpesviruses, influenza virus, and HIV. Foscarnet is approved for the treatment of AIDS patients with CMV retinitis and for acyclovir-resistant mucocutaneous HSV infections in immunocompromised patients. It acts by blocking the pyrophosphate receptor site of CMV DNA polymerase. Viral resistance is attributable to structural alterations in this enzyme. Foscarnet inhibits herpesviruses and cytomegaloviruses that are resistant to acyclovir and ganciclovir. It is administered intravenously in doses adjusted for renal function and with hydration to establish sufficient diuresis.

Foscarnet bioavailability is approximately 20%. Because it can bind with calcium and other divalent cations, foscarnet becomes deposited in bone and may be detectable for many months. Distribution follows a 3-compartment model and produces peak serum concentrations of approximately 30 pg/mL. It is eliminated by both glomerular filtration and tubular secretion, with 80%–90% of the administered dose appearing unchanged in the urine. Dosage adjustment is required in persons with impaired renal function. Treatment may be limited by nephrotoxicity in up to 50% of patients; other side effects include hypocalcemia and neurotoxicity.

Cidofovir (Vistide, formerly known as HPMPC) is a third agent approved for the treatment of CMV retinitis, and it is approved only for that use. Cidofovir is a cytidine nucleoside analogue active against herpesviruses, poxviruses, polyomaviruses, papillomaviruses, and adenoviruses. The mechanism of action is inhibition of DNA synthesis, and resistance is through mutations in DNA polymerase. The prolonged intracellular half-life of an active metabolite allows once-weekly dosing during induction, with dosing every 2 weeks thereafter. The primary side effect is renal toxicity, which can be decreased by IV prehydration and by both pretreatment and posttreatment with high-dose probenecid. Ocular side effects include uveitis and hypotony. Cidofovir does not have direct cross-resistance with acyclovir, ganciclovir, or foscarnet, although some virus isolates may have multiple resistances and even develop triple resistance. Cidofovir was shown to inhibit CMV replication when administered intravitreally in a small series of patients. Dosage administered was 20 μg/0.1 mL. Long-lasting suppression of CMV retinitis was noted, with an average time to progression of 55 days. Cidofovir is the second-line therapy for complications after smallpox vaccination (vaccinia virus) and has been used in selected studies for varicella-zoster retinitis, as well as adenoviral keratoconjunctivitis.

Zidovudine (azidothymidine [AZT]) is a thymidine nucleoside analogue with activity against HIV. Zidovudine becomes phosphorylated to monophosphate, diphosphate, and triphosphate forms by cellular kinases in infected and uninfected cells. It has 2 primary methods of action:

1. The triphosphate acts as a competitive inhibitor of viral reverse transcriptase.
2. The azido group prevents further chain elongation and acts as a DNA chain terminator.

Zidovudine inhibits HIV reverse transcriptase at much lower concentrations than those needed to inhibit cellular DNA polymerases. It is currently indicated as treatment for some stages of HIV infection.

Zidovudine is administered orally in doses of 1500 mg/day and is approximately 60% bioavailable, with 40% metabolized by first pass. Peak concentrations occur within 30–90 minutes to give steady-state peak concentrations of 0.05–1.5 fg/mL. Zidovudine is about 40% protein-bound. CSF concentrations vary widely and range from 25% to 100% of serum values. Zidovudine enters the brain, phagocytic cells, liver, muscle, and placenta. Plasma half-life is approximately 1 hour. Intravenous dosage is 1–2 mg/kg 4 times a day.

Fluorouracil is a fluorinated pyrimidine nucleoside analogue that blocks production of thymidylate and interrupts normal cellular DNA and RNA synthesis. Its primary action may be to cause cellular thymine deficiency and resultant cell death. The effect of fluorouracil is most pronounced on rapidly growing cells, and its use as an antiviral agent is primarily related to destruction of infected cells (warts) by topical application.

Acyclovir for the prevention of recurrent herpes simplex virus eye disease. Herpetic Eye Disease Study Group. *N Engl J Med.* 1998;339(5):300–306.

Oral acyclovir for herpes simplex virus eye disease: effect on prevention of epithelial keratitis and stromal keratitis. Herpetic Eye Disease Study Group. *Arch Ophthalmol.* 2000;118(8): 1030–1036.

Medications for *Acanthamoeba* Infections

Acanthamoeba is a genus of ubiquitous, free-living amebae that inhabit soil, water, and air. Their appearance as corneal pathogens has increased due to a number of factors, including the increased use of contact lenses. The species responsible for corneal infections, which include *A polyphaga, A castellanii, A hatchetti,* and *A culbertsoni,* exist as both trophozoites and double-walled cysts. Because of the variations among species of *Acanthamoeba,* no single drug is effective in treating all *Acanthamoeba* keratitis. Polyhexamethylene biguanide (0.02% solution) is a non–FDA-approved disinfectant and the first-line agent with lowest minimal amebicidal concentration. Medications that are effective include chlorhexidine, neomycin, polymyxin B-neomycin-gramicidin mixtures, natamycin 5% topical suspension, imidazoles such as miconazole (powder compounded to 1% topical solution), systemic imidazoles and triazoles, propamidine isethionate 0.1% drops (Brolene; not approved in the United States), and topical dibromopropamidine 0.15% ointment (not approved in the United States). See BCSC Section 8, *External Disease and Cornea,* for updated treatment recommendations.

Kumar R, Lloyd D. Recent advances in the treatment of Acanthamoeba keratitis. *Clin Infect Dis.* 2002;35(4):434–441.

O'Day DM, Head WS. Advances in the management of keratomycosis and Acanthamoeba keratitis. *Cornea.* 2000;19(5):681–687.

Seal DV. Acanthamoeba keratitis update—incidence, molecular epidemiology and new drugs for treatment. *Eye.* 2003;17(8):893–905.

Sudesh S, Laibson PR. The impact of the herpetic eye disease studies on the management of herpes simplex virus ocular infections. *Curr Opin Ophthalmol.* 1999;10(4):230–233.

van Rooij J, Rijneveld WJ, Remeijer L, et al. Effect of oral acyclovir after penetrating keratoplasty for herpetic keratitis: a placebo-controlled multicenter trial. *Ophthalmology.* 2003;110(10):1916–1919.

Local Anesthetics

Local anesthetic agents are used extensively in ophthalmology. Topical preparations yield corneal and conjunctival anesthesia for comfortable performance of examination techniques such as tonometry, gonioscopy, removal of superficial foreign bodies, corneal scraping for bacteriologic studies, and paracentesis, as well as for use of contact lenses associated with fundus examination and laser procedures. Topical and intracameral anesthesia has gained increasing acceptance in cataract, pterygium, and glaucoma surgery. Local retrobulbar and eyelid blocks yield excellent anesthesia and akinesia for intraocular and orbital surgery (Tables 17-18, 17-19).

The local anesthetic agents used in ophthalmology are tertiary amines linked by either ester or amide bonds to an aromatic residue. Because the protonated form is far more soluble and these compounds undergo hydrolysis more slowly in acidic solutions, local anesthetic agents are supplied in the form of their hydrochloride salts. When exposed to tissue fluids at pH 7.4, approximately 5%–20% of the anesthetic agent molecules will be in the unprotonated form, as determined by the pK_a (8.0–9.0) of the individual agent. The more lipid-soluble unprotonated form penetrates the lipid-rich myelin sheath and cell membrane of axons. Once inside, most of the molecules are again protonated. The protonated form gains access to and blocks the sodium channels on the inner wall of the cell membrane and increases the threshold for electrical excitability. As increasing numbers of sodium channels are blocked, nerve conduction is impeded and finally blocked.

After administration of a local anesthetic, nerve fibers that are small or unmyelinated are blocked most quickly because their higher discharge rates open sodium channel gates more frequently and because conduction can be prevented by the disruption of a shorter length of axon. The action potential in unmyelinated fibers spreads continuously along the axon; in myelinated fibers, the action potential spreads by saltation. Therefore, only a short length of an unmyelinated fiber need be functionally interrupted, whereas 1 or more nodes must be blocked in a myelinated fiber. In larger myelinated fibers, the nodes are farther apart.

Clinically, local anesthetics first block the poorly myelinated and narrow parasympathetic fibers (as evidenced by pupil dilation) and sympathetic fibers (vasodilation), followed by sensory fibers (pain and temperature), and finally the larger and more

Table 17-18 Regional Anesthetics

Generic (Trade)	Concentration (%) Maximum Dose	Onset of Action	Duration of Action	Major Advantages/ Disadvantages
Bupivacaine* (Sensorcaine, Marcaine)	0.25%–0.75%	5–11 min	480–720 min (with epinephrine)	Long duration of action/increased toxicity to the extraocular muscles
Lidocaine* (Xylocaine, Anestacaine)	0.5%–2% (500 mg)	4–6 min	40–60 min; 120 min (with epinephrine)	Spreads readily without hyaluronidase
Mepivacaine* (Carbocaine)	2% (500 mg)	3–5 min	120 min	Duration of action greater without epinephrine
Procaine† (Novocain)	1%–2% (500 mg)	7–8 min	30–45 min; 60 min (with epinephrine)	Short duration; poor absorption from mucous membranes

* Amide-type compound
† Ester-type compound

Table 17-19 Topical Anesthetic Agents

Generic Name	Trade Name	Strength
Cocaine		1%–4%
Fluorescein sodium/benoxinate	Fluress	0.25%; 0.4%
	Flurox	
	Available generically	
Fluorescein sodium/proparacaine	Fluoracaine	0.25%; 0.5%
	Flucaine	
Lidocaine	Topical solution	4%
	Viscous gel	2%
Proparacaine	Alcaine	0.5%
	Parcaine	0.5%
	Ophthetic	0.5%
	Available generically	0.5%
Tetracaine	Altacaine	0.5%
	Tetravisc	0.5%
	Available generically	0.5%

myelinated motor fibers (akinesia). The optic nerve, enclosed in a meningeal lining, is often not blocked by retrobulbar injections.

Amide local anesthetics are preferred to ester agents for retrobulbar blocks because the amides have a longer duration of action and less systemic toxicity. However, this duration of action is limited by diffusion from the site of injection because amide agents are not metabolized locally but are metabolized and inactivated in the liver, primarily by dealkylation.

Ester agents are susceptible to hydrolysis by serum cholinesterases in ocular vessels as well as by metabolism in the liver. Toxicity of ester anesthetics may occur at lower doses when serum cholinesterase levels are low because of treatment with echothiophate eye-drops or a hereditary serum cholinesterase deficiency.

The toxic manifestations of local anesthetics are generally related to dose. However, patients with severe hepatic insufficiency may have symptoms of toxicity with either amide or ester local anesthetics, even at lower doses. These manifestations include restlessness and tremor that may proceed to convulsions, and respiratory and myocardial depression. Central nervous system stimulation can be counteracted by IV diazepam; respiratory depression calls for ventilatory support.

Because local anesthetics block sympathetic vascular tone and dilate vessels, a 1:200,000 concentration of epinephrine is frequently added to shorter-acting agents to retard vascular absorption. Such use of epinephrine raises circulating catecholamine levels and may result in systemic hypertension and cardiac arrhythmias.

Topically applied anesthetics disrupt intercellular tight junctions, resulting in increased corneal epithelial permeability to subsequently administered agents (ie, dilating drops). They also interfere with corneal epithelial metabolism and repair and thus cannot be used for chronic pain relief. Because topical anesthetics can become drugs of abuse that can eventually lead to chronic pain syndromes and vision loss, they should not be dispensed to patients.

Lidocaine (Xylocaine) is an amide local anesthetic used in strengths of 0.5%, 1%, and 2% (with or without epinephrine) for injection and 2%–4% for topical mucosal anesthesia, although it is off-label for topical cataract surgery. It yields a rapid (5-minute) retrobulbar or eyelid block that lasts 1–2 hours. The topical solution, applied to the conjunctiva with a cotton swab for 1–2 minutes, reduces the discomfort of subconjunctival injections. Topical lidocaine is preferable to cocaine or proparacaine as the agent for conjunctival biopsy because it has less effect on epithelial morphology. Lidocaine is also extremely useful for suppressing cough during ocular surgery. The maximum safe dose of the 2% solution for local injection is 15 mL in adults. A common side effect is drowsiness.

Mepivacaine (Carbocaine) is an amide agent used in strengths of 1%–3% (with or without a vasoconstrictor). It has a rapid onset and lasts about 2–3 hours. The maximum safe dose is 25 mL of a 2% solution.

Bupivacaine (Marcaine) is an amide agent that has a slower onset of action than does lidocaine. It may yield relatively poor akinesia but has the advantage of long duration of action, up to 8 hours. It is available in 0.25%–0.75% solutions (with or without epinephrine) and is frequently administered in a mixture with lidocaine or mepivacaine to achieve a rapid, complete, and long-lasting effect. The maximum safe dose is 25 mL of a 0.75% solution.

The following agents are commonly used for topical anesthesia of the ocular surface. Because of their higher lipid solubilities, these agents have a more rapid onset than other agents; thus the initial discomfort caused by the drops is shortened. Proparacaine (eg, Ophthaine, Ophthetic) is an ester topical anesthetic available as a 0.5% solution. The least irritating of the topical anesthetics, it has a rapid onset of approximately 15 seconds and lasts about 20 minutes. Used without a preservative, proparacaine reportedly does not inhibit the growth of *Staphylococcus*, *Candida*, or *Pseudomonas* and thus might be preferred to other agents for corneal anesthesia prior to obtaining a scraping for culture from a corneal ulcer. Its structure is different enough from the other local anesthetics that cross-sensitization apparently does not occur.

Benoxinate is an ester topical anesthetic available in a 0.4% solution with fluorescein (Fluress) for use in tonometry. It has an onset and duration similar to that of proparacaine.

Tetracaine is an ester topical anesthetic available in 0.5% solution (Altacaine) and is approved for short-duration ocular surface procedures. It has a longer onset of action and duration of action than proparacaine has and causes more extensive corneal epithelial toxicity.

Topical Anesthetics in Anterior Segment Surgery

The first modern use of topical anesthetics was Koller's use of cocaine in 1884. Since then, synthetic drugs have become available; cocaine is no longer used because of the potential risk of side effects and drug abuse. Tetracaine 0.5% or 1% (amethocaine) and proparacaine 0.5% are short-acting (20 minutes) and are the least toxic of the regional and topical anesthetics to the corneal epithelium. Lidocaine 4% for injection (Lignocaine) can be used topically, as can 2% lidocaine jelly. Bupivacaine 0.5% and 0.75% have a longer duration of action but an increased risk of associated corneal toxicity.

Technique

The aim of topical anesthetics is to block the nerves that supply the superficial cornea and conjunctiva—namely, the long and short ciliary, nasociliary, and lacrimal nerves. Patients should be warned that they will experience some stinging upon application of the drops onto the surface of the cornea.

Because visual perception is not lost, the patient is asked to focus on the source of the light, the intensity of which is subsequently reduced.

Topical anesthetics may be combined with subconjunctival anesthetics. This combination is well tolerated by patients and allows subconjunctival and scleral manipulations to be carried out.

Topical anesthetics can be augmented with a blunt cannula sub-Tenon infusion of anesthetic as a primary anesthetic or intraoperatively in patients who become intolerant of topical anesthetics.

Intraocular lidocaine

Recently, intraocular lidocaine has been used to provide analgesia during surgery. The solution used is 0.3 mL of 1% isotonic, nonpreserved lidocaine administered intracamerally. No side effects have been reported, except for possible transient retinal toxicity if lidocaine is injected posteriorly in the absence of a posterior capsule. Lidocaine obviates the need for intravenous and regional anesthetic supplementation in most patients. Adequate anesthesia is obtained in approximately 10 seconds. As with topical techniques, the ability of the patient to cooperate during surgery is desirable. Contrasting studies have shown no difference with and without intracameral lidocaine as a supplement to topical anesthetics. Because of unreliable patient cooperation, topical and intracameral anesthetics should be used cautiously, if at all, in patients with deafness, dementia, and severe photophobia.

Crandall AS. Anesthesia modalities for cataract surgery. *Curr Opin Ophthalmol.* 2001;12(1): 9–11.

Crandall DC. Pharmacology of ocular anesthetics. In: Tasman W, Jaeger EA, eds. *Duane's Foundations of Clinical Ophthalmology.* Vol 3. Philadelphia: Lippincott; 1999:1–22.

Kansal S, Moster MR, Gomes MC, Schmidt CM Jr, Wilson RP. Patient comfort with combined anterior sub-Tenon's, topical, and intracameral anesthesia versus retrobulbar anesthesia in trabeculectomy, phacotrabeculectomy, and aqueous shunt surgery. *Ophthalmic Surg Lasers.* 2002;33(6):456–462.

Roberts T, Boytell K. A comparison of cataract surgery under topical anaesthesia with and without intracameral lignocaine. *Clin Experiment Ophthalmol.* 2002;30(1):19–22.

Varga JH, Rubinfeld RS, Wolf TC, et al. Topical anesthetic abuse ring keratitis: report of four cases. *Cornea.* 1997;16(4):424–429.

Purified Neurotoxin Complex

Botulinum toxin type A (Botox, formerly called Oculinum) is produced from cultures of the Hall strain of *Clostridium botulinum.* It blocks neuromuscular conduction by binding to receptor sites on motor nerve terminals, entering the nerve terminals and inhibiting the release of acetylcholine. Botulinum toxin type A injections provide effective relief of the excessive, abnormal contractions associated with benign essential blepharospasm and hemifacial spasm. Cosmetic use of botulinum toxin, specifically in the treatment of glabellar folds, has gained popularity as well. Botulinum is approved to treat strabismus, possibly by inducing an atrophic lengthening of the injected muscle and a corresponding shortening of the muscle's antagonist.

Dutton JJ, Fowler AM. Botulinum toxin in ophthalmology. *Focal Points: Clinical Modules for Ophthalmologists.* San Francisco: American Academy of Ophthalmology; 2007, module 3.

Harrison AR. Chemodenervation for facial dystonias and wrinkles. *Curr Opin Ophthalmol.* 2003;14(5):241–245.

Scott AB. Botulinum toxin treatment of strabismus. *Focal Points: Clinical Modules for Ophthalmologists.* San Francisco: American Academy of Ophthalmology; 1989, module 12.

Medications for the Dry Eye

Artificial tear preparations (demulcents) and emollients form an occlusive film over the corneal surface to lubricate and protect the eye from drying. The active ingredients in demulcent preparations are polyvinyl alcohol, cellulose, and methylcellulose and their derivatives: hydroxypropyl cellulose, hydroxyethylcellulose, hydroxypropyl methylcellulose (HPMC), and carboxymethylcellulose. One demulcent is glycerin 0.3% or 1% variously combined with polysorbate 80, HPMC, PEG-400, and dextran 70. Polycarophil is available in combination with dextran 70 and PEG-400. Hydroxypropyl methylcellulose is available alone in 0.3%, 0.2%, and 0.5% solutions, and in formulation with glycerin or dextran 70 or PEG-400, or a combination of these additives. Polyvinyl alcohol may be used alone or with either povidone or a combination of PEG-400 and dextrose. Hydroxypropyl methylcellulose with dextran 70 and propylene glycol with PEG-400 are 2 additional lubricating agents.

The viscosity of artificial tears varies in part due to the concentration of the wetting agent. For example, carboxymethylcellulose is available in 0.25%, 0.5%, and 1% solutions; the increasing viscosity of these solutions is aimed at the increasing severity of dry-eye symptoms.

Multidose preparations contain preservatives, including benzalkonium chloride, EDTA (ethylenediaminetetraacetic acid), methylparaben, polyquad, potassium sorbate, propylparaben, Purite, sodium perborate, and sorbic acid. Although there was significant toxicity with the early preservatives such as thimerosal, the newest generation of ophthalmic preservatives is virtually nontoxic. Unpreserved unit-dose preparations eliminate the cytotoxic effects of preservatives.

Ocular emollients are ointments prepared with sterile petrolatum, liquid lanolin, mineral oil, methylparaben, and polyparaben. Ophthalmic lubricating ointments are useful for easing the symptoms of severe dry eye and exposure keratopathy, as well as for nighttime use in dry eye and nocturnal lagophthalmos.

Kunert KS, Tisdale AS, Gipson IK. Goblet cell numbers and epithelial proliferation in the conjunctiva of patients with dry eye syndrome treated with cyclosporine. *Arch Ophthalmol.* 2002;120(3):330–337. [Erratum appears in *Arch Ophthalmol.* 2002;120(8):1099.]

Kunert KS, Tisdale AS, Stern ME, Smith JA, Gipson IK. Analysis of topical cyclosporine treatment of patients with dry eye syndrome: effect on conjunctival lymphocytes. *Arch Ophthalmol.* 2000;118(11):1489–1496.

Pflugfelder SC. Antiinflammatory therapy for dry eye. *Am J Ophthalmol.* 2004;137(2):337–342.

Small DS, Acheampong A, Reis B, et al. Blood concentrations of cyclosporin A during long-term treatment with cyclosporin A ophthalmic emulsions in patients with moderate to severe dry eye disease. *J Ocul Pharmacol Ther.* 2002;18(5):411–418.

Preservative-free topical cyclosporine emulsion 0.05% (Restasis) has been developed to target the inflammatory etiology of dry eye. Because cyclosporine is poorly water-soluble, it is prepared in a glycerin, castor oil, polysorbate 80 emulsion. Studies have shown that twice-daily dosing with this agent has negligible systemic absorption and side effects. A measurable repopulation of goblet cells and a decrease in conjunctival epithelial cell turnover and the number of lymphocytes have been demonstrated by biopsy. Patients reported a decrease in their subjective dry-eye complaints and had measurable increases in Schirmer wetting at 6 months. The oily vector is marketed separately as the tear supplement Refresh Endura.

Future development of medications for dry eye should be aimed at providing nourishment for the keratoconjunctival surface as well as revitalizing the tear-secreting system. (See also BCSC Section 8, *External Disease and Cornea.*)

Hyperosmolar Agents

Hyperosmolar agents are used to decrease corneal and epithelial edema. One such agent is sodium chloride (Muro 128), which is available without a prescription in a 2% or 5% solution or as an ointment. Products such as these are used for the treatment of corneal edema from Fuchs dystrophy, other causes of endothelial dysfunction, prolonged edema postoperatively, and recurrent erosion syndrome.

Ocular Decongestants

Common agents such as naphazoline, oxymetazoline, tetrahydrozoline, and phenyleph-rine hydrochloride are used as topical drops to cause temporary vasoconstriction of conjunctival vessels. Possible side effects include rebound vasodilation and conjunctival hyperemia. These medications can be abused by patients and can cause ocular surface toxicity. Although they are available as over-the-counter preparations, patients should be instructed not to use them on a chronic basis.

Irrigating Solutions

Sterile isotonic solutions are for general ophthalmic use. Depending on the solution, non-prescription ocular irrigating solutions may contain sodium chloride, potassium chloride, calcium chloride, magnesium chloride, sodium acetate, sodium citrate, boric acid, sodium borate, and sodium phosphate. They are preserved with EDTA, benzalkonium chloride, and sorbic acid. Sterile, physiologically balanced, preservative-free salt solutions (BSS and BSS PLUS) are isotonic to eye tissues and are used for intraocular irrigation during surgical procedures. Glucose glutathione bicarbonate solution (BSS PLUS) has been shown to cause less change in the corneal endothelial morphology postoperatively and to augment the postoperative endothelial pump function. It is not routinely used due to cost concerns, but it may be used in patients who preoperatively are noted to have compromised corneas.

Diagnostic Agents

Fluorescein 2%, lissamine green 1%, and rose bengal, as impregnated paper strips, are examples of solutions commonly used in the examination and diagnosis of external ocular diseases. The first 2 stains outline the defects of the conjunctival and corneal epithelium, whereas the rose bengal indicates abnormal devitalized epithelial cells. For the study of retinal and choroidal circulation as well as abnormal changes in the RPE, sodium fluo-rescein solution in concentrations of 5%, 10%, or 25% is injected intravenously. Fundus fluorescein angiography is helpful in diagnosing various vascular diseases and neoplastic disorders. Fluorescein dye can also be used in anterior segment angiography to demon-strate anterior segment vascular disorders.

Indocyanine green, a tricarbocyanine type of dye, is approved to study choroidal vas-culature in a variety of choroidal and retinal disorders. Typically, 25 mg of dye is injected as IV solution. Indocyanine green angiography is particularly helpful in identifying and delineating poorly defined choroidal neovascular membranes in AMD. Indocyanine green and trypan blue dye are useful in delineating the anterior capsule during phacoemulsifica-tion of mature cataracts. Whereas indocyanine green may be constituted off-label for this use, the FDA has approved trypan blue for use as an anterior capsule stain during surgery.

Matsuda M, Kinoshita S, Ohashi Y, et al. Comparison of the effects of intraocular irrigating solutions on the corneal endothelium in intraocular lens implantation. *Br J Ophthalmol.* 1991;75(8):476–479.

McDermott M, Snyder R, Slack J, Holley G, Edelhauser H. Effects of intraocular irrigants on the preserved human corneal endothelium. *Cornea.* 1991;10(5):402–407.

Saini JS, Jain AK, Sukhija J, Gupta P, Saroha V. Anterior and posterior capsulorhexis in pediatric cataract surgery with or without trypan blue dye: randomized prospective clinical study. *J Cataract Refract Surg.* 2003;29(9):1733–1737.

Werner L, Pandey SK, Escobar-Gomez M, Hoddinott DS, Apple DJ. Dye-enhanced cataract surgery. Part 2: learning critical steps of phacoemulsification. *J Cataract Refract Surg.* 2000;26(7):1060–1065.

Viscoelastic Agents

Viscoelastic agents possess certain chemical and physical properties that include the capacity to resist flow and deformation. Viscoelastics for ophthalmic use must also be inert, isosmotic, sterile, nonpyrogenic, nonantigenic, and optically clear. In addition, they must be sufficiently hydrophilic to allow easy dilution and irrigation from the eye. Naturally occurring and synthetic compounds include sodium hyaluronate, chondroitin sulfate, hydroxypropyl methylcellulose, and polyacrylamide and are available in a variety of concentrations. Combined chondroitin sulfate/sodium hyaluronate materials are also available. Viscoelastic agents protect ocular tissues, such as the corneal endothelium and epithelium, from surgical trauma; help to maintain intraocular space; and facilitate tissue manipulation. Thus, they are indispensable tools in cataract or glaucoma surgery, penetrating keratoplasty, anterior segment reconstruction surgery, and retinal surgery. (See also the discussions of hyaluronic acid and vitreous collagen cross-linking in Chapter 12 of this volume and BCSC Section 11, *Lens and Cataract.*)

Fibrinolytic Agents

Tissue plasminogen activator (tPA), urokinase, and streptokinase are all fibrinolytic agents. tPA is a naturally occurring serine protease with a molecular mass of 68 kD. Because tPA is normally present at a higher concentration in the aqueous humor of the human eye than it is in blood, it is less toxic to ocular tissues and is specific for dissolution of fibrin clots. tPA has been used successfully in the resolution of fibrin clots after vitrectomy, keratoplasty, and glaucoma filtering procedures. These drugs are not approved by the FDA for ocular use and are therefore used with an off-label application.

Tripathi RC, Tripathi BJ, Park JK, et al. Intracameral tissue plasminogen activator for resolution of fibrin clots after glaucoma filtering procedures. *Am J Ophthalmol.* 1991;111(2):247–248.

Thrombin

Thrombin, a sterile protein substance, is approved to control hemorrhage from accessible capillaries and small venules, as would be seen with standard surface incisions. Its use in maintaining hemostasis during complicated intraocular surgery is off-label, as this requires injection. Intravitreal thrombin has been used to control intraocular hemorrhage during vitrectomy. The addition of thrombin (100 units/mL) to the vitrectomy infusate significantly shortens intraocular bleeding time, and thrombin produced by DNA recombinant techniques minimizes the degree of postoperative inflammation. Thrombin causes significant ultrastructural corneal endothelial changes when human corneas are perfused with 1000 units/mL.

Antifibrinolytic Agents

Antifibrinolytic agents, such as ε-aminocaproic acid and tranexamic acid, inhibit the activation of plasminogen. These agents may be used systemically to treat cases of hemorrhage secondary to excessive fibrinolysis and to prevent recurrent hyphema, which most commonly occurs 2–6 days after the original hemorrhage. They are contraindicated in the presence of active intravascular clotting, such as diffuse intravascular coagulation (DIC), as they can increase the tendency for thrombosis. They should not be used in pregnancy, in patients with coagulopathies or on platelet inhibition therapy, or in patients with renal or hepatic disease. Patients with larger hyphemas and those with delayed presentation are at a higher risk for rebleeding, but patients with early presentation and those with smaller hyphemas are at a low risk for rebleeding. The use of ε-aminocaproic acid is usually reserved for patients at a higher risk of rebleeding.

ε-Aminocaproic acid is used in a dosage of 50–100 mg/kg every 4 hours, up to 30 g daily. Possible adverse reactions include nausea, vomiting, muscle cramps, conjunctival suffusion, nasal congestion, headache, rash, pruritus, dyspnea, tonic toxic confusional states, cardiac arrhythmias, and systemic hypotension. Gastrointestinal side effects are similar with doses of either 50 or 100 mg/kg. The drug should be continued for a full 5–6 days to achieve maximal clinical effectiveness. Topical ε-aminocaproic acid may be an attractive alternative to systemic delivery in the treatment of traumatic hyphema, but the efficacy of topical treatment has been questioned. Optimal topical concentration to maximize aqueous levels and minimize corneal epithelial toxicity is 30% ε-aminocaproic acid in 2% carboxypolymethylene.

Tranexamic acid (Cyklokapron) is another antifibrinolytic agent used off-label to reduce the incidence of rebleeding after traumatic hyphema. It is 10 times more potent in vitro than is ε-aminocaproic acid. The usual dosage is 25 mg of tranexamic acid/kg 3 times daily for 3–5 days. Gastrointestinal side effects are rare.

Karkhaneh R, Naeeni M, Chams H, Abdollahi M, Mansouri MR. Topical aminocaproic acid to prevent rebleeding in cases of traumatic hyphema. *Eur J Ophthalmol.* 2003;13(1):57–61.

Shiuey Y, Lucarelli MJ. Traumatic hyphema: outcomes of outpatient management. *Ophthalmology.* 1998;105(5):851–855.

Corneal Storage Medium

The corneal storage medium helps to prolong the viability of donor corneas to be used for transplantation. The main components of the various kinds of media include a bicarbonate-buffered minimum essential medium (MEM) or a hybrid medium of MEM/TC 199, chondroitin sulfate, and dextran (to retard proteoglycan loss during storage and reduce intraoperative and postoperative rebound swelling), as well as gentamicin sulfate or other antibiotics used as prophylactic agents. Corneal tissue storage can be prolonged with the addition of recombinant growth factors such as epidermal growth factor and with antioxidants, insulin, adenosine triphosphate precursors, anticollagenases, and antiproteases.

Vitamin Supplements and Antioxidants

Nonprescription vitamin supplements have enjoyed increased popularity because of their antioxidant properties and are used for intermediate-to-severe AMD. The Age-Related Eye Disease Study (AREDS) is discussed in depth in BCSC Section 12, *Retina and Vitreous.*

Interferon

A naturally occurring species-specific defense against viruses, interferon is synthesized intracellularly and increases resistance to virus infection. Synthetic analogues such as polyinosinic acid–polycytidylic acid have been used to induce patients to form their own interferon.

Topically administered interferon has been found to be ineffective in the treatment of epidemic keratoconjunctivitis caused by adenovirus. In herpes simplex keratitis patients, however, interferon used in conjunction with acyclovir showed significantly quicker healing time than treatment with acyclovir alone (5.8 vs 9.0 days). Interferon has also been found to speed the healing of an epithelial defect when used in combination with trifluridine. The dosage of interferon (30 million IU/mL) was 2 drops per day for the first 3 days of treatment. Interferon alone has little effect on the treatment of herpes simplex keratitis. In combination, however, it seems to act as a topical adjuvant to traditional antiviral therapy in resistant herpes simplex keratitis.

Interferon has also been shown to inhibit vascular endothelial cell proliferation and differentiation. It is particularly effective in the treatment of juvenile pulmonary hemangiomatosis, which used to be a fatal condition before the development of interferon. Intralesional administration of interferon has been reported to be especially effective in ocular Kaposi sarcoma.

Growth Factors

Growth factors are a diverse group of proteins that act at autocrine and paracrine levels to affect various cellular processes, including metabolic regulation, tissue differentiation, cell growth and proliferation, maintenance of viability, and changes in cell morphology.

The growth factors are synthesized in a variety of cells and have a spectrum of target cells and tissues. Various growth factors have been found in retina, vitreous humor, aqueous humor, and corneal tissues. These include

- epidermal growth factor
- fibroblast growth factors

- transforming growth factor βs
- vascular endothelial growth factor
- insulin-like growth factors

These growth factors are capable of diverse, synergistic, and sometimes antagonistic biologic activities.

Under normal physiologic conditions, the complex and delicate coordination of the effects of and the interactions among growth factors maintains the homeostasis of intraocular tissues. The net effect of a growth factor depends on its bioavailability, which is determined by its concentration, its binding to carrier proteins, the level of its receptor in the target tissue, and the presence of other complementary or antagonistic regulatory factors.

Pathologically, the breakdown of blood–ocular barriers disrupts the balance among growth factors in the ocular media and tissues and may result in various abnormalities. The disruption in the balance among isoforms of transforming growth factor βs, basic fibroblast growth factor, vascular endothelial growth factor, and insulin-like growth factors is suspected to cause ocular neovascularization. Transforming growth factor βs and platelet-derived growth factor are implicated in the pathogenesis of proliferative vitreoretinopathy and in the excessive proliferation of Tenon capsule fibroblasts, which can result in the scarring of the glaucoma filtration bleb. Increased concentrations of insulin-like growth factors in plasmoid aqueous humor may be responsible for the abnormal hyperplastic response of the lens epithelium and corneal endothelium seen in inflammatory conditions and in traumatic insults to the eye.

Identifying growth factors and understanding their mechanisms of action in the eye offer great potential for providing the ophthalmologist with new methods for manipulation of and intervention in ocular disorders. Epidermal growth factor and fibroblast growth factor can accelerate corneal wound repair after surgery, chemical burns, or ulcers and can increase the number of corneal endothelial cells. Fibroblast growth factor has also been shown to delay the process of retinal dystrophy in Royal College of Surgeons rats.

Vascular endothelial growth factor (VEGF), also known as vasculotropin, deserves special mention. It is a dimeric, heparin-binding polypeptide mitogen and has 4 isoforms that are generated from alternative splicing of mRNA. The VEGF gene is widely expressed in actively proliferating vascular tissue and is implicated in the pathogenesis of various neovascular retinopathies such as diabetes mellitus and age-related choroidal neovascularization (CNV).

Intravitreal injections of VEGF inhibitors are used in the treatment of wet macular degeneration. Patients with CNV who have been treated with anti-VEGF have shown a slower loss of vision, especially moderate (>3 lines of vision lost) to severe vision loss (>6 lines lost) and, in some cases, an improvement in vision. Pegaptanib (Macugen), the first approved agent, requires intravitreal injections every 6 weeks for up to 2 years and shows a decrease in efficacy in the second year of treatment. Subsequent agents have largely supplanted pegaptanib. Ranibizumab (Lucentis) is approved, and bevacizumab (Avastin) is being used off-label, for the treatment of wet age-related macular degeneration.

Ranibizumab is given as an intravitreal injection of 0.5 mg (0.05 mL) monthly, with a possible decrease to every 3 months after 4 injections.

Bartlett JD, Jaanus SD, eds. *Clinical Ocular Pharmacology.* 5th ed. St Louis: Butterworth-Heinemann/Elsevier; 2008.

Brunton LL, Lazo JS, Parker KL, eds. *Goodman & Gilman's the Pharmacological Basis of Therapeutics: Digital Edition.* 11th ed. New York: McGraw-Hill; 2006.

Eyetech Study Group. Anti-vascular endothelial growth factor therapy for subfoveal choroidal neovascularization secondary to age-related macular degeneration: phase II study results. *Ophthalmology.* 2003;110(5):979–986.

Fraunfelder FT, Fraunfelder FW. *Drug-Induced Ocular Side Effects.* 5th ed. Boston: Butterworth-Heinemann; 2001.

Krzystolik MG, Afshari MA, Adamis AP, et al. Prevention of experimental choroidal neovascularization with intravitreal anti-vascular endothelial growth factor antibody fragment. *Arch Ophthalmol.* 2002;120(3):338–346.

Micromedex® Healthcare Series. n.d. Thomson Micromedex, Greenwood Village, CO. http://www.thomsonhc.com. Accessed 24 January 2006.

Murray L. *Drug Topics Red Book Update.* Montvale, NJ: Thomson PDR; 2007.

Murray L, ed. *Physicians' Desk Reference.* 58th ed. Montvale, NJ: Thomson PDR; 2004.

Physicians' Desk Reference for Ophthalmic Medicines. 35th ed. Montvale, NJ: Thomson PDR; 2007.

U.S. Food and Drug Administration. Drugs@FDA: FDA Approved Drug Products. 2007. Available at: http://www.accessdata.fda.gov/scripts/cder/drugsatfda/. Accessed September 2007.

The authors would like to thank Joan Murhammer, RPh, from the Drug Information Center at the University of Iowa Hospitals and Clinics for her invaluable assistance in updating the information on available medications marketed in the United States.

Basic Texts

Anatomy

Beard C, Quickert MH. *Anatomy of the Orbit: A Dissection Manual*. 3rd ed. Birmingham, AL: Aesculapius; 1988.

Bron AJ, Tripathi RC, Tripathi BJ, eds. *Wolff's Anatomy of the Eye and Orbit*. 8th ed. London: Chapman & Hall; 1997.

Duke-Elder S, Wybar KC, eds. *The Anatomy of the Visual System*. St Louis: Mosby; 1976. *System of Ophthalmology*; vol 2.

Dutton JJ. *Atlas of Clinical and Surgical Orbital Anatomy*. Philadelphia: Saunders; 1994.

Fine BS, Yanoff M. *Ocular Histology: A Text and Atlas*. 2nd ed. Hagerstown, MD: Harper & Row; 1979.

Hogan MJ, Alvarado JA, Weddell JE. *Histology of the Human Eye: An Atlas and Textbook*. Philadelphia: Saunders; 1971.

Miller NR, Newman NJ, Biousse V, Kerrison JB, eds. *Walsh and Hoyt's Clinical Neuro-Ophthalmology*. 6th ed. Philadelphia: Lippincott Williams & Wilkins; 2004.

Snell RS, Lemp MA. *Clinical Anatomy of the Eye*. 2nd ed. Malden, MA: Wiley-Blackwell; 1998.

Tasman W, Jaeger EA, eds. *Duane's Ophthalmology*. Philadelphia: Lippincott Williams & Wilkins; 2007.

Zide BM, ed. *Surgical Anatomy Around the Orbit: The System of Zones*. Philadelphia: Lippincott Williams & Wilkens; 2006.

Zide BM, Jelks GW, eds. *Surgical Anatomy of the Orbit*. New York: Raven Press; 1985.

Embryology

Jakobiec FA, ed. *Ocular Anatomy, Embryology, and Teratology*. Philadelphia: Harper & Row; 1982.

O'Rahilly R, Müller F. *Human Embryology and Teratology*. 3rd ed. New York: Wiley-Liss; 2001.

Genetics

Merin S. *Inherited Eye Diseases: Diagnosis and Management*. 2nd ed. Boca Raton, FL: Taylor & Francis; 2005.

Nussbaum RL, McInnes RR, Huntington FW. *Thompson & Thompson Genetics in Medicine*. 7th ed. Philadelphia: Elsevier/Saunders; 2007.

Traboulsi EI, ed. *Genetic Diseases of the Eye*. New York: Oxford University Press; 1998.

Biochemistry and Metabolism

Berman ER. *Biochemistry of the Eye.* Perspectives in Vision Research. New York: Springer; 1991.

Kaufman PL, Alm A, eds. *Adler's Physiology of the Eye.* 10th ed. Philadelphia: Elsevier/ Mosby; 2003.

Tombran-Tink J, Barnstable CJ. *Retinal Degenerations: Biology, Diagnostics, and Therapeutics.* Totowa, NJ: Humana Press; 2007.

Ocular Pharmacology

Brunton LL, ed. *Goodman and Gilman's The Pharmacological Basis of Therapeutics.* 11th ed. New York: McGraw-Hill; 2006.

Bartlett JD, Jaanus SD, eds. *Clinical Ocular Pharmacology.* 5th ed. St Louis: Elsevier/ Butterworth-Heinemann; 2008.

Zimmerman TJ, Karanjit K, Mordechaie S, Fechtner RD, eds. *Textbook of Ocular Pharmacology.* 3rd ed. Philadelphia: Lippincott Williams & Wilkins; 1997.

Related Academy Materials

Focal Points: Clinical Modules for Ophthalmologists

For information on Focal Points modules, go to http://one.aao.org/CE/Educational Products/FocalPoints.aspx.

Ahmed M, Foster CS. Steroid therapy for ocular inflammatory disease (Module 7, 2006).

Hertle RW, Kowal LM, Yeates KO. The ophthalmologist and learning disabilities (Module 2, 2005).

Oester A, Baffi JZ, Balamurali BK. Pharmacotherapy targeting ocular neovascularization (Module 7, 2008).

Sheth BP. Drugs and pregnancy (Module 7, 2007).

Stead SW, Bell SN. Ocular anesthesia (Module 3, 2001).

Wygnanski-Jaffe T, Levin AV. Introductory genetics for the ophthalmologist (Module 5, 2005).

Print Publications

Arnold AC, ed. *Basic Principles of Ophthalmic Surgery* (2006).

Jordan DR, Anderson RA. *Surgical Anatomy of the Ocular Adnexa: A Clinical Approach.* Ophthalmology Monograph 9 (1996).

Parke DW II, ed. *The Profession of Ophthalmology: Practice Management, Ethics, and Advocacy* (2005).

Rockwood EJ, ed. *ProVision: Preferred Responses in Ophthalmology.* Series 4. Self-Assessment Program (2007).

Traboulsi EI. *A Compendium of Inherited Disorders and the Eye.* Ophthalmology Monograph 18. Published by Oxford University Press, in cooperation with the American Academy of Ophthalmology (2005).

Wilson FM II, ed. *Practical Ophthalmology: A Manual for Beginning Residents.* 5th ed. (2005).

Online Materials

For Preferred Practice Patterns and Complementary Therapy Assessments, go to http://one.aao.org/CE/PracticeGuidelines/default.aspx.

Basic and Clinical Science Course (Sections 1–13); http://one.aao.org/CE/Educational Products/BCSC.aspx

Clinical Education Cases; http://one.aao.org/CE/EducationalContent/Cases.aspx

Clinical Education and Ethics Courses; http://one.aao.org/CE/EducationalContent/Courses.aspx

Focal Points modules; http://one.aao.org/CE/EducationalProducts/FocalPoints.aspx

Maintenance of Certification Exam Study Kit, version 2.0 (2007); http://one.aao.org/CE/MOC/default.aspx

Rockwood EJ, ed. *ProVision: Preferred Responses in Ophthalmology.* Series 4. Self-Assessment Program, 2-vol set (2007); http://one.aao.org/CE/EducationalProducts/Provision.aspx

Preferred Practice Patterns

Preferred Practice Patterns are available at http://one.aao.org/CE/PracticeGuidelines/PPP.aspx.

Preferred Practice Patterns Committee. *Comprehensive Adult Medical Eye Evaluation* (2005).

Preferred Practice Patterns Committee, Pediatric Ophthalmology/Strabismus Panel. *Pediatric Eye Evaluations* (2007).

Preferred Practice Patterns Committee. *Summary Benchmarks for Preferred Practice Patterns* (2008).

Complementary Therapy Assessments

Complementary Therapy Assessments are available at http://one.aao.org/CE/PracticeGuidelines/Therapy.aspx.

Complementary Therapy Task Force. *Acupuncture for Ocular Conditions and Headaches* (2003).

Complementary Therapy Task Force. *Antioxidant Supplements and Age-Related Macular Degeneration* (2002).

Complementary Therapy Task Force. *Antioxidant Vitamin and Mineral Supplements and Cataract Prevention and Progression* (2002).

Complementary Therapy Task Force. *Ginkgo Biloba Extract and Ocular Conditions* (2002).

Complementary Therapy Task Force. *Marijuana in the Treatment of Glaucoma* (2003).

Complementary Therapy Task Force. *Nutritional Supplements: Perioperative Implications for Eye Surgery* (2003).

Complementary Therapy Task Force. *Vision Therapy for Learning Disabilities* (2001).

CDs/DVDs

Basic and Clinical Science Course (Sections 1–13) (CD-ROM, 2009).

Guyton DL. *Retinoscopy and Subjective Refraction* (DVD; reviewed for currency 2007).

Movaghar M, Lawrence MG. *Eye Exam: The Essentials.* From *The Eye Exam and Basic Ophthalmic Instruments* (DVD, 2004; reviewed for currency 2007).

Tang R. *Ocular Manifestations of Systemic Disease.* From *Eye Care Skills: Presentations for Physicians and Other Health Care Professionals* (CD-ROM; reviewed for currency 2005).

To order any of these materials, please order online at www.aao.org/store or call the Academy's Customer Service toll-free number 866-561-8558 in the U.S. If outside the U.S., call 415-561-8540 between 8:00 AM and 5:00 PM PST.

Credit Reporting Form

Basic and Clinical Science Course, 2011–2012
Section 2

The American Academy of Ophthalmology is accredited by the Accreditation Council for Continuing Medical Education to provide continuing medical education for physicians.

The American Academy of Ophthalmology designates this enduring material for a maximum of 15 *AMA PRA Category 1 Credits™*. Physicians should claim only credit commensurate with the extent of their participation in the activity.

If you wish to claim continuing medical education credit for your study of this Section, you may claim your credit online or fill in the required forms and mail or fax them to the Academy.

To use the forms:

1. Complete the study questions and mark your answers on the Section Completion Form.
2. Complete the Section Evaluation.
3. Fill in and sign the statement below.
4. Return this page and the required forms by mail or fax to the CME Registrar (see below).

To claim credit online:

1. Log on to the Academy website (www.aao.org/cme).
2. Select Review/Claim CME.
3. Follow the instructions.

Important: These completed forms or the online claim must be received at the Academy by June 2013.

I hereby certify that I have spent _____ (up to 15) hours of study on the curriculum of this Section and that I have completed the study questions.

Signature: _____
                                                                        Date

Name: _____

Address: _____

City and State: _____   Zip: _____

Telephone: (_____) _____   Academy Member ID# _____
             area code

Please return completed forms to: **Or you may fax them to:** 415-561-8575
American Academy of Ophthalmology
P.O. Box 7424
San Francisco, CA 94120-7424
Attn: CME Registrar, Customer Service

2011–2012
Section Completion Form

Basic and Clinical Science Course

Answer Sheet for Section 2

Question	Answer	Question	Answer	Question	Answer
1	a b c d	19	a b c d	37	a b c d
2	a b c d	20	a b c d	38	a b c d
3	a b c d	21	a b c d	39	a b c d
4	a b c d	22	a b c d	40	a b c d
5	a b c d	23	a b c d	41	a b c d
6	a b c d	24	a b c d	42	a b c d
7	a b c d	25	a b c d	43	a b c d
8	a b c d	26	a b c d	44	a b c d e
9	a b c d	27	a b c d	45	a b c d
10	a b c d	28	a b c d	46	a b c d
11	a b c d	29	a b c d	47	a b c d
12	a b c d	30	a b c d		
13	a b c d	31	a b c d		
14	a b c d	32	a b c d e		
15	a b c d	33	a b c d		
16	a b c d	34	a b c d		
17	a b c d	35	a b c d		
18	a b c d	36	a b c d		

Section Evaluation

Please complete this CME questionnaire.

1. To what degree will you use knowledge from BCSC Section 2 in your practice?

   ☐ Regularly

   ☐ Sometimes

   ☐ Rarely

2. Please review the stated objectives for BCSC Section 2. How effective was the material at meeting those objectives?

   ☐ All objectives were met.

   ☐ Most objectives were met.

   ☐ Some objectives were met.

   ☐ Few or no objectives were met.

3. To what degree is BCSC Section 2 likely to have a positive impact on health outcomes of your patients?

   ☐ Extremely likely

   ☐ Highly likely

   ☐ Somewhat likely

   ☐ Not at all likely

4. After you review the stated objectives for BCSC Section 2, please let us know of any additional knowledge, skills, or information useful to your practice that were acquired but were not included in the objectives.

5. Was BCSC Section 2 free of commercial bias?

   ☐ Yes

   ☐ No

6. If you selected "No" in the previous question, please comment.

7. Please tell us what might improve the applicability of BCSC to your practice.

Study Questions

Although a concerted effort has been made to avoid ambiguity and redundancy in these questions, the authors recognize that differences of opinion may occur regarding the "best" answer. The discussions are provided to demonstrate the rationale used to derive the answer. They may also be helpful in confirming that your approach to the problem was correct or, if necessary, in fixing the principle in your memory.

1. Which bone is not part of the orbital floor?
   a. maxilla
   b. palatine
   c. greater wing of the sphenoid
   d. zygomatic

2. Which structure does not pass through the annulus of Zinn?
   a. superior division of cranial nerve III
   b. cranial nerve IV
   c. nasociliary branch of cranial nerve V (V_1)
   d. optic nerve

3. Which extraocular muscle originates from the annulus of Zinn?
   a. levator palpebrae superioris
   b. superior oblique
   c. lateral rectus
   d. inferior oblique

4. Which of the rectus muscles inserts closest to the limbus?
   a. lateral rectus
   b. medial rectus
   c. superior rectus
   d. inferior rectus

5. Regarding the stratified layers of the neurosensory retina, which is a true membrane?
   a. external limiting membrane
   b. internal limiting membrane
   c. inner plexiform layer
   d. None of the above are true membranes.

6. The air–tear interface at the surface of the cornea is responsible for approximately what percentage of the refractive power of the human eye?
   a. 25%
   b. 33%
   c. 50%
   d. 66%

7. Which of the following structures is not part of the uveal tract of the eye?

   a. iris

   b. ciliary body

   c. choroid

   d. neurosensory retina

8. Which of the following cranial nerves exits from the dorsal aspect of the midbrain?

   a. CN III (oculomotor)

   b. CN IV (trochlear)

   c. CN V (trigeminal)

   d. CN VI (abducens)

9. The optic nerve averages what total length?

   a. 10 mm

   b. 20 mm

   c. 40 mm

   d. 80 mm

10. An expanding lesion of the cavernous sinus is least likely to affect which of the following?

   a. internal carotid artery

   b. cranial nerve III

   c. ophthalmic division of cranial nerve V (V_1)

   d. mandibular division of cranial nerve V (V_3)

11. Aneurysms that affect the oculomotor nerve (CN III) commonly occur at the junction of which 2 arteries?

   a. internal and external carotid arteries

   b. anterior cerebral and anterior communicating arteries

   c. basilar and posterior cerebral arteries

   d. posterior communicating and internal carotid arteries

12. The human lens is derived from which embryonic tissue?

   a. neuroectoderm

   b. neural crest cells

   c. surface ectoderm

   d. mesoderm

13. All of the following structures include neural crest cell–derived tissue except:

   a. trabecular meshwork

   b. iris stroma

   c. ciliary epithelium

   d. corneal endothelium

14. Which is not true of homeobox genes?

    a. They are about 180 base pairs long.

    b. They control the activity of subordinate genes.

    c. They are found only in mammals.

    d. The *PAX6* gene is a homeobox gene that appears to be a master control gene for the development of the eye.

15. Which of the following disorders is not associated with a defect in a mitochondrial gene?

    a. Leber hereditary optic neuropathy (LHON)

    b. chronic progressive external ophthalmoplegia (CPEO)

    c. neuropathy, ataxia, and retinitis pigmentosa (NARP)

    d. retinoblastoma

16. Which of the following is not correct about retinoblastoma?

    a. It may be associated with chromosome 13 long arm (13q14) deletion syndrome.

    b. It affects between 1 and 15,000–34,000 live births in the United States.

    c. Approximately 50% of patients with hereditary retinoblastoma have a family history of the disease.

    d. The hereditary pattern of familial retinoblastoma is autosomal dominant, but the defect is autosomal recessive at a cellular level.

17. A certain ocular disorder is found to occur more often in males than females, but affected males do not transmit the disorder. However, virtually every son and daughter of an affected female inherits the trait. What is the most likely mode of inheritance of this disorder?

    a. autosomal dominant

    b. autosomal recessive

    c. X-linked recessive

    d. mitochondrial

18. Mutations in the rhodopsin gene are associated with which inherited ocular disease?

    a. juvenile glaucoma

    b. Leber optic neuropathy

    c. retinitis pigmentosa

    d. Stargardt disease

19. Mitochondrial inheritance is based on which of the following?

    a. paternal mitochondria

    b. maternal mitochondria

    c. acquired mitochondria

    d. de novo mitochondria

20. Linkage analysis is a method that determines which of the following?

    a. paternity

    b. type of inheritance

    c. how often a medication should be given

    d. the proximity of 1 gene to another

21. Many of the genes encoded in the mitochondrial genome are important for which of the following processes?

    a. cell motility

    b. proteasomal degradation

    c. energy metabolism

    d. autophagy

22. *PAX6* mutations are associated with

    a. aniridia

    b. optic nerve hypoplasia

    c. renal hypoplasia

    d. corneal granular dystrophy

23. Which of the following pairs accurately describes the cell type that makes the tear-layer component?

    a. goblet cells—lipid layer

    b. meibomian glands—mucin layer

    c. gland of Krause—aqueous layer

    d. gland of Wolfring—mucin layer

24. Which of the following immunoglobulins is found in the tear film?

    a. IgA

    b. IgM

    c. IgE

    d. IgD

25. Which of the following is a true basement membrane?

    a. Bowman's layer

    b. zonule of Zinn

    c. Descemet's membrane

    d. anterior border layer of iris

26. Descemet's membrane is principally made from

    a. type I collagen

    b. type II collagen

    c. type III collagen

    d. type IV collagen

27. The main corneal mechanism for holding the LASIK flap in place after surgery is
    a. endothelial–Descemet's membrane interaction
    b. endothelial pump
    c. Bowman's layer–stromal adhesions
    d. stromal collagen adhesions

28. Which of the following lens proteins is not found in the human lens?
    a. α-crystallin
    b. β-crystallin
    c. γ-crystallin
    d. ε-crystallin

29. Photoreceptor cones have 1 of 3 visual pigments, with absorptive maxima of 570 nm, 540 nm, and 440 nm. Which of these would absorb blue light the most?
    a. 570 nm
    b. 540 nm
    c. 440 nm
    d. none of the above

30. Cone density is greatest in which area of the retina?
    a. macula
    b. peripapillary region
    c. arcuate regions
    d. peripheral retina

31. Which vitamin is most critical for the photoreceptor response to light?
    a. A
    b. B
    c. C
    d. D

32. Pharmacologic principles apply differently to the elderly because
    a. hepatic perfusion and enzymatic activity increase with age
    b. renal function decreases with age
    c. the elderly have more albumin relative to weight
    d. the elderly have more body water relative to weight
    e. the elderly have less body fat relative to weight

33. Clinical effects of direct-acting muscarinic agents (miotics) include all *except* which of the following?
    a. increased myopia
    b. decreased range of accommodation
    c. central anterior chamber shallowing
    d. reduced night vision

34. Which of the following is a direct-acting cholinergic agent?
    a. pilocarpine (Isopto Carpine, Pilocar, Pilostat)
    b. echothiophate iodide (Phospholine Iodide)
    c. physostigmine (Eserine Salicylate)
    d. demecarium bromide (Humorsol)

35. Which of the following statements is correct about cocaine?
    a. It directly stimulates adrenergic receptors.
    b. It directly stimulates muscarinic receptors.
    c. It blocks re-uptake of norepinephrine.
    d. It blocks adrenergic receptors.

36. Systemic side effects of oral carbonic anhydrase inhibitors include all *except* which of the following?
    a. paresthesias
    b. weight loss
    c. hyperkalemia
    d. metabolic alkalosis

37. Which of the following is not a mast-cell stabilizer or antihistamine?
    a. lodoxamide tromethamine (Alomide)
    b. cromolyn sodium (Crolom)
    c. olopatadine hydrochloride (Patanol)
    d. ketorolac tromethamine (Acular)

38. Antiviral agents include all *except* which of the following?
    a. trifluridine (Viroptic)
    b. amphotericin B
    c. vidarabine
    d. acyclovir

39. Which of the following local/regional anesthetic agents has the longest duration of effect?
    a. lidocaine
    b. procaine
    c. bupivacaine
    d. mepivacaine

40. A retrobulbar anesthetic is least likely to produce anesthesia of cranial nerve
    a. II
    b. III
    c. IV
    d. VI

41. Factors that influence drug penetration of the cornea include all of the following *except:*

    a. concentration

    b. drop volume

    c. pH

    d. vehicle

42. Which of the following statements about drug penetration is correct?

    a. Drugs with a higher percentage of charged molecules, or ionic forms, penetrate more rapidly.

    b. Drugs with higher lipid solubility have better penetration of cell membranes.

    c. Preserved medication has a decreased ocular penetration and may require a higher concentration of the active drug.

    d. Most drugs obtain a higher ocular penetration in ointment form than in solution.

43. Timolol 0.5% has how many milligrams (mg) per drop, given 20 drops per milliliter (mL)?

    a. 1 mg

    b. 0.75 mg

    c. 0.50 mg

    d. 0.25 mg

44. Which of the following series correctly depicts the relative duration of drug action?

    a. atropine>homatropine>scopolamine>cyclopentolate>tropicamide

    b. atropine>scopolamine>homatropine>cyclopentolate>tropicamide

    c. cyclopentolate>tropicamide>scopolamine>homatropine>atropine

    d. homatropine>cyclopentolate>tropicamide>scopolamine>atropine

    e. homatropine>atropine>scopolamine>cyclopentolate>tropicamide

45. Which of the following agents are associated with corneal complications, including melting and corneal perforations?

    a. topical alpha agonists

    b. topical steroids

    c. topical carbonic anhydrase inhibitors

    d. topical nonsteroidal anti-inflammatory drugs

46. Which of the following is a potential side effect of tetracyclines?

    a. depression of prothrombin

    b. inhibition of bactericidal antibiotics

    c. decreased efficacy of oral contraceptives

    d. all of the above

47. Which of the following is the only agent to have a significant effect on postsurgical endophthalmitis?

    a. preoperative preparation of the eye with topical povidone-iodine

    b. intracameral vancomycin

    c. intracameral aminoglycosides

    d. subconjunctival fluoroquinolones

Answers

1. **c.** The greater wing of the sphenoid is part of the lateral wall of the orbit.

2. **d.** Cranial nerve IV passes through the superior orbital fissure but not through the annulus of Zinn.

3. **c.** The lateral rectus. The superior, inferior, medial, and lateral recti muscles all arise from the annulus of Zinn.

4. **b.** The 4 recti muscle insertions form the spiral of Tillaux, with the medial rectus inserting closest to the limbus, at 5.5 mm, and the superior rectus most distal from the limbus, at 7.7 mm.

5. **d.** None of the above. The inner and outer limiting membranes are not true membranes.

6. **d.** The adult human eye has a focusing power of approximately 60 diopters (60 D). The air–tear interface of the cornea is responsible for approximately 40 D, and the lens contributes approximately 20 D of power.

7. **d.** The neurosensory retina. The uveal tract is the main vascular compartment of the eye and consists of the iris, ciliary body, and choroid.

8. **b.** Cranial nerve IV exits from the dorsal midbrain. It also has the longest intracranial course of any cranial nerve, approximately 75 mm.

9. **c.** 40 mm. The intraorbital portion averages 25 mm in length; however, the total nerve also consists of intraocular, intracanalicular, and intracranial portions.

10. **d.** The mandibular division of cranial nerve V (V_3) does not pass through the cavernous sinus.

11. **d.** Aneurysms at the junction of the posterior communicating and internal carotid arteries may affect CN III (oculomotor).

12. **c.** Surface ectoderm. One of the earliest events of embryogenesis is the determination of lens development. The underlying mesoderm signals a region of surface ectoderm to become the lens. The lens becomes apparent by 27 days' gestation.

13. **c.** Ciliary epithelium is derived from the optic cup, which is an extension of the forebrain.

14. **c.** Homeobox genes are found across the entire plant and animal kingdom.

15. **d.** The hereditary pattern in familial retinoblastoma is autosomal dominant. The other 3 conditions appear to be a result of a defect in mitochondrial genes.

16. **c.** Only about 10% of patients with hereditary retinoblastoma have a family history of the disease. The remaining 90% appear to have a new mutation in their germ cells.

17. **d.** The inheritance pattern of mitochondrial disease might superficially resemble that of an X-linked trait. Maternal transmission, however, differs from X-linked inheritance in that all the offspring of affected females (both daughters and sons) can inherit the trait but only daughters can pass it on.

18. **c.** More than 70 different mutations are known to cause retinitis pigmentosa.

19. **b.** A significant number of disorders associated with the eye or visual system involve mitochondrial deletions or mutations. Mitochondrial disease should be considered whenever the inheritance pattern of a trait suggests maternal transmission.

20. **d.** Linkage is the major exception or modification to the law of independent assortment. Nonallelic genes located reasonably close together on the same chromosome tend to be transmitted together more frequently than by chance alone; thus, they are said to be linked.

21. **c.** Mitochondrial genes are important in the production of peptides, which are involved in the mitochondrial respiratory chain and ATP synthase.

22. **a.** A *PAX6* mutation is associated with aniridia.

23. **c.** Goblet cells make the mucin layer and meibomian glands make the lipid layer. Glands of Krause and Wolfring produce the aqueous layer.

24. **a.** IgA and IgG are found in the tear film.

25. **c.** Descemet's membrane is a true basement membrane produced by the corneal endothelium.

26. **d.** Descemet's membrane is a 10-μm-thick basement membrane between the endothelium and posterior corneal stroma. Type IV collagen is the most abundant collagen in Descemet's membrane. Type I collagen, however, is the major collagen component of the corneal stroma.

27. **b.** The endothelial pump is responsible for generating the negative hydrostatic pressure that is necessary for holding the LASIK flap in place after surgery.

28. **d.** ε-Crystallin is a taxon-specific crystallin, which is found only in a phylogenetically restricted group of species.

29. **c.** Blue light is predominantly absorbed by cones that absorb the shorter wavelengths (ie, 440 nm).

30. **a.** Cone photoreceptor density is greatest in the macular region of the retina.

31. **a.** Vitamin A, a metabolic precursor of 11-*cis*-retinaldehyde, is most necessary for the light-induced photoreceptor response.

32. **b.** Compared with younger patients, older patients have less lean body mass due to a decrease in muscle bulk, less body water and albumin, and an increase in relative adipose tissue. These physiologic differences alter tissue binding and drug distribution. Human renal function decreases with age. Hepatic perfusion and enzymatic activity are also affected by age.

33. **b.** Miotic agents constrict the pupillary sphincter and the ciliary muscle. Increasing myopia and decreased central anterior chamber are a result of ciliary muscle contraction. Pupillary constriction causes decreased night vision but increases the range of accommodation (pinhole effect).

34. **a.** In this list, pilocarpine (Isopto Carpine, Pilocar, Pilostat) is the only direct-acting cholinergic agent.

35. **c.** Cocaine blocks re-uptake of norepinephrine at adrenergic receptor terminals. This increases the adrenergic response but does not directly stimulate or block receptor response.

36. **d.** Oral carbonic anhydrase inhibitors can have many systemic side effects, one being a systemic metabolic acidosis, not alkalosis.

37. **d.** Ketorolac tromethamine (Acular) is a nonsteroidal anti-inflammatory agent. Each of the others is a mast-cell stabilizer and an antihistamine, or they combine the effects of both.

38. **b.** Amphotericin B is an antifungal agent.

39. **c.** Bupivacaine has the longest duration of effect (8–12 hours) of the local/regional agents listed.

40. **c.** The fourth cranial nerve (CN IV) is located outside the muscle cone in the orbit and is least likely to be affected by injection of retrobulbar anesthetics.

41. **b.** When a 50-μL drop is delivered from the usual commercial dispenser, the volume of the tear lake rises from 7 μL to only 10 μL in the blinking eye of an upright patient. Thus, changing the volume of the drop does not enhance the absorption of medication.

42. **b.** Studies of the permeability of isolated corneas to families of chemical compounds show that lipid solubility is more important than water solubility in promoting penetration.

43. **d.** A 0.5% solution has 0.5 gram/100 milliliters (mL), or 5 milligrams (mg)/milliliter. As there are approximately 20 drops per milliliter, there are 5 mg/20 drops. So, 5 mg/20 drops = 0.25 mg/1 drop. If this drop is given bilaterally, there is up to 0.50 mg of active agent available for systemic absorption.

44. **b.** The duration of action of atropine is 7–14 days, scopolamine is 4–7 days, homatropine is 3 days, cyclopentolate is 2 days, and tropicamide is 4–6 hours.

45. **d.** Both diclofenac and ketorolac have been associated with corneal complications, including melting and perforation. The preponderance of patients were found to be on generic diclofenac, which was subsequently removed from the US market.

46. **d.** Tetracyclines may depress prothrombin, thus prolonging the bleeding in patients on anticoagulation medication. As bacteriostatic drugs, tetracyclines may inhibit bacterial medications and should not be used concurrently. They also may decrease the efficacy of oral contraceptives.

47. **a.** Topical povidone-iodine solution (Betadine 5%) exhibits broad-spectrum antimicrobial activity when used to prepare the surgical field and rinse the ocular surface. It has been shown to have a significant effect on postsurgical endophthalmitis.

Index

(*f* = figure; *t* = table)